Handbook of
ORTHODONTICS

For Elsevier
Commissioning Editor: Alison Taylor
Development Editor: Carole McMurray, Hannah Kenner
Project Manager: Bryan Potter
Designer: George Ajayi
Illustration Manager: Jennifer Rose and Gillian Richards

Handbook of
ORTHODONTICS

by

Martyn T Cobourne BDS (Hons) FDSRCS (Eng), FDSRCS (Ed), MSc,
MOrth RCS (Eng), FDSOrth RCS, PhD, FHEA
Reader and Hon Consultant in Orthodontics, King's College London Dental Institute,
Guy's and St Thomas' NHS Foundation Trust, UK

Andrew T DiBiase BDS (Hons), FDSRCS (Eng), MSc, MOrthRCS (Eng),
FDSOrth RCS
Consultant Orthodontist, East Kent Hospitals University NHS Foundation Trust, UK

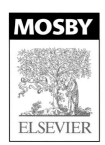

Edinburgh   London   New York   Oxford   Philadelphia   St Louis   Sydney   Toronto 2009

MOSBY
ELSEVIER

First published 2010
  Reprinted 2010

ISBN: 978 0 7234 34504

British Library Cataloguing in Publication Data
A catalogue record for this book is available from the British Library

Library of Congress Cataloging in Publication Data
A catalog record for this book is available from the Library of Congress

Notice
Knowledge and best practice in this field are constantly changing. As new research and experience broaden our knowledge, changes in practice, treatment and drug therapy may become necessary or appropriate. Readers are advised to check the most current information provided (i) on procedures featured or (ii) by the manufacturer of each product to be administered, to verify the recommended dose or formula, the method and duration of administration, and contraindications. It is the responsibility of the practitioner, relying on their own experience and knowledge of the patient, to make diagnoses, to determine dosages and the best treatment for each individual patient, and to take all appropriate safety precautions. To the fullest extent of the law, neither the Publisher nor the Authors assume any liability for any injury and/or damage to persons or property arising out or related to any use of the material contained in this book.

Neither the Publisher nor the Authors assume any responsibility for any loss or injury and/or damage to persons or property arising out of or related to any use of the material contained in this book. It is the responsibility of the treating practitioner, relying on independent expertise and knowledge of the patient, to determine the best treatment and method of application for the patient.

The Publisher

 ELSEVIER your source for books, journals and multimedia in the health sciences
www.elsevierhealth.com

The publisher's policy is to use paper manufactured from sustainable forests

Printed in China

Preface

We were delighted to be given the opportunity of writing a textbook on the subject of orthodontics and have attempted to synthesise our thoughts on what is a complex, but extremely rewarding speciality of dentistry. However, this was accompanied by a degree of trepidation. The practice of orthodontics is often described as being more art than science, controversies continue to rage on many aspects of clinical practice and if you ask two or more specialists for an opinion, there is rarely a complete consensus. We have tried to keep this in mind during the preparation of this book, but are aware that not all of the contents will be universally accepted.

Orthodontics is a continuously evolving speciality and new innovations are constantly being developed. Whilst we have described many of these, we have deliberately concentrated on those principles and techniques that have the most robust evidence base. There is currently a trend within clinical orthodontics for more and more spectacular claims to be made about treatment efficiency, primarily by manufacturers of the 'latest and best' appliances. This is something we have tried to avoid, preferring to adopt a more traditional approach.

A firm understanding of the basic sciences is an important platform for any orthodontist and we make no apology for describing craniofacial development, growth and disease in some detail. If the underlying biology is on your side, orthodontic treatment is often more straightforward, but unfortunately this is by no means guaranteed. Ultimately, the underlying biology of the patient will always be the winner; however, by attempting to understand it, the orthodontist at least gives themselves a chance of coming a very close second! There have been many exciting developments in these subjects over the last two decades and we believe that practitioners should be aware of them. Within these chapters we have extensively referenced the OMIM website (Online Mendelian Inheritance in Man), which provides the reader with an excellent and comprehensive database of human genes and genetic disorders (http://www.ncbi.nlm.nih.gov/omim).

We have also attempted to write a book that will appeal to all students of orthodontics, but with such a wide potential audience, there will inevitably be some areas that are more relevant to the reader than others. We would therefore kindly request that some leeway be afforded to us if certain sections are found to be more useful than others. Finally, we would like to acknowledge the many excellent teachers and textbooks that we were fortunate enough to be exposed to during our own training. Inevitably, they have left their collective mark on us and we apologise in advance if there is any unwitting repetition of their ideas within the pages of this book.

London and Canterbury, 2009

MTC
ATD

Acknowledgements

We are extremely grateful to our many colleagues who have been kind enough to source and donate figures used in this book. We have acknowledged individual sources in the relevant figure legends, but are particularly grateful to Christoph Huppa, Evelyn Sheehy and Zahra Kordi who made great efforts on our behalf to locate relevant clinical pictures. We would also like to thank a number of people who kindly proof-read and made numerous comments on the text within various chapters; Raymond Edler and Sue Mildenhall for the relevant sections on contemporary treatment of cleft palate; Peter Kesling, who cast his expert eye over sections relating to Tip-Edge mechanics; Eric Whaites, who advised on the complex and controversial subject of radiation protection and Oliver Bowyer, who read several draft chapters and gave relevant feedback from the perspective of an orthodontic trainee. We would like to thank James Abbott who constructed many of the removable appliances illustrated in the book and Padhraig Fleming, Paul Scott and Saba Quereshi for numerous figures and their support.

At Elsevier, we would like to thank Michael Parkinson, who had enough faith in our original proposal to commission the book in the first place; our development editors, Hannah Kenner and Carole McMurray who cheerfully dealt with the original manuscript and our project manager Bryan Potter, who set the book up and happily accommodated our multiple last-minute changes.

Finally, we would like to acknowledge the immense help and assistance provided by our wives Jackie and Sarah. Not only for their expert proof-reading and checking of all things related to orthodontic theory (Jackie) and English grammar (Sarah); but also for putting up with our three-year preoccupation with this project—particularly as two (soon-to-be three) children have been born during the writing and production of this book.

This book is dedicated to Jackie and Miles; Sarah, Wilf, Arthur and Stanley; and to the memory of David DiBiase.

Contents

1 Occlusion and malocclusion

Orthodontics is the speciality of dentistry concerned with the management and treatment of malocclusion. In the majority of cases, a malocclusion does not in itself represent a disease state, but rather a variation from what is considered ideal. It is therefore important for the orthodontist to have a clear definition of ideal occlusion, as this will form a basis for diagnosis and treatment planning.

Ideal occlusion

The ideal relationship of the teeth can be defined in terms of static (or morphological) and functional occlusion. Edward Angle (Box 1.1) felt the key to normal occlusion was the relative anteroposterior position of the first permanent molars, which he used to define the dental arch relationship. He also recognized the importance of good cuspal interdigitation to provide mutual support for the teeth in function (Angle, 1899). Almost one hundred years after Angle, Lawrence Andrews redefined the concept of an ideal static occlusion by describing it in terms of six individual keys, including an updated ideal relationship for the first molars (Andrews, 1972) (Box 1.2).

Orthodontists have traditionally based their treatment upon these static goals, with little consideration for the dynamics of occlusion or temporomandibular joints and associated musculature that forms the masticatory system. However, over the past few decades there has been a greater interest in the principles of gnathology and aspects of an occlusion in function (Table 1.1). Much has been written about what constitutes an ideal functional occlusion and why it is important (Box 1.3); however, an essential concept is one of mutual protection, whereby teeth of the anterior and posterior dentitions protect each other in function. Mutual protection is thought to be achieved in the presence of:

- An immediate and permanent posterior disclusion in lateral and protrusive contact with no associated non-working side interferences (tooth contacts); this is achieved by the presence of canine guidance or group function in lateral excursion (Fig. 1.1) and incisal guidance in protrusion. Thus, the anterior teeth protect the posteriors;
- Multiple, simultaneous and bilateral contacts of the posterior teeth in intercuspal position (ICP) with the incisor teeth slightly out of contact; thus, the posterior teeth protect the anteriors; and
- ICP (or centric occlusion, CO) coincident with the retruded contact position (RCP) (or centric relation, CR) but with some limited freedom for the mandible to move slightly forwards in the sagittal and horizontal planes from ICP.

In reality, an ideal static or functional occlusion is rarely found in Western societies (Fig. 1.1), which have a high occurrence of various traits of malocclusion.

> ### Box 1.1   Edward Hartley Angle
>
> Edward Angle was an American dentist born in 1855. Originally trained as a prosthodontist, he developed an interest in occlusion and was instrumental in developing orthodontics as a specialty of dentistry. Amongst his many achievements, including developing the principles upon which most modern fixed appliances are based, Angle proposed a classification of malocclusion that is still relevant today. He suggested that normal occlusion was based fundamentally around the position of the first permanent molar teeth. If these teeth were in the correct relationship and the remaining teeth occupied a smoothly curved line of occlusion, a normal occlusion would result. Angle's molar classification is still used today but it is now realized that first molar position is not immutable and the position these teeth come to occupy in the dental arch can be influenced by the environment.

> ### Table 1.1   Occlusal definitions
>
> - Retruded contact position (RCP) or centric relation (CR) is the position of the mandible in relation to the maxilla with the condylar head in its terminal hinge axis (uppermost and foremost within the glenoid fossa).
> - Intercuspal position (ICP) or centric occlusion (CO) is the occlusion that occurs with the teeth in a position of maximum intercuspation.
> - Canine guidance is present when contact is maintained on the working side canine teeth during lateral excursion of the mandible.
> - Group function is present when contacts are maintained between several teeth on the working side during lateral excursion of the mandible.
> - Non-working side interferences are occlusal contacts present on the non-working side during lateral excursion of the mandible.

Classification of malocclusion

Malocclusion can be defined as an appreciable deviation from the ideal that may be considered aesthetically or functionally unsatisfactory. Malocclusion has been described in numerous ways, ranging from specific classifications to indices of treatment need and outcome. Unlike a disease process, when the presence of specific features classifies the disease, a wide range of occlusal traits can constitute a malocclusion. However, within this spectrum, certain features can be identified for the purpose of classification, which allows communication and a basis for diagnosis. For any classification to be of use it needs to be simple, objective and reliable.

Molar classification

Angle classified occlusion according to the molar relationship and this remains the most internationally recognized classification of malocclusion. When looking at ideal occlusion, Angle found that the mesiobuccal cusp of the upper first permanent molar should occlude with the sulcus between the mesial and distal buccal cusps of the lower

Box 1.2 Andrews Six Keys of Occlusion

KEY 1		**Key 1** **Molar relationship** - the distal surface of the distal marginal ridge of the upper first permanent molar occludes with the mesial surface of the mesial marginal ridge of the lower second molar. The mesio-buccal cusp of the upper first permanent molar falls within the groove between the mesial and middle cusps of the lower first permanent molar
KEY 2		**Key 2** **Crown angulation or mesio-distal tip** - the gingival portion of the long axis of each tooth crown is distal to the occlusal portion of that axis. The degree of tip varies with each tooth type
KEY 3		**Key 3** **Crown inclination or labio-lingual/bucco-lingual torque** - for the upper incisors the occlusal portion of the crowns labial surface is labial to the gingival portion. In all other crowns, the occlusal portion of the labial or buccal surface is lingual to the gingival portion
KEY 4		**Key 4** **Rotations** - there should be an absence of any tooth rotations within the dental arches
KEY 5		**Key 5** **Spacing** - there should be an absence of any spacing within the dental arches
KEY 6		**Key 6** **Occlusal plane** - the occlusal plane should be flat

first permanent molar (Fig. 1.2). He therefore based his classification of occlusion on this relative mesiodistal position:

- Class I—the position of the dental arches is normal, with first molars in normal occlusion.
- Class II—the relations of the dental arches are abnormal, with all the mandibular teeth occluding distal to normal. Angle recognized two subdivisions under class II:
  - Class II division 1—upper incisors are protruding;
  - Class II division 2—upper incisors are lingually inclined.
- Class III—the relations of the dental arches are also abnormal, with all mandibular teeth occluding mesial to normal.

In clinical practice, it is common to describe molar relationships in terms of half or even a third of a tooth unit of a class II or class III relationship (Fig. 1.2). However, a

Box 1.3   How important is an ideal functional occlusion?

Advocates of an ideal functional occlusion claim it is necessary to avoid temporomandibular dysfunction, periodontal breakdown and long-term occlusal instability. Indeed, it has been suggested that orthodontic treatment is indicated in all young adults in whom the occlusion is not functionally optimal. These criteria would mean treating most of the population, as an ideal functional occlusion is not very common. For example, as many as 75% of subjects have been described as having non-working side contacts (Tipton & Rinchuse, 1991), whilst a difference of greater than 2 mm has been reported between RCP and ICP for up to 40% of orthodontic patients (Hidaka et al., 2002). So does this matter? Whilst artificially creating non-working side interferences can increase the signs and symptoms of temporomandibular dysfunction (Christensen and Rassouli, 1995), the results of occlusal equilibration, when an idealized functional occlusion is created, are equivocal. Canine guidance has been reported to reduce electromyographic (EMG) activity of the muscles of mastication (Christensen and Rassouli, 1995) but the reproducibility of EMG is open to question (Cecere et al., 1996). There does appear to be a relationship between temporomandibular dysfunction and large slides from RCP into ICP (Solberg et al., 1979) although the correlations between other traits of malocclusion and temporomandibular dysfunction are generally weak (Egermark-Eriksson et al., 1981). So by treating to an ideal functional occlusion does it eliminate or reduce temporomandibular dysfunction? Unfortunately, there is a lack of evidence to support this, or the claim that it results in greater long-term stability (Luther, 2007a, b). Therefore, while any treatment should aim for an ideal functional occlusion, if it is not achieved, there do not appear to be long-term serious consequences to the patient.

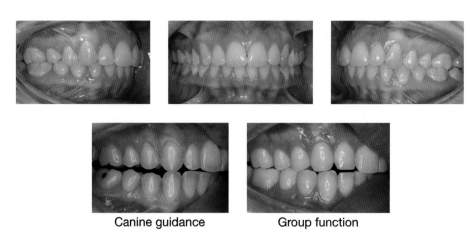

Canine guidance   Group function

Figure 1.1 Ideal untreated occlusion. The incisor, canine and molar relationship are class I, the dental arches are well aligned and there are no transverse discrepancies. In lateral excursion there should be either canine guidance or group function.

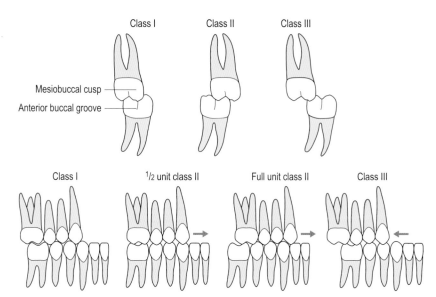

Figure 1.2 The Angle molar classification. The buccal segment occlusion can be further defined in relation to the degree of mesial or distal occlusion and this is usually measured in units of tooth space.

basic premise of the Angle classification is that the first permanent molars hold a fixed position within the dental arch, which is not necessarily the case. Early loss of deciduous teeth can influence their position and distort the molar relationship and this classification can also be difficult to apply when there is an asymmetric molar relationship. These problems can lead to low levels of inter-examiner agreement (Gravely and Johnson, 1974).

Canine classification

The canine relationship also provides a useful anteroposterior occlusal classification:
- Class I—the maxillary permanent canine should occlude directly in the embrasure between mandibular canine and first premolar.
- Class II—the maxillary permanent canine occludes in front of the embrasure between mandibular canine and first premolar.
- Class III—the maxillary permanent canine occludes behind the embrasure between mandibular canine and first premolar.

   Similarly to the molar relationship, the severity of the canine relationship can also be described in terms of tooth units and can be inappropriately influenced by local factors such as crowding (Fig. 1.2).

Incisor classification

A more clinically relevant method of classifying malocclusion is based upon the relationship of the maxillary and mandibular incisors. This represents a truer reflection of the underlying skeletal base relationship and also highlights what is often of most concern to the patient. It is essentially the Angle classification, as applied to the incisor

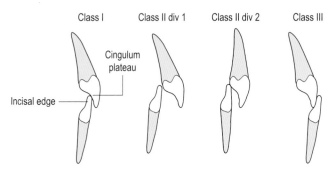

Figure 1.3 British Standards Institute incisor classification.

teeth, and is defined upon the relationship of the mandibular incisor tip to the cingulum plateau of the maxillary central incisors (Fig. 1.3), being included in the British Standards Institute's *Glossary of Dental Terms*:

- Class I—the lower incisor tips occlude or lie below the cingulum plateau of the upper incisors
- Class II—the lower incisor tips occlude or lie posterior to the cingulum plateau of the upper incisors. This classification is further subdivided into:
  - Class II division 1—the overjet is increased with upright or proclined upper incisors;
  - Class II division 2—the upper incisors are retroclined, with a normal or occasionally increased overjet.
- Class III—the lower incisor tips occlude or lie anterior to the cingulum plateau of the upper incisors.

Confusion can arise when the upper incisors are upright or retroclined, but with an increased overjet. This has led to the introduction of a class II intermediate classification (Williams and Stephens, 1992):

- Class II intermediate—the lower incisor edges lie posterior to the cingulum plateau of the upper central incisors. The upper incisors are upright or slightly retroclined and the overjet lies between 5 and 7-mm.

In reality, an increased overjet with retroclined upper incisors is within the descriptive range of class II division 2.

Prevalence of malocclusion

Malocclusion has been described as a disease of Western societies, and certainly within developed polygenic societies, certain occlusal traits such as crowding are more common. Indeed, from data generated by population studies, the presence of one or more traits of malocclusion is very common. In the USA, noticeable incisor irregularity is present in the majority of adults, with only 34% having well-aligned mandibular incisors and 45% well-aligned maxillary incisors. In addition, about 20% of the American population has a marked deviation from the ideal sagittal jaw relationship, with 2% of these being disfiguring and at the limit for orthodontic correction (Proffit et al, 1998). Within the UK, the last Child Dental Health Survey found around 35% of 12 year olds with a definite need for orthodontic treatment on dental health or aesthetic grounds, which increased to 43% when those already in treatment were included (Chestnutt et al, 2006).

Ethnicity also has a significant bearing on malocclusion. Class II problems are commoner in white populations of northern European descent, whilst class III malocclusion is a common trait amongst Chinese and Japanese societies. Amongst African-Caribbean populations, anterior open bite is more common than in Caucasians who, in turn, have a greater proportion of increased overbite.

Aetiology of malocclusion

A malocclusion should be regarded as a developmental condition and does not represent a single entity. Rather, it is the sum of a number of complex occlusal traits, which demonstrate multifactorial inheritance. Although in certain cases specific factors and pathologies can be identified as the cause of a malocclusion; in the majority, the aetiology is less clear. In each individual there is a close interaction between genetics and the environment during development and growth of both the jaws and dentition; it is at this interface that the aetiology of malocclusion lies (Box 1.4).

Evolutionary trends
Comparison of large population studies with archaeological records confirms that malocclusion has become more common over the past 1000 years. In fact, epidemiological data show that the increase in human occlusal variation has been rapid, taking place within a couple of generations, occasionally even from one generation to the next (Weiland et al, 1997). A rapid change such as this would imply a significant contribution from a changing environment, such as has occurred with increasingly urbanized and industrialized societies (Corruccini, 1984). It has been hypothesized that

---

Box 1.4   Nature versus nurture?

How much a malocclusion is due to the genetic makeup of an individual or the environmental influence upon growth and dental development is the key to understanding the aetiology of malocclusion. The forefathers of modern orthodontics thought that malocclusion was a disease of civilization and that by re-establishing normal jaw function and occlusion; a stable treatment result would be achieved. With a greater understanding of genetics and inheritance, as well as the introduction of cephalometric radiography, it was thought that malocclusion resulted from inherited factors. Therefore, treatment became directed at correcting malocclusion within the existing facial skeleton and soft tissue envelope; both cephalometric and clinical treatment goals were developed, often based around the position of the mandibular incisor teeth. More recently, as science has moved away from simple Mendelian genetics, there has been a shift back to examining the environmental causes of malocclusion. This has also led to renewed interest in treatments that attempt to modify jaw growth.

Figure 1.4 Well-interdigitated class I dentition showing diet-related occlusal interproximal wear.

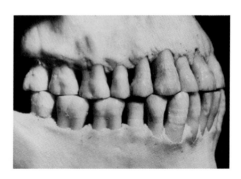

dietary changes in modern societies, with increased consumption of soft, energy-rich food, has resulted in less interproximal wear between the teeth. Research on aboriginal and stone aged populations has demonstrated this lack of attrition as a possible cause of malocclusion, particularly crowding (Begg, 1954). However, it has been shown that the amount of tooth material lost in each quadrant by interproximal wear is not more than 2 to 3-mm (Fig. 1.4).

A soft diet may also result in underdevelopment of the jaws and a lack of arch space, leading to crowding. According to this hypothesis, hard diet requires vigorous mastication, stimulating the growth of facial bones, particularly in the transverse dimension of the maxilla and mandible. Tooth wear is merely a by-product, brought about by diet-related attrition and high masticatory activity, and has only a minor effect on tooth alignment. Experimental studies have shown that dietary consistency and masticatory activity affect not only the masticatory muscles, but also many aspects of bone growth, including bone size and mass, internal bone structure, and craniofacial size and morphology (Varrela, 2006).

Genetic influences
Genetically homogenous societies exhibit low levels of malocclusion compared to heterogeneous societies and a significant genetic component appears to exist for many individual dental and occlusal anomalies. Early animal experiments initially put forward a compelling argument for a genetic component to malocclusion, based upon inbreeding of dogs, culminating in gross facial deformity. It later emerged that these studies were flawed, merely segregating mutations for specific traits such as achondroplasia, which are present in many breeds of small dog, but rare in humans.

Until recently, most information on the relative contribution of genetic factors to malocclusion has been gained from family studies and the twin method. Monozygotic twins are genetically identical, whereas dizygotic twins only share 50% of their genetic makeup. Therefore, by comparing the differences in occlusal traits between pairs in both groups, some indication of the genetic influence on a particular trait is given; the larger the difference, the greater the genetic effect (Corruccini et al, 1990). This assumes that the environmental effects are similar for both groups.

Many developmental dental anomalies have been shown to occur together and have a strong familial trend. An example of this is development of a palatally impacted maxillary canine, which is more common in females and certain ethnic groups and is often associated with microdont or absent lateral incisors (Peck et al, 1994). Similarly, jaw growth appears to be mostly genetically determined. A higher correlation has been shown between patients and immediate family than in unrelated subjects for class II division 1 malocclusion, which supports a polygenetic inheritance, particularly in relation to mandibular retrognathia. However, environmental factors, such as lower lip position and digit sucking, can also play a part. Mandibular prognathism, found in class III malocclusions, seems to have a high genetic predisposition, as demonstrated by the high familial inheritance and variation amongst different ethnic groups. More robust evidence for this exists from studies of siblings and first degree relatives (Litton et al, 1970; Watanabe et al, 2005).

Dental arch size and form seems to be more subject to environmental influences (Cassidy et al, 1998). Dental crowding represents a discrepancy between the size of the teeth and the size of the dental arch. Tooth development, including the size, form and presence of teeth within a dentition, is under strong genetic influence. However, the main aetiological factor in crowding appears to be arch size as opposed to tooth size (Howe et al, 1983).

Large population studies have also investigated the influence of population admixture and inbreeding on malocclusion. Generally, the results of these epidemiological studies have shown a greater genetic influence on skeletal relations and arch size and a lower heritability of dental variables such as overbite, molar relationships and crowding, suggesting a greater environmental influence. The importance of hereditary factors also appears to increase with severity of the malocclusion. Although craniofacial form and growth may be under genetic control, the reason that siblings often present with similar malocclusions is probably related to their similar responses to environmental influences. Therefore, while malocclusion appears to be acquired, the underlying genetic control of craniofacial form will tend to divert siblings into similar physiological responses, resulting in the development of similar malocclusions (King et al, 1993).

These studies have also shown that malocclusion does not follow simple Mendelian inheritance, but rather polygenetic or epigenetic transmission, when the interaction of genes with each other and the environment during development determine the phenotypic variation of the trait. Therefore, each would have an additive effect, showing variation along a continuous scale for traits of a malocclusion, which is exactly what happens. Theoretically, in genetically isolated communities, alleles for these traits may be expressed more frequently, giving an indication which have a greater genetic component. Island studies investigating the effects of inbreeding on malocclusion support this polygenetic theory of transmission for certain traits such as overjet and overbite (Lauc et al, 2003).

Environmental factors

The developing dentition is under the influence of resting soft tissue pressure form, and function: lying in a position of muscular balance or equilibrium (Proffit, 1978). Teeth erupt under the influence of the lips and cheeks on one side and the tongue on the other. Abnormal soft tissue patterns seen in those with persistent digit-sucking habits or lip incompetence, with the lower lip trapped behind the upper incisors in function, may predispose to an increased overjet. An alteration in tooth position can also arise when there is a change in this balance of force. Possible causes may be physiological, habitual or pathological and may impact on the lips, cheeks, tongue and periodontal tissues.

Physiological factors

A physiological adaptation can take place in the presence of a skeletal base discrepancy. When teeth erupt, they do so under the influence of soft tissue pressure from the lips, cheeks and tongue. There is a tendency, most notably in the labial segments, for them to upright or procline towards teeth in the opposing arch. This is most often seen in class III skeletal cases, with proclination of the upper incisors and retroclination of the lowers (Fig. 1.5).

Soft tissue envelope

The zone of balance between the lips and cheeks and tongue can in part dictate where the teeth sit. If the forces are imbalanced it can result in tooth movement. Many children have lip incompetence:

- If the lower lip rests behind the upper incisor, this may predispose to an increased overjet and is described as a lip trap (Fig. 1.6).
- In a small percentage of patients there appears to be hyperactivity of the mentalis muscle, resulting in retroclination of the lower incisors and described as a strap-like lower lip (Fig. 1.7).
- Similarly, a high lower lip position is thought to contribute to retroclination of the upper incisors in a class II division 2 relationship (Fig. 1.8).

In cases with anterior open bite, an anterior oral seal on swallowing is created by the tongue coming forward to fill the gap. This is an adaptive behaviour, secondary to the malocclusion. Occasionally, a tongue thrust is the primary cause of the malocclusion: the so-called endogenous (primary) tongue thrust. Although often described,

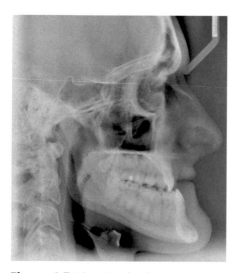

Figure 1.5 Class III malocclusion showing incisor dentoalveolar compensation. The mandibular incisors have retroclined in an attempt to achieve a class I incisor relationship in the presence of a class III skeletal base.

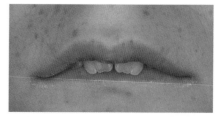
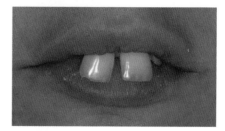

Figure 1.6 Lip trap contributing to an increase in overjet.

this is a rare phenomenon and is probably related to the anterior resting position of the tongue as opposed to excessive activity.

Mouth breathing

Children with nasopharyngeal obstruction associated with enlarged adenoids have been shown to have longer faces and smaller mandibles compared to controls (Fig. 1.9) (Linder-Aronson, 1970).

Neonates by necessity are nasal breathers to allow suckling but most pre-adolescent children adopt a posture with their lips habitually apart at rest. This resolves in many cases, due to greater vertical growth of the lips compared to the lower facial skeleton, particularly in boys. Total experimental obstruction of the nasal airway in primates and humans results in a change of head posture, with the neck being extended and a downward and backward growth rotation of the mandible occurring. Following adenoidectomy for children with severe nasopharyngeal obstruction, a greater horizontal rather than vertical growth pattern has been described (Linder-Aronson et al, 1986; Woodside et al, 1991). In humans, total obstruction of the nasal airway is rare and many children, even with some nasal blockage and lip incompetence,

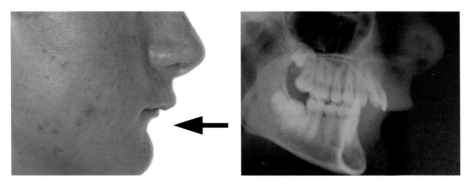

Figure 1.7 Strap-like lower lip.

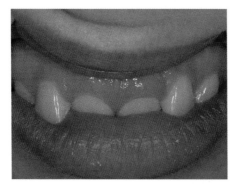

Figure 1.8 A high lower lip position retroclining the upper central incisors and proclining the upper lateral incisors in a class II division 2 incisor relationship (the upper lip has been retracted).

Figure 1.9 Child with increased facial height and lip incompetence with a history of nasal blockage and mouth breathing. This appearance has been described as an adenoidal face.

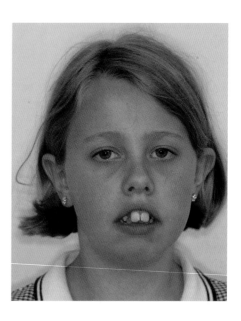

do breathe through their noses. It is therefore impossible to generalize on a normal population using data gathered from extremes. The question still remains whether partial nasal blockage is an aetiological factor in malocclusion, as the situation appears more complex than a simple form–function interaction (Vig, 1998).

Muscular activity

Conditions associated with a loss of muscle tone, such as muscular dystrophy and certain types of cerebral palsy, result in a downward and backward rotation of the mandible, an increased lower face height and an anterior open bite (Fig. 1.10). Adults with increased anterior face height have reduced bite force and also a different composition of muscle fibres in the masseter, which implicates muscles as a primary cause of malocclusion (Hunt et al, 2006). However, in children with similar skeletal makeup, the bite force is the same as children with normal face height, implying that the loss in force may develop with, as opposed to causing, a malocclusion (Proffit & Fields, 1983).

Sucking habits

Children can indulge in a variety of non-nutritive sucking habits during their early years, which in the majority of cases involve the use of dummies and/or digits. Dummy sucking is more common in the first few years of life but quite rare beyond the age of five years. In contrast, digit sucking is more prevalent in children over five, being seen in around 10% of this population (Brenchley, 1991). Both these habits can influence the developing dental arches and occlusion if continued beyond the second year of life, with the severity of the effects being related primarily to the type, frequency, intensity and duration of the habit:

- Increased maxillary arch length and prognathism;
- Narrowing of the maxillary arch and widening of mandibular arch width;
- Posterior crossbite;

- Maxillary incisor proclination, spacing and increased overjet;
- Reduced overbite and anterior open bite; and
- Class II buccal segments.

In general terms, dummy sucking is more commonly associated with a symmetrical open bite and posterior crossbite, having a greater effect on the deciduous dentition than digit sucking (Duncan et al, 2007). Digit sucking tends to produce an asymmetric open bite and increased overjet and can have a more significant influence on the mixed and permanent dentitions (Fig. 1.10). The changes in overjet and overbite arise because of the direct affect of the habit on incisor position; whilst a lowering of tongue position away from the upper arch, increased pressure from the cheeks and an absence of tooth contact in the buccal segments contribute to the development of a posterior crossbite. Significantly, many of these occlusal changes can persist well beyond cessation of the habit and if it is continued into the mixed dentition they can be permanent.

Pathology

A number of pathological conditions can contribute directly to a malocclusion, causing either skeletal discrepancies or more local effects upon the dentition.

Childhood fractures of jaws

The condyle is the commonest site of fracture in the mandible during childhood and many go undiagnosed. In severe cases with bilateral fracture and dislocation from the glenoid fossa, an anterior open bite can be one of the presenting features due to a loss in ramus height. A long-term sequelae of early trauma to the mandibular condyle can be asymmetry, with an ipsilateral decrease in ramus height and deviation of the chin point to the affected side (Fig. 1.11). The severity of outcome is in part related to the age at the time of injury. However, a high percentage of children sustaining a condylar fracture have normal mandibular growth due to the reparative capacity of the condyle, even when displaced from the glenoid fossa.

Juvenile rheumatoid arthritis

An inflammatory arthritis occurring before the age of 16 years and involving the temporomandibular joints can result in the development of a severe class II malocclusion due to restricted growth of the mandible (Fig. 1.12).

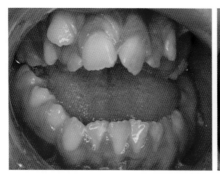 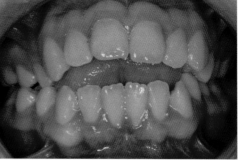

Figure 1.10 Anterior open bite related to cerebral palsy (left) and persistent digit-sucking habit (right).

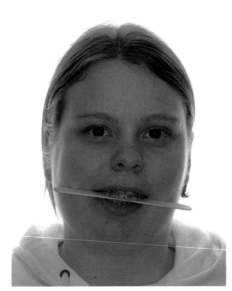

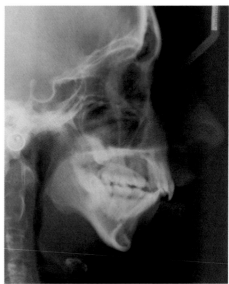

Figure 1.11 Mandibular asymmetry in an adult following fracture of the condyles as a child.

Figure 1.12 Lateral skull radiograph of patient with a history of juvenile rheumatoid arthritis.

Excessive growth hormone

Overproduction of growth hormone from an anterior pituitary tumour causes gigantism in children and acromegaly in adults. In both circumstances, the patient presents with a worsening class III malocclusion characterized by mandibular excess (Fig. 1.13).

Periodontal disease

With the loss of alveolar bone that occurs due to periodontal disease, teeth become more susceptible to influence from the soft tissue envelope that surrounds them. Any change in this balance that occurs with age can result in tooth movement. This is commonly seen when upper incisors escape control of the lower lip, resulting in an increase in the overjet and spacing (Fig. 1.14).

Dentoalveolar trauma

Trauma to the primary maxillary incisors can result in displacement of the tooth into the developing tooth bud of the permanent successor. Damage to the crown or dilaceration of the root can occur, resulting in failure of eruption and impaction of the tooth. Loss of a permanent incisor due to trauma can result in space loss and shift in the dental centre line in crowded dentitions (Fig. 1.15).

Early loss of primary teeth

Although water fluoridation and dental education has significantly reduced the incidence of caries in children, the enforced loss of primary teeth due to caries still remains a major aetiological factor in the development of a local malocclusion. In a crowded dentition, the early loss of deciduous teeth can result in space loss, increased crowding and deviations of the dental centre lines.

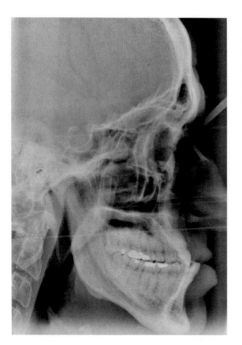

Figure 1.13 Lateral skull radiograph showing a class III malocclusion in an adult resulting from excessive growth hormone secondary to a pituitary tumour. Note the indistinct and enlarged borders of the pituitary fossa.

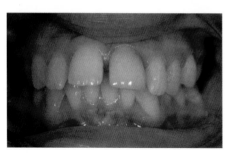

Figure 1.14 Proclination and spacing of the upper labial segment resulting from periodontal bone loss.

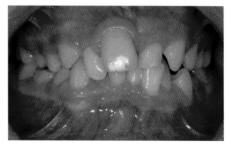

Figure 1.15 Loss of UL1 through trauma with subsequent space loss and a shift in the dental centreline.

Benefits of orthodontic treatment

For any elective medical intervention there should be a clear list of benefits for the patient and these should outweigh any potential risks. It is clear that orthodontic treatment can provide significant cosmetic advantages to a patient. However, it has proved difficult to provide strong evidence in support of the widely assumed belief that treatment can also improve the oral health and psychological well-being of an individual.

Resistance to caries and periodontal disease

Dental caries is endemic in most developed societies and the primary aetiological factors are the presence of cariogenic flora in dental plaque and the frequent intake of refined sugars. The disease process can be controlled with good diet and oral hygiene and is unrelated to the presence or absence of a malocclusion. There is some evidence that straight teeth and a normal overjet are easier to keep clean (Addy et al, 1986; Davies et al, 1988) and that recipients of orthodontic treatment have lower plaque scores (Davies et al, 1991), but this may be more related to the modification of behaviour during treatment rather than the actual presence of straight teeth.

The primary aetiological factor in periodontal disease is dental plaque and the principle way to avoid this condition is maintaining good oral hygiene, not orthodontic treatment. However, there are two specific areas where orthodontic treatment can help to prevent periodontal breakdown:

- Correction of an anterior crossbite with associated recession on a lower incisor; and
- Correction of a deep and traumatic overbite.

Improved masticatory efficiency

Evidence to suggest that having a class I occlusion improves masticatory efficiency is weak. It is perfectly possible to survive without teeth on a Western diet, as many people do, and whilst orthodontic treatment can be beneficial in correcting functional problems such as crossbites, it is unlikely to make a significant difference to masticatory efficiency. One exception is the correction of an anterior open bite when patients are unable to incise food except by biting into it with their posterior teeth.

Prevention or cure of temporomandibular joint dysfunction

The aetiology of temporomandibular joint dysfunction remains controversial, which explains in part the large variety of modalities used to treat it. At the very least, the aetiology is considered to be multifactorial. The relationship between malocclusion and temporomandibular dysfunction has been explored extensively, mostly in large epidemiological studies, and whilst some traits of a malocclusion have been shown to have a correlation with the signs and symptoms of joint dysfunction (Table 1.2), these are very weak (Egermark-Eriksson et al, 1983).

Improvement in speech

Speech patterns are established very early in life and in most cases a long time before eruption of the permanent dentition. Some speech problems are related to certain traits of a malocclusion, such as anterior open bite and a lisp, but treating the malocclusion will not guarantee resolution of the problem.

Table 1.2 Occlusal features associated with temporomandibular dysfunction

- Anterior open bite.
- Deep overbite.
- Class II and III molar relationships.
- Posterior crossbite with displacement.

Prevention of trauma

An increased overjet is a risk factor for trauma to the upper incisors (Jarvinen, 1978). As a consequence, a high percentage of patients with a class II division 1 incisor relationship present with damaged upper incisors. Correction of the incisor relationship will theoretically reduce the vulnerability of these teeth to damage following trauma. Unfortunately most incidences of trauma occur soon after eruption of the permanent incisors and prior to the age when orthodontics is usually started.

Psychological benefits

In its original constitution the World Health Organization defined health as 'a state of complete physical, social and mental well-being and not merely the absence of disease and infirmity'. Therefore, even though a malocclusion is not a disease state, the benefits of treating it should be considered in terms of both the social and mental well-being of an individual. Certain occlusal traits, such as an increased overjet, can lead to a reduction in self-esteem and can be a target for teasing. More severe malocclusions associated with facial disfigurement, such as those seen in cleft lip and palate, have been shown to have a profound and long-lasting psychological impact. However, longitudinal studies have demonstrated little objective evidence to support the assumption that orthodontic treatment can improve long-term psychological health of the individual (Kenealy et al, 2007).

More recently work has focused on the impact malocclusion can have on quality of life for individuals. Certain occlusal traits such as an increased overjet and spacing appear to have some negative impact in children and their families (Johal et al, 2007), whilst in adults severe skeletal problems that require surgical correction can have a profound impact on individual quality of life.

Risks of orthodontic treatment

Orthodontic treatment is not without risk. These risks can arise as a direct consequence of placing an appliance or be secondary to the treatment itself.

Risks from appliances

The principle risks arise from the use of fixed appliances and these can affect the teeth, periodontium and soft tissues.

Enamel decalcification

The incidence of demineralization during fixed appliance therapy is high and can result in the development of enamel opacities on the labial surfaces of the teeth. Incidences of up to 50% of patients undergoing fixed appliance therapy have been reported (Gorelick et al, 1982). The main aetiological factors are poor oral hygiene and a diet high in refined sugars. In combination and over the long-term, these factors will inevitably result in demineralization and permanent marking of the teeth (Fig. 1.16). Excellent oral hygiene and a non-cariogenic diet are therefore a prerequisite to orthodontic treatment involving fixed appliances. During treatment, the chances of developing enamel opacities can be reduced by the regular use of topical fluoride supplements. The use of a 0.05% sodium fluoride mouthwash on a daily basis will significantly reduce the incidence of white spot lesions (Benson et al, 2005) and fluoride-releasing

Figure 1.16 Generalized demineralization following orthodontic treatment with fixed appliances.

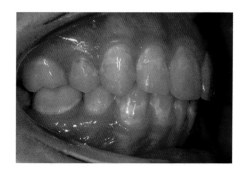

bonding agents such as glass ionomer will reduce caries levels experienced during treatment (Derks et al, 2004).

Enamel fracture

The removal of a fixed appliance bonded to enamel carries a small risk of fracture at the enamel–dentinal junction if bracket bond strengths are too high. In reality, bond strengths used are considerably lower than this and at debond, failure usually occurs at the bracket base–cement junction. An exception to this proved to be some early ceramic bracket systems; manufacturers were concerned with failure of the bracket bond during treatment and enhanced the mechanical bonding chemically. This resulted in excessive bond strengths and a significant risk of enamel fracture on debonding. Modern ceramic bracket bases are designed with features that facilitate easier debonding, which reduces the risk of enamel fracture.

Root resorption

External root resorption is an almost universal finding following orthodontic treatment, but this is usually not clinically significant and has no influence on long-term health of the teeth. Severe root resorption, when more than a quarter of the root length is lost, has been reported to occur in less than 3% of orthodontic patients (Fig. 1.17) (Sameshima and Sinclair, 2004). The greatest amount and severity of root resorption is seen in the anterior maxillary region, especially the maxillary lateral incisors. There is a genetic tendency and ethnic susceptibility, with Asian patients having a lower incidence. The greatest association with root resorption appears to be the duration of treatment and the distance the teeth must move (Linge and Linge, 1991; Segal et al, 2004). Other risk factors associated with a higher incidence of root resorption include:

- Unusually shaped roots, including blunted, pipette-shaped and short roots;
- History of dentoalveolar trauma;
- Excessive orthodontic force;
- Movement of teeth without occlusal contact;
- Intrusive forces;
- Reduction of large overjets by distal movement of anterior teeth; and
- Pushing apices of teeth into cortical bone.

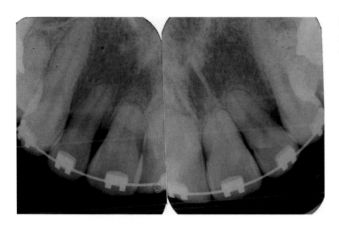

Figure 1.17 Severe root resorption during orthodontic treatment.

Pain and damage to the pulp
Orthodontic treatment, especially with fixed appliances, can be painful. However, this pain usually subsides within a few days of appliance activation and can be controlled with analgesia. The use of excessive force or pushing the apex of teeth through the cortical plate can result in a loss of vitality. Teeth with a history of trauma are more susceptible to vitality loss during treatment but in most cases there is no obvious cause. Fortunately, loss of vitality is a rare complication of orthodontics.

Gingivitis
Gingival irritation is inevitable with the use of fixed appliances, especially the placement of bands and this is exacerbated by poor oral hygiene, which can result in gingival hyperplasia. Gingival health improves significantly following the removal of appliances, with a reduction in probing depths mainly due to shrinkage of hyperplastic tissues (Fig. 1.18). Certain medications such as antiepileptic drugs and immunosuppressants in combination with poor oral hygiene can result in extensive gingival hyperplasia that can require gingival surgery following appliance removal.

Alveolar bone loss
A small loss of alveolar bone height following orthodontic treatment has been reported in relation to teeth adjacent to extraction sites but there appears to be no long-term effect on periodontal health from orthodontic treatment (Zachrisson and Alnaes, 1974). An exception to this is orthodontic treatment in patients with active periodontal disease because this can rapidly increase bone loss. Periodontal disease should be treated, stable and well maintained in these patients prior to commencing orthodontic treatment.

Oral ulceration
Aphthous ulceration in susceptible individuals is common with fixed appliances, particularly during the early stages of treatment. This can be exacerbated if archwires are not cut or bent back and left protruding from molar tubes (Fig. 1.19).

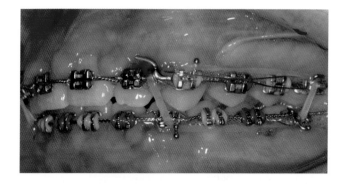

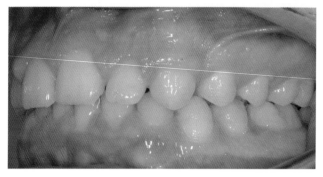

Figure 1.18 Gingival hyperplasia during orthodontic treatment and subsequent improvement on removal of the appliance.

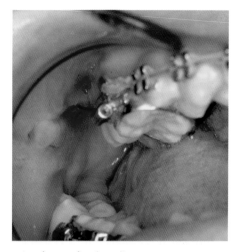

Figure 1.19 Oral ulceration from a fixed appliance.

Allergic reaction

Orthodontic wires and brackets contain nickel and nickel allergy is increasing in frequency. Its prevalence has been reported to be approximately 10% in the USA and Europe, being more common in females. It is usually a Type IV allergic reaction related to wearing jewellery or watches and body piercing. Fortunately oral reactions are rare although prolonged exposure to nickel-containing oral appliances may increase sensitivity to nickel (Bass et al, 1993). Intraoral signs are non-specific and have been reported to include erythematous areas and severe gingivitis despite good oral hygiene.

Headgear injury

A number of intra- and extraoral injuries have been reported with the use of headgear, particularly the risk of ocular penetration. The majority of these injuries occur as a result of the inner bow of the headgear detaching from the molar bands at night. Headgear injury is discussed further in Chapter 5.

Generalized risks associated with orthodontic treatment

A number of more general risks have been proposed with regard to orthodontic treatment, in particular causing damage to the facial profile or temporomandibular joints. A great deal of controversy surrounds these claims and currently there is little robust evidence in the literature to support them. In contrast, it is well recognized that the final tooth positions achieved following orthodontic treatment can relapse and it is important for any orthodontic patient to understand that absolute stability cannot be guaranteed without permanent retention.

Facial aesthetics

The position of the dentition within the soft tissues of the face has an impact on facial aesthetics. Over-retraction of the incisor dentition, especially in relation to mid-arch premolar extractions, has been criticized for flattening facial profiles, especially in relation to the position of the lips. Conversely, excessive proclination of the incisor teeth in association with arch expansion can result in a poor facial appearance. The relationship between incisor movement and soft tissue changes are complex. There have been numerous, mostly retrospective studies, assessing facial change following orthodontic treatment, and although the extraction of teeth produces slightly more retrusive profiles than non-extraction treatment, in the majority of cases the facial changes are seen as beneficial by both lay and professional judges, irrespective of whether teeth were extracted.

Temporomandibular joint dysfunction

There have been claims and successful litigation in relation to orthodontic treatment and the exacerbation of symptoms associated with temporomandibular joint dysfunction. However, there is currently a lack of robust evidence linking orthodontics and particularly the extraction of permanent teeth to these signs and symptoms. Orthodontic treatment has not been shown to be a causative factor in the development of temporomandibular dysfunction later in life, regardless of whether teeth are extracted (Dibbets and van der Weele, 1991; Kremenak et al, 1992a, b; Mohlin et al, 2004; Sadowsky et al, 1991). However, it is important that any signs and symptoms of temporomandibular dysfunction are recorded prior to treatment and that attention is paid to the functional occlusion at the end of treatment.

Relapse

Longitudinal studies have shown a high potential for relapse following the correction of certain occlusal traits, which include:

- Rotated teeth;
- Lower incisor crowding;
- Changes in position of the lower incisors;
- Expansion of the lower intercanine width; and
- Spacing.

The appearance of increased dental crowding later in life has been found to occur in untreated individuals and as such, should be regarded as an age-related change rather than relapse.

Failure of treatment

Successful orthodontic treatment requires significant cooperation and compliance, which some patients find difficult. This is less of a problem with adult patients who are generally highly motivated towards treatment, but in children and adolescents high discontinuation rates have been reported. Clearly, a patient who fails to complete a course of treatment may end up with an occlusal result that is unsatisfactory or even worse than the presenting malocclusion, particularly if permanent teeth have been extracted and space closure has not been completed.

Provision of orthodontic treatment

Given the high prevalence of malocclusion within the general population and increasing demand for treatment, attempts have been made to develop indices for prioritization of orthodontic treatment provision within healthcare systems (Box 1.5). This is especially relevant where dental health services are subsidized by the government as part of a national health service, such as in the UK and Scandinavia.

Index of Treatment Need (IOTN)

The IOTN was developed within the UK (Brook and Shaw, 1989) where the majority of orthodontic treatment has been provided within a state-funded health service and this has proved to be the most widely used and recognized index. Based on the Swedish National Board for Welfare Index (Linder-Aronson, 1974), it defines need for treatment, both in terms of dental health benefits and aesthetic handicapping and has been shown to be reproducible and reliable over time (Cooper et al, 2000). The IOTN is split into Dental Health and Aesthetic components.

Dental Health Component (DHC)

The DHC has five categories, defining treatment need from none (Grade 1) to a great need (Grade 5). The following characteristics are scored for each individual:

- Missing teeth;
- Overjet;
- Crossbites;
- Displacement of contact points (crowding); and
- Overbite.

Box 1.5 Limitations of occlusal indices

The use of indices to quantify the need for orthodontic treatment is controversial and far from being universally accepted. Indeed, the American Association of Orthodontics does not recognize any index as a scientifically valid measurement of the need for orthodontic treatment (Shaw et al., 1995). An ideal index has a number of requirements:

- Reliability and reproducibility;
- Validity;
- Acceptability to both professionals and the public;
- Objectivity; and
- Simple to apply.

Certainly the Index of Treatment Need (IOTN) has been shown to be reproducible and simple to apply; however, criticism regarding its validity has been made. Does it measure the need for orthodontic treatment? The perceived need depends upon many factors, only one of which is the malocclusion. These factors can include the country of origin of the clinician and the system of remuneration under which they are employed (Richmond and Daniels, 1998a). Similar differences have been found regarding what constitutes acceptable treatment (Richmond and Daniels, 1998b). The Dental Health Component (DHC) reflects our current understanding of the health risks of a malocclusion, although the correlations between dental disease and certain traits of a malocclusion are very weak. In addition, little allowance is made for facial aesthetics and the psychological impact of a malocclusion, both of which are often reasons that treatment is sought. The Aesthetic Component, which should in part allow for these factors, although validated among professionals, correlates poorly with lay opinion as to what constitutes a need for treatment (Hunt et al., 2002). As the desire for orthodontic treatment is primarily driven by the perception of a patient regarding their own dental aesthetics, future indices may well incorporate patient factors into their scoring systems.

The DHC is hierarchical, for each individual the highest score is found and recorded, irrespective of any other features within the malocclusion. The five categories are further subdivided using letters, which describe the feature of the malocclusion that has been scored (Table 1.3).

Aesthetic Component

This records the aesthetic handicapping of the malocclusion and is based on a series of ten photographs, which show a graduated decrease in dental aesthetics (Fig. 1.20). A score is given from 0 to 10 based upon the perceived aesthetic impairment of an individual's malocclusion, not morphological similarities with the photographs. A high-level agreement has been found between scores given by professionals and those given by patients.

Table 1.3 Dental health component of the IOTN

Grade 1—No treatment required

1.	Extremely minor malocclusions, including displacements less than 1 mm

Grade 2—Little need for treatment

2.a	Increased overjet > 3.5 mm but ≤ 6 mm (with competent lips)
2.b	Reverse overjet greater than 0 mm but ≤ 1 mm
2.c	Anterior or posterior crossbite with ≤ 1 mm discrepancy between RCP and ICP
2.d	Displacement of teeth > 1 mm but ≤ 2 mm
2.e	Anterior or posterior open bite > 1 mm but ≤ 2 mm
2.f	Increased overbite ≥ 3.5 mm (without gingival contact)
2.g	Prenormal or postnormal occlusions with no other anomalies (up to $\frac{1}{2}$ a unit of discrepancy)

Grade 3—Borderline need for treatment

3.a	Increased overjet > 3.5 mm but ≤ 6 mm (incompetent lips)
3.b	Reverse overjet greater than 1 mm but ≤ 3.5 mm
3.c	Anterior or posterior crossbites with > 1 mm but ≤ 2 mm discrepancy between RCP and ICP
3.d	Displacement of teeth > 2 mm but ≤ 4 mm
3.e	Lateral or anterior open bite > 2 mm but ≤ 4 mm
3.f	Increased and incomplete overbite without gingival or palatal trauma

Grade 4—Treatment required

4.a	Increased overjet > 6 mm but ≤ 9 mm
4.b	Reverse overjet > 3.5 mm with no masticatory or speech difficulties
4.c	Anterior or posterior crossbites with > 2 mm discrepancy between RCP and ICP
4.d	Severe displacements of teeth > 4 mm
4.e	Extreme lateral or anterior open bites > 4 mm
4.f	Increased and complete overbite with gingival or palatal trauma
4.h	Less extensive hypodontia requiring pre-restorative orthodontics or orthodontic space closure to obviate the need for a prosthesis
4.l	Posterior lingual crossbite with no functional occlusal contact in one or more buccal segments
4.m	Reverse overjet > 1 mm but < 3.5 mm with recorded masticatory and speech difficulties
4.t	Partially erupted teeth, tipped and impacted against adjacent teeth
4.x	Existing supernumerary teeth

Grade 5—Treatment required

5.a	Increased overjet > 9 mm
5.h	Extensive hypodontia with restorative implications (more than one tooth missing in any quadrant requiring pre-restorative orthodontics)

Table 1.3 Dental health component of the IOTN—cont'd

5.i	Impeded eruption of teeth (apart from 3rd molars) due to crowding, displacement, the presence of supernumerary teeth, retained deciduous teeth and any pathological cause
5.m	Reverse overjet > 3.5 mm with reported masticatory and speech difficulties
5.p	Defects of cleft lip and palate
5.s	Submerged deciduous teeth

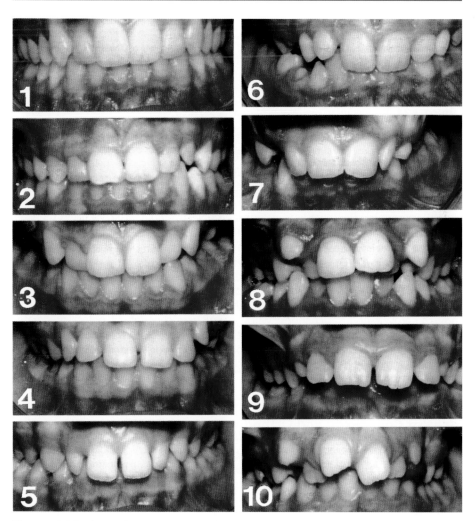

Figure 1.20 The aesthetic component of the IOTN. The SCAN scale was first published in 1987 by the European Orthodontic Society (Evans R and Shaw W, Preliminary evaluation of an illustrated scale for dental attractiveness. Eur J Orthod 9: 314–318). IOTN aesthetic and dental health components reproduced courtesy of Orthocare.

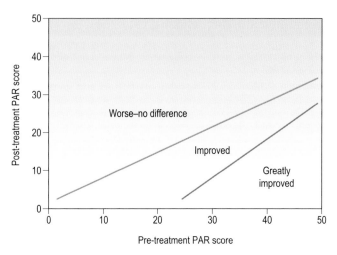

Figure 1.21 Nomogram of pre- and post-treatment PAR scores.

Monitoring orthodontic treatment

The outcome of orthodontic treatment can be recorded in terms of occlusal changes and an attempt has been made to give this an objective numeric score using the Peer Assessment Rating (PAR) (Richmond et al, 1992a, b). This gives an accumulative score, indicating the extent of deviation from a normal functioning occlusion assessed from dental study casts. There is no maximum cut-off level, and the pre- and post-treatment models should be assessed, which gives a percentage score for the change with treatment. A reduction in the weighted PAR score of less than 30% is considered to show occlusal changes that are worse or no different. A reduction of greater than 30% shows improved occlusal changes, whilst a PAR reduction of 22 points or greater indicates a greatly improved occlusal result. This can be plotted on a nomogram (Fig. 1.21), which is divided into three sections: upper (worse–no difference), middle (improved) and lower (greatly improved). This is useful when looking at the outcome of multiple patients, as it gives an indication of the quality of treatment an individual or group of individuals is providing.

Index of Complexity and Orthodontic Need (ICON)

Based on the IOTN and PAR indices a single index, the Index of Complexity and Need (ICON), has been developed to measure both treatment need and outcome of treatment (Daniels and Richmond, 2000). By combining five occlusal traits (IOTN Aesthetic Component, crossbite, upper arch crowding and spacing, buccal segment antero-posterior relationships, and anterior vertical relationship) with different weightings, a numeric score is given that can be used to ascertain need for treatment, the complexity of the treatment and the improvement resulting from treatment. This has been shown to be reproducible for treatment need and complexity but less so for outcome, due to low levels of agreement between examiners as to what constitutes acceptable treatment (Richmond and Daniels, 1998a, b).

Further reading

CLARK JR AND EVANS RD (2001). Functional occlusion: I. A review. *J Orthod* 28: 76–81.
DAVIES S AND GRAY RM (2001). What is occlusion? *Br Dent J* 191: 235–8, 241–245.
DAVIES SJ, GRAY RM, SANDLER PJ ET AL (2001). Orthodontics and occlusion. *Br Dent J* 191: 539–542, 545–549.

References

ADDY M, DUMMER PM, GRIFFITHS G ET AL (1986). Prevalence of plaque, gingivitis and caries in 11–12-year-old children in South Wales. *Community Dent Oral Epidemiol* 14: 115–118.
ANDREWS LF (1972). The six keys to normal occlusion. *Am J Orthod* 62: 296–309.
ANGLE EH (1899). Classification of malocclusion. *Dental Cosmos* 41: 248–264.
BASS JK, FINE H AND CISNEROS GJ (1993). Nickel hypersensitivity in the orthodontic patient. *Am J Orthod Dentofacial Orthop* 103: 280–285.
BEGG PR (1954). Stone age man's dentition. *Am J Orthod* 40: 298–312.
BENSON PE, SHAH AA, MILLETT DT ET AL (2005). Fluorides, orthodontics and demineralization: a systematic review. *J Orthod* 32: 102–114.
BRENCHLEY ML (1991). Is digit sucking of significance? *Br Dent J* 171: 357–362.
BROOK PH AND SHAW WC (1989). The development of an index of orthodontic treatment priority. *Eur J Orthod* 11: 309–320.
CASSIDY KM, HARRIS EF, TOLLEY EA ET AL (1998). Genetic influence on dental arch form in orthodontic patients. *Angle Orthod* 68: 445–454.
CECERE F, RUF S AND PANCHERZ H (1996). Is quantitative electromyography reliable? *J Orofac Pain* 10: 38–47.
CHESTNUTT IG, BURDEN DJ, STEELE JG ET AL (2006). The orthodontic condition of children in the United Kingdom, 2003. *Br Dent J* 200: 609–612;quiz 638.
CHRISTENSEN LV AND RASSOULI NM (1995). Experimental occlusal interferences. Part I. A review. *J Oral Rehabil* 22: 515–520.
COOPER S, MANDALL NA, DIBIASE D ET AL (2000). The reliability of the Index of Orthodontic Treatment Need over time. *J Orthod* 27: 47–53.
CORRUCCINI RS (1984). An epidemiologic transition in dental occlusion in world populations. *Am J Orthod* 86: 419–426.
CORRUCCINI RS, TOWNSEND GC, RICHARDS LC ET AL (1990). Genetic and environmental determinants of dental occlusal variation in twins of different nationalities. *Hum Biol* 62: 353–367.
DANIELS C AND RICHMOND S (2000). The development of the index of complexity, outcome and need (ICON). *J Orthod* 27: 149–162.
DAVIES TM, SHAW WC, ADDY M ET AL (1988). The relationship of anterior overjet to plaque and gingivitis in children. *Am J Orthod Dentofacial Orthop* 93: 303–309.
DAVIES TM, SHAW WC, WORTHINGTON HV ET AL (1991). The effect of orthodontic treatment on plaque and gingivitis. *Am J Orthod Dentofacial Orthop* 99: 155–161.
DERKS A, KATSAROS C, FRENCKEN JE ET AL (2004). Caries-inhibiting effect of preventive measures during orthodontic treatment with fixed appliances. A systematic review. *Caries Res* 38: 413–420.
DIBBETS JM AND VAN DER WEELE LT (1991). Extraction, orthodontic treatment, and craniomandibular dysfunction. *Am J Orthod Dentofacial Orthop* 99: 210–219.
DUNCAN K, MCNAMARA C, IRELAND AJ (2007) Sucking habits in childhood and the effects on the primary dentition: findings of the Avon Longitudinal Study of Pregnancy and Childhood. *Int J Paediatr Dent* 18: 178–188.
EGERMARK-ERIKSSON I, CARLSSON GE AND INGERVALL B (1981). Prevalence of mandibular dysfunction and orofacial parafunction in 7-, 11- and 15-year-old Swedish children. *Eur J Orthod* 3: 163–172.

EGERMARK-ERIKSSON I, INGERVALL B AND CARLSSON GE (1983). The dependence of mandibular dysfunction in children on functional and morphologic malocclusion. *Am J Orthod* 83: 187–194.

GORELICK L, GEIGER AM AND GWINNETT AJ (1982). Incidence of white spot formation after bonding and banding. *Am J Orthod* 81: 93–98.

GRAVELY JF AND JOHNSON DB (1974). Angle's classification of malocclusion: an assessment of reliability. *Br J Orthod* 1: 79–86.

HIDAKA O, ADACHI S AND TAKADA K (2002). The difference in condylar position between centric relation and centric occlusion in pretreatment Japanese orthodontic patients. *Angle Orthod* 72: 295–301.

HOWE RP, MCNAMARA JA Jr AND O'CONNOR KA (1983). An examination of dental crowding and its relationship to tooth size and arch dimension. *Am J Orthod* 83: 363–373.

HUNT N, SHAH R, SINANAN A ET AL (2006). Northcroft Memorial Lecture 2005: Muscling in on malocclusions: Current concepts on the role of muscles in the aetiology and treatment of malocclusion. *J Orthod* 33: 187–197.

HUNT O, HEPPER P, JOHNSTON C ET AL (2002). The Aesthetic Component of the Index of Orthodontic Treatment Need validated against lay opinion. *Eur J Orthod* 24: 53–59.

JARVINEN S (1978). Incisal overjet and traumatic injuries to upper permanent incisors. A retrospective study. *Acta Odontol Scand* 36: 359–362.

JOHAL A, CHEUNG MY AND MARCENE W (2007). The impact of two different malocclusion traits on quality of life. *Br Dent J* 202: E2.

KENEALY PM, KINGDON A, RICHMOND S ET AL (2007). The Cardiff dental study: a 20-year critical evaluation of the psychological health gain from orthodontic treatment. *Br J Health Psychol* 12: 17–49.

KING L, HARRIS EF AND TOLLEY EA (1993). Heritability of cephalometric and occlusal variables as assessed from siblings with overt malocclusions. *Am J Orthod Dentofacial Orthop* 104: 121–131.

KREMENAK CR, KINSER DD, HARMAN HA ET AL (1992a). Orthodontic risk factors for temporomandibular disorders (TMD). I: Premolar extractions. *Am J Orthod Dentofacial Orthop* 101: 13–20.

KREMENAK CR, KINSER DD, MELCHER TJ ET AL (1992b). Orthodontics as a risk factor for temporomandibular disorders (TMD). II. *Am J Orthod Dentofacial Orthop* 101: 21–27.

LAUC T, RUDAN P, RUDAN I ET AL (2003). Effect of inbreeding and endogamy on occlusal traits in human isolates. *J Orthod* 30: 301–308; discussion 297.

LINDER-ARONSON S (1970). Adenoids. Their effect on mode of breathing and nasal airflow and their relationship to characteristics of the facial skeleton and the denition. A biometric, rhino-manometric and cephalometro-radiographic study on children with and without adenoids. *Acta Otolaryngol Suppl* 265: 1–132.

LINDER-ARONSON S (1974). Orthodontics in the Swedish Public Dental Health Service. *Trans Eur Orthod Soc*: 233–240.

LINDER-ARONSON S, WOODSIDE DG AND LUNDSTROM A (1986). Mandibular growth direction following adenoidectomy. *Am J Orthod* 89: 273–284.

LINGE L and LINGE BO (1991). Patient characteristics and treatment variables associated with apical root resorption during orthodontic treatment. *Am J Orthod Dentofacial Orthop* 99: 35–43.

LITTON SF, ACKERMANN LV, ISAACSON RJ AND SHAPIRO BL (1970). A genetic study of Class 3 malocclusion. *Am J Orthod* 58: 565–577.

LUTHER F (2007a). TMD and occlusion part I. Damned if we do? Occlusion: the interface of dentistry and orthodontics. *Br Dent J* 202: E2; discussion 38–39.

LUTHER F (2007b). TMD and occlusion part II. Damned if we don't? Functional occlusal problems: TMD epidemiology in a wider context. *Br Dent J* 202: E3; discussion 38–39.

MOHLIN BO, DERWEDUWEN K, PILLEY R ET AL (2004). Malocclusion and temporomandibular disorder: a comparison of adolescents with moderate to severe dysfunction with those without signs and symptoms of temporomandibular disorder and their further development to 30 years of age. *Angle Orthod* 74: 319–327.

PECK S, PECK L AND KATAJA M (1994). The palatally displaced canine as a dental anomaly of genetic origin. *Angle Orthod* 64: 249–256.

PROFFIT WR (1978). Equilibrium theory revisited: factors influencing position of the teeth. *Angle Orthod* 48: 175–186.

PROFFIT WR AND FIELDS HW (1983). Occlusal forces in normal- and long-face children. *J Dent Res* 62: 571–574.

PROFFIT WR, FIELDS HW Jr AND MORAY LJ (1998). Prevalence of malocclusion and orthodontic treatment need in the United States: estimates from the NHANES III survey. *Int J Adult Orthodon Orthognath Surg* 13: 97–106.

RICHMOND S AND DANIELS CP (1998a). International comparisons of professional assessments in orthodontics: Part 1—Treatment need. *Am J Orthod Dentofacial Orthop* 113: 180–185.

RICHMOND S AND DANIELS CP (1998b). International comparisons of professional assessments in orthodontics: Part 2—treatment outcome. *Am J Orthod Dentofacial Orthop* 113: 324–328.

RICHMOND S, SHAW WC, O'BRIEN KD ET AL (1992a). The development of the PAR Index (Peer Assessment Rating): reliability and validity. *Eur J Orthod* 14: 125–139.

RICHMOND S, SHAW WC, ROBERTS CT ET AL (1992b). The PAR Index (Peer Assessment Rating): methods to determine outcome of orthodontic treatment in terms of improvement and standards. *Eur J Orthod* 14: 180–187.

SADOWSKY C, THEISEN TA AND SAKOLS EI (1991). Orthodontic treatment and temporomandibular joint sounds—a longitudinal study. *Am J Orthod Dentofacial Orthop* 99: 441–447.

SAMESHIMA GT AND SINCLAIR PM (2004). Characteristics of patients with severe root resorption. *Orthod Craniofac Res* 7: 108–114.

SEGAL GR, SCHIFFMAN PH AND TUNCAY OC (2004). Meta analysis of the treatment-related factors of external apical root resorption. *Orthod Craniofac Res* 7: 71–78.

SHAW WC, RICHMOND S AND O'BRIEN KD (1995). The use of occlusal indices: a European perspective. *Am J Orthod Dentofacial Orthop* 107: 1–10.

SOLBERG WK, WOO MW AND HOUSTON JB (1979). Prevalence of mandibular dysfunction in young adults. *J Am Dent Assoc* 98: 25–34.

TIPTON RT AND RINCHUSE DJ (1991). The relationship between static occlusion and functional occlusion in a dental school population. *Angle Orthod* 61: 57–66.

VARRELA J (2006). Masticatory function and malocclusion: A clinical perspective. *Semin Orthod* 12: 102–109.

VIG KW (1998). Nasal obstruction and facial growth: the strength of evidence for clinical assumptions. *Am J Orthod Dentofacial Orthop* 113: 603–611.

WATANABE M, SUDA N AND OHYAMA K (2005). Mandibular prognathism in Japanese families ascertained through orthognathically treated patients. *Am J Orthod Dentofacial Orthop* 128: 466–470.

WEILAND FJ, JONKE E AND BANTLEON HP (1997). Secular trends in malocclusion in Austrian men. *Eur J Orthod* 19: 355–359.

WILLIAMS AC and STEPHENS CD (1992). A modification to the incisor classification of malocclusion. *Br J Orthod* 19: 127–130.

WOODSIDE DG, LINDER-ARONSON S, LUNDSTROM A ET AL (1991). Mandibular and maxillary growth after changed mode of breathing. *Am J Orthod Dentofacial Orthop* 100: 1–18.

ZACHRISSON BU AND ALNAES L (1974). Periodontal condition in orthodontically treated and untreated individuals. II. Alveolar bone loss: radiographic findings. *Angle Orthod* 44: 48–55.

2 Prenatal development of the craniofacial region

During evolution, modern humans split from their last common ancestor with the apes around seven million years ago. Since that time, *Homo sapiens* have acquired features that make them unique as a species and separate them from other primates:

- An erect posture and bipedalism;
- Expansion of the cerebral hemispheres, with an accompanying increase in brain size and development of higher intelligence;
- Modification of the hand to allow apposition between thumb and fingers; and
- Descent of the larynx relative to the cranial base and the concomitant development of speech and language.

Many of these evolutionary changes are reflected in the form and function of the craniofacial region (Fig. 2.1). The essential morphology of the head and face is fundamental to being human and the development of this region is complicated, beginning early in life and requiring the coordinated growth and interaction of all primary cell populations within the embryo.

Embryonic origins of the head and neck

The early embryo is derived from three primary germ layers of tissue (Table 2.1):

- Ectoderm (first germ layer);
- Endoderm (second germ layer); and
- Mesoderm (third germ layer).

There is also a further contribution from the neural crest (or fourth germ layer). Ectoderm and endoderm are derived from the epiblast and hypoblast, two fundamental cell populations within the bilaminar disc of the early embryo (Fig. 2.2). Mesoderm is produced during the process of gastrulation and the conversion of a bilaminar embryo into one with three primary tissue layers (Fig. 2.3).

In mammals, neural crest cells arise during formation of the neural tube and migrate extensively throughout the embryo in four overlapping domains:

- Cranial;
- Cardiac;
- Trunk; and
- Sacral.

Cranial neural crest cells provide the building blocks for generating much of the skeleton and connective tissue of the head, in addition to the cranial ganglia and peripheral nerves innervating these skeletal structures. In the developing head, neural

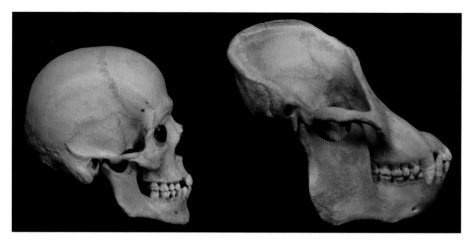

Figure 2.1 Comparison of a human (left) and orangutan (right) skull. In the human skull, the cranium is enlarged and the forehead is upright above the eyes, reflecting the expansion of the frontal lobes. The human face is therefore positioned downwards and backwards relative to the forebrain.

crest cells arising from the forebrain and midbrain regions populate the upper face, whilst those from the posterior midbrain and hindbrain migrate into the pharyngeal arch system (see Fig. 2.14). Cranial neural crest cells interact with ectodermal and mesodermal cell populations present within these regions, leading to the formation of craniofacial bones, cartilages and connective tissue (Fig. 2.4).

The prechordal plate—a molecular organizer for the brain and face

A region of fundamental importance for early development of the brain and face is the prechordal plate, an area of thickened endoderm that lies beneath the future forebrain of the early embryo (Fig. 2.5).

The prechordal plate acts as a true head organizer, producing molecular signals that pattern the forebrain and subdivide the eyefield into two. In the absence of normal signalling from this region, holoprosencephaly (HPE) or cyclopia can occur. In the most severe cases, the lower forebrain does not form and the upper part remains as a single undivided vesicle, rather than developing into paired cerebral hemispheres (Muenke & Beachy, 2000). This lack of midline development within the central nervous system has important consequences for the face, with a spectrum of facial deformity reflecting the severity of the brain malformation. Failure of forebrain division leads to a lack of separation of the optic primordia and the formation of a single cyclopic eye, which becomes situated below a rudimentary midline facial proboscis or nose-like structure (see Fig. 13.21).

Table 2.1 Embryonic origins of the head and neck

Ectoderm

Skin
Hair
Sebaceous glands
Anterior lobe of the pituitary gland
Oral epithelium
Tooth enamel
Nasal and olfactory epithelium
External auditory canal

Neural tube

Forebrain
Midbrain
Hindbrain
Cervical spinal cord

Cranial neural crest

Sensory ganglia
Sympathetic ganglia (V, VII, IX, X)
Parasympathetic ganglia of neck
Schwann cells
Meninges
  Dura mater
  Pia mater
  Arachnoid mater
Pharyngeal arch cartilages
Dermal skull bones
Connective tissue of:
  Cranial musculature
  Adenohypophysis
  Lingual glands
  Thymus
  Thyroid
  Parathyroid
Vascular and dermal smooth muscles
Odontoblasts and pulp of the teeth
Corneal endothelium and stroma
Melanocytes and melanopores
Epidermal pigment cells
Carotid body type I cells
C cells of ultimopharyngeal body

Endoderm

Pharynx
  Thyroid
Pharyngeal pouches
  I Tympanic cavity
     Pharyngotympanic tube
  II Tonsillar recess
  III Thymus
     Inferior parathyroid
  IV Superior parathyroid
     Ultimopharyngeal body

Mesoderm

Head mesoderm
  Craniofacial musculature
Paraxial mesoderm
  Axial neck skeleton and basal occipital bone

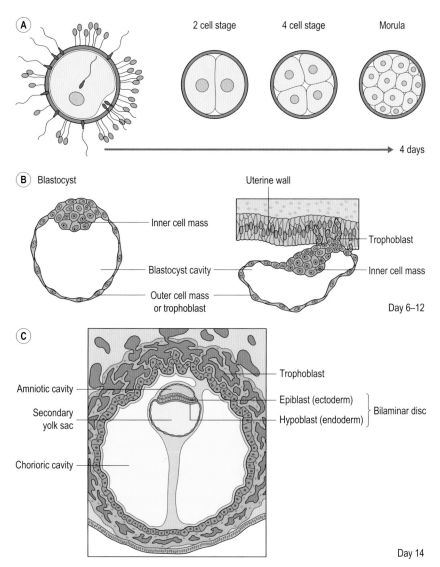

Figure 2.2 Early development of the embryo. (A) Following fertilization, the zygote undergoes a series of mitotic cell divisions to produce a sixteen cell morula. (B) The cells within the morula are quickly organised into outer and inner cell masses and the early embryo is known as a blastocyst. Cells of the outer cell mass form the trophoblast, which mediates implantation of the blastocyst into the uterine wall and contributes to the placenta. The inner cell mass forms the embryo itself. (C) During implantation, the inner cell mass differentiates into two layers; the epiblast (future ectoderm) and hypoblast (future endoderm), which together form the bilaminar disc of the early embryo. Redrawn from Sandler TW (ed.) (2003), *Langman's Medical Embryology*, 9th edn (Baltimore: Lippincott Williams and Wilkins).

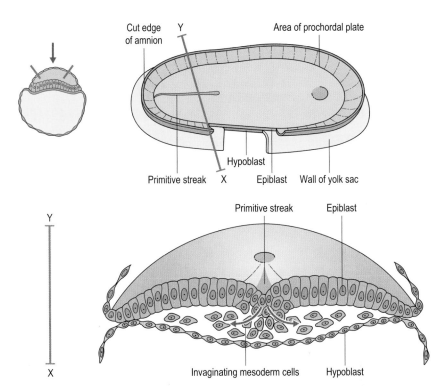

Figure 2.3 Gastrulation. During the third week of embryonic development, the third germ layer or mesoderm is formed by the process of gastrulation. Cells of the epiblast migrate through the primitive streak, a raised structure on the surface of the epiblast, and detach to position themselves between epiblast and hypoblast and form the mesodermal cell layer. Redrawn from Sandler TW (ed.) (2003), *Langman's Medical Embryology*, 9th edn (Baltimore: Lippincott Williams and Wilkins).

Early organization of the craniofacial region

Primary architecture of the craniofacial region is established during early development and is based upon segmentation (Fig. 2.6). At the future head end of the human embryo, the neural tube is segmented into three vesicles, which will form:
- Forebrain;
- Midbrain; and
- Hindbrain.

  On the lateral side of the head are the pharyngeal arches, which form:
- Neck;
- Pharynx; and
- Jaws.

  In the upper region of the head is the frontonasal process, which surrounds the early forebrain and will form:
- The upper face.

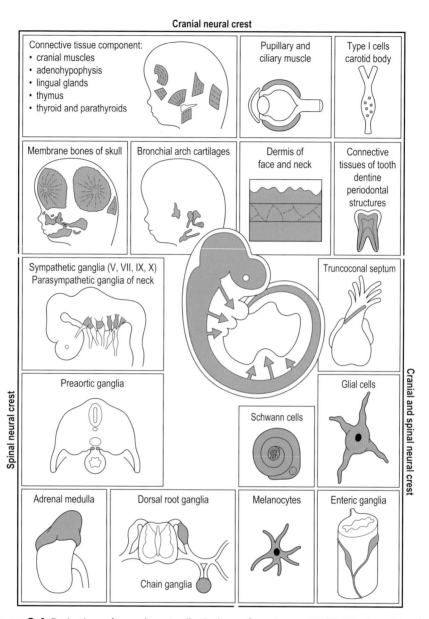

Figure 2.4 Derivatives of neural crest cells. Redrawn from Larsen WJ (1998). *Essentials of Human Embryology* (Edinburgh: Churchill Livingstone).

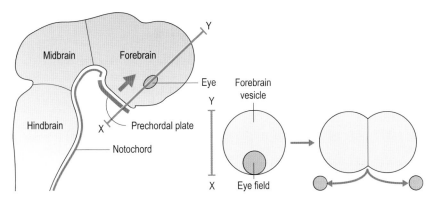

Figure 2.5 Signalling from the prechordal plate is important for patterning ventral regions of the early forebrain and producing bilateral subdivision of the eyefield. Sonic hedgehog (SHH) signalling from the prechordal plate plays an important role in this process.

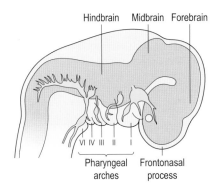

Figure 2.6 Segmentation of the craniofacial region in the early embryo. The neural tube is segmented into forebrain, midbrain and hindbrain vesicles; the frontonasal process is situated over the developing forebrain and the segmented pharyngeal arches are situated ventrally.

In the lower region of the head is the first pharyngeal arch, which will form:

- The midface; and
- The lower face.

The pharyngeal arches

In humans there are six pharyngeal arches, which appear progressively during the fourth week of embryonic development. Each arch is covered externally by ectoderm and internally by endoderm, whilst a core of mesodermal tissue exists within. As development proceeds, this central core becomes infiltrated by cranial neural crest cells that migrate into the arches from their site of origin adjacent to the roof of the neural tube. The junction of each arch is in close proximity with its neighbour, producing a pharyngeal cleft of ectoderm externally and a pouch of endoderm internally (Fig. 2.7).

The pharyngeal arches give rise to a number of structures within the head and neck (Fig. 2.8):

- The first pharyngeal arch produces the jaws and dentition;
- The second pharyngeal arch forms the suprahyoid apparatus of the neck;
- The third pharyngeal arch contributes to the infrahyoid region;

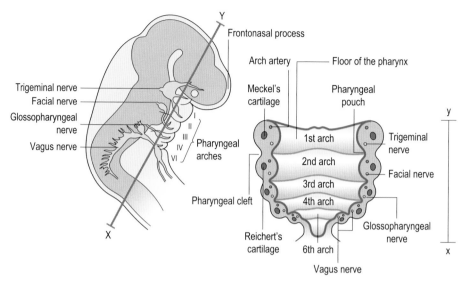

Figure 2.7 The pharyngeal arches. Each arch is covered externally by ectoderm and internally by endoderm. Within each arch is a core of mesoderm, which becomes progressively infiltrated with migrating neural crest cells. In addition, a characteristic nerve, cartilage and artery are situated within each arch.

- The fourth and sixth pharyngeal arches form the laryngeal structures; and
- The fifth pharyngeal arch is the exception, rapidly degenerating after formation and making no contribution towards any permanent structures in the human.

The embryonic tissue components within each arch give rise to specific structures:

- Ectoderm produces the skin and sensory neurons of the lower face and neck;
- Endoderm forms the mucosal lining of the pharynx and associated endocrine organs (thyroid, parathyroid and thymus) of the neck;
- Cranial neural crest cells produce most of the skeletal and connective tissues within the head and neck; and
- Mesoderm produces the associated craniofacial musculature, cardiac outflow tract and endothelial cells of the pharyngeal arch arteries.

Within the pharyngeal arch system are also characteristic sets of bilaterally symmetrical arteries, nerves and cartilages. Those associated with the first two arches make contributions to the maxillary and stapedial arteries in the adult, whilst those within the lower pharyngeal arches are responsible for generating major arteries within the neck and cardiothoracic region. Neural crest cells that migrate into the third and fourth pharyngeal arches are known collectively as the cardiac neural crest, these cells making an important contribution to remodelling of the pharyngeal arch arteries and to the formation of a functional cardiac outflow tract and cardiothoracic vascular system. Any disruption within the embryonic pharyngeal region can have serious implications for normal development, which is exemplified by a group of related disorders known as the 22q11 deletion syndromes (Box 2.1).

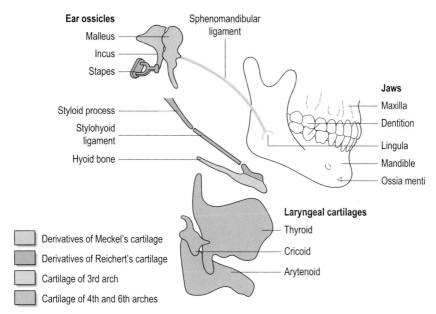

Figure 2.8 Skeletal derivatives of the pharyngeal arches. The first arch gives rise to the upper and lower jaws, the dentition, the malleus and incus (middle ear ossicles) and sphenomandibular ligament. The second arch gives rise to the styloid process, stylohyoid ligament, stapes (middle ear ossicle) and the lesser cornu and upper part of the body of the hyoid bone. The third arch gives rise to the greater cornu and lower part of the body of the hyoid bone. The fourth arch gives rise to the laryngeal cartilages. Those structures formed by the pharyngeal arch cartilages are indicated in colour. Redrawn from Wendell-Smith CP, Williams RL, Treadgold S (1984), *Basic Human Embryology*, 3rd edn (London: Pitman Publishing).

Box 2.1   TBX1: a mediator of normal pharyngeal arch development

T-box genes encode a large group of transcription factors and TBX1 is thought to be a key player in the aetiology of the DiGeorge (DGS; OMIM 601362) and Velocardiofacial (VCFS; OMIM 192430) or 22q11 Deletion syndromes (22q11DS). These syndromes form part of a group of related human dysmorphic disorders that result from deletion or rearrangement of a large region of chromosome 22q11 (Baldini, 2005; Scambler, 2000). 22q11DS subjects are characterized by defects in the cardiac outflow tract and aortic arch, thymic and parathyroid aplasia or hypoplasia, and anomalies of the craniofacial region, which include micrognathia, cleft palate and a characteristic facial appearance. The principle clinical phenotypes present within these syndromes are thought to result from an absence of normal pharyngeal pouch signalling and localized disruption of neural crest migration within the pharyngeal arch system.

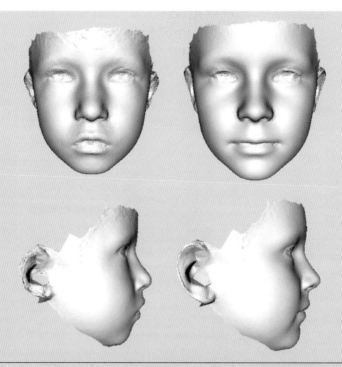

Three-dimensional facial scans of individuals with 22q11DS (left) and control subjects (right) aged between 2 weeks and 24 years. The 22q11DS face is only subtly different from the average, but careful examination reveals an exaggerated length of the nose, with a narrow nares and nasal base, but fullness above the tip. The eyes are upslanted and the ears cupped or unusual in shape (Hammond et al, 2005). Reproduced with kind permission of Professor Peter Hammond, Institute of Child Health, University College London.

The candidacy of *TBX1* for 22q11DS has been based upon its location within the deleted region of chromosome 22, its expression domain in endoderm and mesoderm of the developing pharyngeal arches and the finding that mice generated with a targeted deletion in *Tbx1* exhibit a spectrum of phenotypic effects encompassing most of the common 22q11DS malformations (Lindsay et al, 2001). More recent genetic experiments in mice, designed to ablate the function of *Tbx1* in different regions of the early pharynx at different developmental time points, have provided clues as to the role of this transcription factor during patterning and differentiation of the pharyngeal arch derivatives. In particular, *Tbx1* activity influences the proliferation and expansion of endoderm lining the embryonic pharynx; a role that facilitates normal segmentation of the pharyngeal arches and the formation of structures derived from these regions.

Development of the face

Development of the face is a dynamic process, relying upon complex tissue interactions that are closely coordinated, both temporally and spatially (Fig. 2.9). Growth and development of this region is driven by neural crest migration and proliferation, which directs the formation and approximation of a series of swellings or processes. Ultimately, these processes fuse with each other to produce seamless regions of ectoderm and the characteristic features of a face. At the molecular level, a host of signalling molecules, transcription factors and extracellular matrix proteins control the cellular activities underlying these processes (Francis-West et al, 2003).

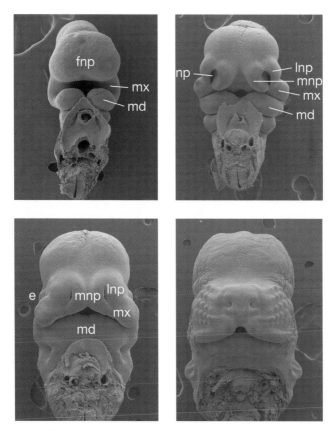

Figure 2.9 Early facial development. Scanning electron micrographs of an early mouse embryo show development of the face from a series of rudimentary processes. In particular, the lateral part of the upper lip is formed from the maxillary processes, whilst the philtrum is derived from the paired medial nasal processes, which fuse in the midline. e, eye; fnp, frontonasal process; md, mandibular process; mx, maxillary process; lnp, lateral nasal process; mnp, medial nasal process; np, nasal placode.

Human facial development begins at approximately four weeks post conception, with the appearance of five processes, which surround the early oral cavity or stomodeum (Table 2.2):

- Frontonasal process;
- Maxillary processes (paired) of the first pharyngeal arch; and
- Mandibular processes (paired) of the first pharyngeal arch.

During the fourth week of development the frontonasal process rapidly enlarges as the underlying forebrain expands into bilateral cerebral hemispheres and the paired mandibular processes unite to provide continuity to the forbearer of the lower jaw and lip.

By five weeks of development, medial and lateral nasal processes form within the enlarged frontonasal process to surround an early ectodermal thickening, the nasal placode. The nasal placode gives rise to highly specialized olfactory receptor cells and nerve fibre bundles innervating the future nasal cavity. As the medial and lateral nasal processes enlarge, the nasal placodes sink into the nasal pits, which demarcates the nostrils.

Medial growth of the maxillary processes dominates subsequent development of the face, resulting first in contact and then fusion with the lateral nasal processes to form:

- Nasolacrimal duct;
- Cheek; and
- Alar base of the future nose.

Further growth towards the midline pushes the lateral nasal processes superiorly and allows fusion of the maxillary processes with the medial nasal processes inferiorly, merging them together in the midline to form:

- Central portion of the nose;
- Upper lip philtrum; and
- Primary palate.

Thus, the upper lip is formed from the maxillary processes laterally and the medial nasal processes in the midline (Jiang et al, 2006).

Posteriorly, from the medial sides of the maxillary process, the secondary palate is formed via growth, elevation and subsequent fusion between the paired palatine processes. These processes also fuse with the nasal septum superiorly and the primary palate anteriorly, ultimately separating the oral and nasal cavities. The essential features of the human face have formed by eight weeks of development.

Development of the pharyngeal region

Endoderm lining the pharyngeal arches, in the form of the pharyngeal pouches, gives rise to a number of important structures associated with the mature pharynx (Fig. 2.10).

- The first pharyngeal pouch forms a small internal projection, the tubotympanic recess, which contributes to the tympanic cavity and pharyngotympanic tube. At its deepest aspect, the tubotympanic recess comes into direct contact with ectoderm of the first pharyngeal cleft at the site of the tympanic membrane or eardrum.
- The second pharyngeal pouch forms the tonsillar fossa and contributes to the epithelial component of the palatine tonsil.

Table 2.2 Building the head and neck

Frontonasal process

Forehead including upper eyelids and conjunctiva

Medial nasal processes

Nose
Upper lip philtrum
Pre-maxilla and incisor teeth

Lateral nasal processes

Ala base of the nose
Nasolacrimal duct

First pharyngeal arch

Muscles of mastication
Mylohyoid
Anterior belly of digastric
Tensor veli palatini
Tensor tympani

Maxillary process

Lower eyelid and conjunctiva
Cheek
Lateral portion of the upper lip
Maxilla
Palatine
Pterygoid
Zygomatic
Squamosal
Alisphenoid
Secondary palate
Canine, premolar and molar teeth

Mandibular process

Lower lip
Mandible and mandibular dentition
Meckel's cartilage: Lingula
                   Ossia menti
                   Sphenomandibular ligament
                   Anterior malleolar ligament
                   Malleus
                   Incus

Second pharyngeal arch

Muscles of facial expression
Posterior belly of digastric
Stylohyoid
Stapedius
Stapes
Styloid process
Stylohyoid ligament
Lesser horn of hyoid bone and upper portion of body of hyoid bone

Third pharyngeal arch

Stylopharyngeus
Greater horn of hyoid bone
Lower portion of body of hyoid bone

Fourth pharyngeal arch

Levator palatini
Pharyngeal constrictors
Laryngeal cartilages

Sixth pharyngeal arch

Intrinsic muscles of the larynx

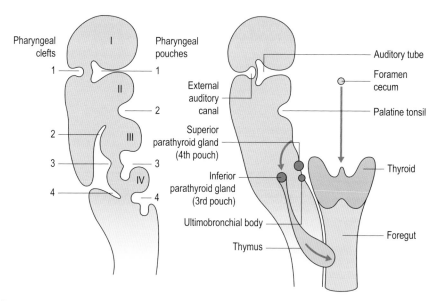

Figure 2.10 Derivatives of the pharyngeal clefts and pouches in the head and neck. Redrawn from Sandler TW (ed.) (2003), *Langman's Medical Embryology*, 9th edn (Baltimore: Lippincott Williams and Wilkins).

- The third pharyngeal pouch possesses both superior and inferior projections, which in conjunction with cranial and cardiac neural crest cells, generate the inferior parathyroid and thymus glands, respectively.
- The fourth pharyngeal pouch gives rise to the superior parathyroid glands.
- The fifth pharyngeal pouch is essentially transitory.
- The ultimobranchial body or lowest of the pharyngeal pouches becomes incorporated within the thyroid gland as parafollicular or C cells.

Externally, there are four pharyngeal clefts, but only one develops into a recognizable structure in the neonate. The first pharyngeal cleft forms the external auditory canal and contributes to the eardrum of the external ear. The remaining pharyngeal clefts are obliterated by downward growth of the second pharyngeal arch, disappearing as the cervical sinus.

The tongue arises from a series of swellings, which appear around the sixth week of development in the floor of the primitive pharynx (Fig. 2.11).

- The lateral lingual swellings and midline tuberculum impar are derived from mesoderm of the first pharyngeal arch and form the anterior two-thirds of the tongue.
- The hypobranchial eminence forms a posterior midline swelling and has contributions from second, third and fourth arch mesoderm to form the posterior third of the tongue.
- The epiglottal swelling is also a derivative of the fourth arch and forms at the most posterior boundary of the tongue, giving rise to the epiglottis of the larynx.

Simultaneously with formation of the tongue, the thyroid gland is formed from a proliferation of endoderm at the foramen cecum, a site between the tuberculum

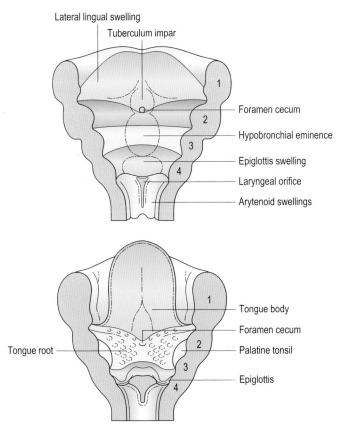

Figure 2.11 Embryonic origins of tongue. The floor of the pharynx gives rise to a series of elevations at around the sixth week of embryonic development, which contribute to the anterior two-thirds and posterior third of the mature tongue. Redrawn from Sandler TW (ed.) (2003), *Langman's Medical Embryology*, 9th edn (Baltimore: Lippincott Williams and Wilkins).

impar and hypobranchial eminence in the pharyngeal floor. Descent of the primitive thyroid into the neck occurs over a period of a few weeks, resulting in the gland assuming its final position below the thyroid cartilage.

Development of the skull

The individual bones that make up the human skull are formed by two basic mechanisms:

- Endochondral bones develop from within a cartilaginous template; and
- Intramembranous bones arise following direct differentiation of mesenchymal cells into osteoblasts.

With the exception of the clavicle, bones with an intramembranous origin are only found in the craniofacial region. Collectively, both endochondral and intramembranous bones of the skull originate from two embryonic cell populations:

- Cranial neural crest; and
- Paraxial mesoderm.

The boundary of these two tissue contributions within the skull lies at the level of the coronal suture.

The skull can also be subdivided on an anatomical basis into two distinct regions:

- Neurocranium; and
- Viscerocranium.

The neurocranium is composed of the cranial vault (or desmocranium), which develops in membrane and surrounds the brain, and the cranial base (or chondrocranium), which develops from a cartilaginous template and forms the base of the skull. The viscerocranium or facial skeleton is also formed in membrane and develops from the facial processes and pharyngeal arches.

The cranial vault (desmocranium)

The cranial vault is formed entirely in membrane, being composed of the following bones:

- Frontal;
- Parietal;
- Squamous temporal; and
- Occipital (above the superior nuchal line).

These bones begin to appear during the fifth week of development and by around seven months ossification has progressed to the extent that they meet each other at specialized joints called sutures.

Sutures are specialized growth sites, which allow coordinated bone growth as the flat bones of the skull are displaced by growth of the brain and sensory capsules. In the neonatal skull, enlarged sutures or fontanelles are found in regions where three or more calvarial bones meet and a metopic suture exists between the initially paired frontal bones (Fig. 2.12). This provides a degree of flexibility to the infant skull, allowing it to pass down the birth canal. Sutures play an important role during postnatal growth of the skull and any form of premature fusion in these joints can lead to craniosynostosis (see Fig. 13.18).

The cranial base (chondrocranium)

The cranial base is formed from a series of individual cartilages that lie between the early brain capsule and foregut, and begin to appear in the sixth week of development (Fig. 2.13). These cartilages form part of the primary cartilaginous skeleton within the embryo and extend from the cranial end of the notochord to the nasal capsule; both in the midline and more laterally.

In the midline, the occipital sclerotomes (which arise from the occipital somites) merge with the parachordal cartilage to form the basilar and condylar regions of the occipital bone. The hypophyseal (postsphenoid) and trabecular (presphenoid) cartilages form the body of the sphenoid bone whilst the trabecular and nasal cartilages form the perpendicular plate and crista galli of the ethmoid bone. Primary cartilages are also situated in the lateral regions of the skull base, the ala temporalis (alisphenoid)

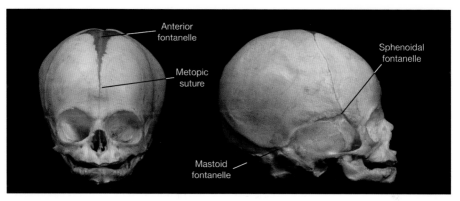

Figure 2.12 The neonatal skull has anterior, posterior (not visible), sphenoidal and mastoid fontanelles.

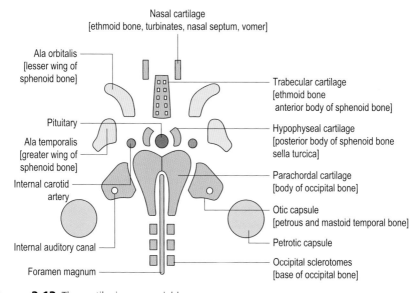

Figure 2.13 The cartilaginous cranial base.

and ala orbitalis (orbitosphenoid), forming the greater and lesser wings of the sphenoid, respectively.

The early cranial base is also characterized by the presence of cartilaginous sensory capsules, which surround the developing sense organs and ultimately contribute to the skull base. The otic capsule contains the vestibular apparatus and cochlear, merging with the lateral part of the parachordal cartilage to form the petrous and mastoid temporal bone. The paired nasal capsules surround the olfactory cells situated at the base of the nasal pits. These cartilages merge with each other and the prechordal cartilage anteriorly to form the nasal cavity.

Facial skeleton (viscerocranium)

The bones of the facial skeleton or viscerocranium develop in membrane from neural crest cells that have migrated into the first and second pharyngeal arches and the facial processes. Ossification centres usually begin to appear within intramembranous condensations from around the seventh week of intrauterine development.

In the maxilla, ossification is first seen in the region of the deciduous canine; whilst in the mandible it occurs lateral to Meckel's cartilage, between the mental and incisive branches of the inferior alveolar nerve. In both jaws, ossification spreads rapidly into the various processes of these bones. The bulk of Meckel's cartilage is resorbed during this process of ossification, but some small regions do persist. Anteriorly, nodular remnants known as the ossia menti become incorporated into the mandibular symphysis; whilst posteriorly, the cartilage extends from the point where the inferior alveolar nerve enters the mandible, back towards the ear and forms a number of structures (see Fig. 2.8):

- Lingula of the mandible;
- First two ossicles of the middle ear (malleus and incus);
- Anterior malleolar ligament (from the perichondrium); and
- Sphenomandibular ligament (from the perichondrium).

Embryonic development of the mandible is further complicated by the formation of three secondary cartilages at around 10 weeks of development:

- Condylar cartilage;
- Coronoid cartilage; and
- Symphyseal cartilage.

These are known as secondary cartilages because they appear after the primary cartilaginous skeleton has been formed within the embryo. Secondary cartilages are found in intramembranous bones within the skulls of many birds and mammals, usually at the site of articulations or muscle attachments. The chondrocytes in secondary cartilage differentiate from progenitor cells within the periosteum of membrane bones. Mechanical stimulation in these regions causes these progenitor cells to differentiate into chondrocytes rather than osteoblasts (Hall, 1984).

Secondary cartilage is distinct from primary cartilage, both structurally and functionally, and can be regarded as an adaptation of intramembranous bone to allow growth in a field of compression. In humans, the coronoid and symphyseal cartilages are essentially transitory, disappearing during the first year of life and playing no significant role in development. However, the condylar cartilage persists until around 20 years of age and is an important centre of postnatal mandibular growth (see Box 3.3). It is the ability of this cartilage to adapt to external functional stimulation that has led many orthodontists to think that clinically significant growth of the mandibular condyle can be stimulated in an adolescent child with the use of a functional appliance.

Molecular regulation of early craniofacial development

In recent years, the advent of molecular biology and the ability to manipulate gene function in vivo has allowed biologists to make significant progress in understanding how embryonic development is controlled at the molecular level. This is particularly true of craniofacial development, where much information has been gathered on how this complex region is constructed within the embryo.

Early development of the head is based upon segmentation

Neural crest cells derived from the hindbrain are essential for normal formation of the face and neck. The early theme of segmentation within the embryonic craniofacial region (seen within the primary vesicles of the neural tube and the pharyngeal arches) is further reiterated in the hindbrain, which is also a segmented structure composed of seven subunits called rhombomeres.

- A key feature of vertebrate craniofacial development is the finding that neural crest cells migrating and forming much of the facial skeleton arise from the same level of neural tube as the rhombomeres whose neurones will ultimately innervate that region.

Thus, the origin of neural crest cells can be traced for different regions of the head:

- Neural crest destined for the first pharyngeal arch migrate essentially from rhombomeres 1 and 2; and
- Neural crest for the second and third pharyngeal arches migrate from rhombomeres 4 and 6, respectively.

The even numbered rhombomeres (2, 4 and 6) contain the exit points for cranial nerves V, VII and IX; which will innervate structures within pharyngeal arches 1, 2 and 3, respectively. Thus, an axial level-specific code exists, established early in development prior to any neural crest migration; cells recognize each other and have a positional identity. Following their migration into the arches they produce the individual skeletal structures that make up the head in an orderly and integrated manner (Fig. 2.14).

Clearly, these mechanisms of craniofacial development are under genetic control. A number of genes and gene families that play a critical role in this process, establishing regional identity within the vertebrate head, have been identified.

Lessons from the fly

The fruitfly *Drosophila melanogaster* has proved to be a useful organism for studying early embryonic development. The *Drosophila* embryo, larva and ultimately, the adult fly is also based upon segmentation (Fig. 2.15). The basic fly body plan consists of:

- Head;
- Three thoracic segments;
- Eight abdominal segments; and
- Tail.

Once these basic segments have been established, a group of genes known as homeotic genes specify their characteristic structure.

- Homeotic genes encode transcription factors and therefore regulate the activity of other genes; and
- Homeotic genes are characterized by a highly conserved sequence called the homeobox, which encodes the region within the transcription factor protein that binds to DNA.

In the fly, homeotic genes are found in a single cluster within two complexes on chromosome 3:

Figure 2.14 Neural crest migration and the formation of head structures. The early neural tube is segmented into forebrain, midbrain and hindbrain, with the hindbrain being further segmented into rhombomeres. Neural crest cells migrate from their point of origin adjacent to the neural tube into the pharyngeal arches and express different combinations of Hox genes according to their axial origin. This migration is specific, neural crest destined for the first pharyngeal arch migrates from rhombomeres 1 and 2 (with a small contribution of crest from the midbrain region), whilst neural crest for the second and third pharyngeal arches migrates from rhombomeres 3 and 4 and 5 and 6, respectively. Rhombomeres 2, 4, 6 and 7 contain the exit points for cranial nerves V, VII, IX and X; these nerves will innervate structures derived from pharyngeal arches 1, 2, 3 and 4, respectively. Thus, early formation of the head is axial specific; neural crest migration is organized according to the region where these cells originate from.

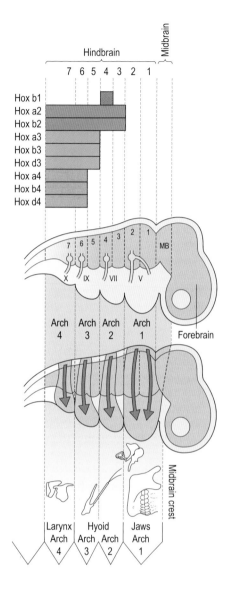

- *Antennapedia* complex; and
- *bithorax* complex.

In addition to their highly conserved structure, homeotic genes also demonstrate another remarkable feature. The axial level within the fly in which each gene functions displays a direct relationship with its position on the chromosome; a term known as colinearity. Those expressed in the most anterior, head end of the fly are found at the furthest end of the chromosome, whilst those in the thorax and abdomen are found progressively further along toward the opposite end. To put this more simply, these genes serve as a molecular representation of the anteroposterior axis of the fly embryo (Fig. 2.15).

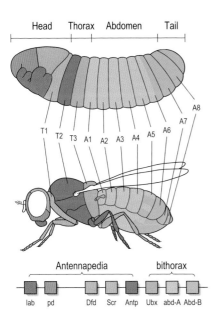

Figure 2.15 The body plan of the fly larva is segmented into a head, thorax, abdomen and tail. Homeotic genes are found within two complexes on fly chromosome 3 (*Antennapedia* and *bithorax*), and are expressed along the body axis of the fly in the order that they appear along this chromosome. Each homeotic gene functions to specify the characteristic anatomical structures that develop within each individual segment.

Homeotic genes provide a combinatorial code for the specification of each regional embryonic segment in the fly embryo. Mutations in these genes can lead to bizarre homeotic transformations where one segment of the fly can assume the phenotype of another. As an example of the power of these genes, one of them, *Antennapedia*, specifies identity of the second thoracic segment; in the dominant mutation of *Antennapedia* this gene becomes expressed inappropriately in the head of the fly. As a result of this, there is a growth of thoracic legs from the head sockets, instead of antenna.

Hox genes and craniofacial development

The genetic control of development is more universal than one might imagine. A family of homeobox-containing genes very closely related to the homeotic genes of *Drosophila* are also found in vertebrates. These genes are called Hox genes and in the mouse and human genomes there are a total of thirty-nine, arranged in four clusters (instead of one in the fly) on four different chromosomes; *Hoxa-d* in mice and *HOXA-D* in man (Fig. 2.16). There are more of them because mice and humans have a structurally more complex body plan than flies. The presence of Hox genes means that humans and flies have a common ancestor. It might have taken several hundred million years of evolution to separate us, but the essential function of the genes that pattern the embryo has been retained.

The expression of Hox genes in the vertebrate embryo can be seen within the neural tube, from the anterior region of the hindbrain through the length of the spinal cord. However, the expression patterns show a very precise spatial restriction. Each Hox gene is expressed in an overlapping domain along the anteroposterior axis of the embryo, but each gene has a characteristic segmental limit of expression at its anterior boundary. In the developing head, this spatially restricted expression pattern is seen in the hindbrain with the anterior limits of Hox gene expression corresponding to rhombomere boundaries. As neural crest cells migrate from rhombomeres of the

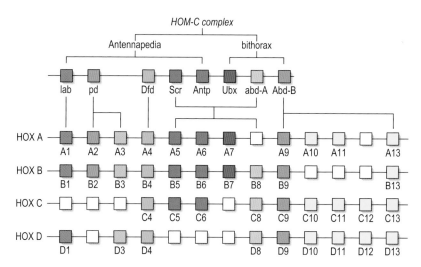

Figure 2.16 HOX genes in man. The 39 human HOX genes are organized within four clusters on four different chromosomes (HOX A-D). They are derived from a single ancestral cluster, from which the single *HOM-C* complex in *Drosophila* is also derived. *HOM-C* is itself composed of two clusters, *Antennapedia* (which contains five genes: *labial, proboscipedia, Deformed, Sex combs reduced, Antennapedia*) and *bithorax* (containing three genes: *Ultrabithorax, abdominal A, Abdominal B*). Cluster duplication during evolution has led to the concept of paralogous groups of Hox genes; thus groups of up to four genes derived from a common ancestral gene can be found. These paralogues can exhibit similar expression domains along the anteroposterior axis of the embryo, leading to redundancy between genes. Diagram adapted from Scott MP (1992), Vertebrate homeobox gene nomenclature. *Cell* 71:551–553.

neural tube into specific pharyngeal arches, the particular combination or code of Hox gene expression characteristic of the rhombomere is retained. Thus, cranial neural crest from each axial level conveys a unique and combinatorial Hox code. This code can be considered to specify form and pattern for the different pharyngeal arch-derived regions of the head and neck (Fig. 2.17).

Patterning the first pharyngeal arch
Neural crest cells destined for the first pharyngeal arch, from which the maxilla and mandible develop, do not express Hox genes related to the homeotic homeobox. Indeed, it has been suggested that this loss of Hox gene expression from the first pharyngeal arch was the event that facilitated the evolution of a jaw. However, skeletal elements derived from the first and second arches are profoundly sensitive to the expression domains of the most anterior Hox gene, *Hoxa2* (whose normal anterior boundary of expression lies at the border of pharyngeal arches 1 and 2) (see Fig. 2.14):
- A loss of *Hoxa2* produces transformation of second arch structures into elements derived from the first pharyngeal arch; and
- *Hoxa2* overexpression into the first arch leads to transformation of first arch skeletal elements into second (Box 2.2).

The first pharyngeal arch also gives rise to the dentition and patterning of the tooth primordia that form along the primitive dental axis of the jaws is also under genetic

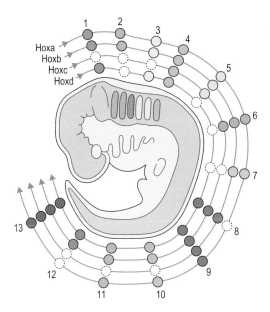

Figure 2.17 Hox gene expression in the mammalian embryo. There are four Hox clusters in mammals (Hoxa-d) situated on four different chromosomes. Those Hox genes that occupy the same position in different clusters are paralogous and in mammals there are thirteen of these paralogous groups. The position of these paralogues on the chromosome reflects their expression along the anteroposterior axis of the embryo (i.e. *Hoxa1* is expressed from the head end, whilst *Hoxa13* begins at the tail end). This complex combinatorial expression of Hox genes represents a genetic blueprint for structure along the embryo. Diagram adapted from Santagati F and Rijli FM (2003), Cranial neural crest and the building of the vertebrate head, *Nat Rev Neurosci* 4:806–818.

Box 2.2   Testing the Hox code

There is now experimental evidence to suggest that Hox genes control the mechanisms that result in morphogenesis of regions in the head and neck. One method of testing the Hox code is via the use of transgenic technology, by either disrupting or overexpressing a particular Hox gene in transgenic mice. Targeted disruption of the *Hoxa2* gene, which is normally expressed in the second pharyngeal arch, leads to a loss of some specific second arch structures such as the stapes. In addition to this, there is also a duplication of proximal first arch structures, which are fused to those that have developed normally (Gendron-Maguire et al, 1993; Rijli et al, 1993). In other words, this gene deletion has produced a type of homeotic transformation. An absence of *Hoxa2* leads to cells of the second arch adopting the identity of a first arch. *Hoxa2* is clearly involved in patterning the second pharyngeal arch and its derivatives. *Hoxa2* overexpression into the first arch leads to transformation of first arch skeletal elements into second (Grammatopoulos et al, 2000). Another Hox gene, *Hoxd4*, is normally expressed in the spinal cord, with an anterior limit of expression at the level of C1. If the expression domain of *Hoxd4* is experimentally extended beyond C1 into the occipital region of the head, the resulting phenotype exhibits transformation of the skull occipital bones into additional cervical vertebrae (Lufkin et al, 1992).

control. Teeth represent a unique series of structures whose differences can be described in terms of changes in both shape and size, these changes being reflected in the position of the tooth within the future dental arch. Thus, in the human dentition central and lateral incisors are found in the anterior region of the dental arch, with canine, premolar and molar teeth situated progressively more posteriorly. Overexpression of *Hoxa2* in the mandibular primordium does not affect tooth development, suggesting that patterning of the dentition and skeletal elements within the pharyngeal arches are independent (James et al, 2002).

If Hox genes do not pattern any of the structures derived from the first pharyngeal arch, either skeletal or dental; which genes are responsible? Subfamilies of homeobox genes, more diverged from the ancestral Hox genes, are expressed in spatially restricted patterns within the first pharyngeal arch and activity of these genes is important for patterning both the jaw skeleton and dentition (see Fig. 4.3).

Giving the jaws identity: Dlx genes

Distal-less (Dlx) genes incorporate a six-gene family of mammalian homeobox genes (*Dlx1–3; 5–7*) that exhibit nested domains of expression in neural crest of the pharyngeal arches during their development (Fig. 2.18). Within the mammalian genome, these genes are arranged in opposing pairs, with each pair having similar domains of expression:

- *Dlx2/1*;
- *Dlx5/6*; and
- *Dlx3/7*.

Dlx2/1 are expressed throughout the proximal-distal axis of the pharyngeal arches, whilst the expression domains of *Dlx5/6* and *Dlx3/7* become progressively more restricted in a distal direction:

- The study of mice with targeted mutations in different combinations of Dlx genes has suggested that a Dlx code of expression might be important in establishing structural identity of the pharyngeal arches; in particular, identity of the maxillary and mandibular processes of the first pharyngeal arch.

Mice with a combined loss of *Dlx1/2* function exhibit subtle anomalies in structures derived from more proximal regions of the pharyngeal arches, in particular the maxillary process of the first pharyngeal arch. Even though they are expressed in the distal pharyngeal arches, the loss of *Dlx1/2* does not seem to affect the patterning of these regions, because of compensatory action by other Dlx genes. However, in mice lacking the function of both *Dlx5* and *Dlx6*, genes that are only expressed in more distal regions of the pharyngeal arches, a homeotic transformation is found to occur; these mice have some conversion of mandibular arch structures to maxillary (Fig. 2.18) (Depew et al, 2002). This is because in essence, a loss of *Dlx5/6* converts the code for a mandible into that for a maxilla. Thus, nested Dlx gene expression appears to play a fundamental role in establishing both the identity of different pharyngeal arches and the identity of the maxillary and mandibular processes of the first pharyngeal arch (Graham, 2002; Schilling, 2003).

Molecular biology of bone formation

Bone formation within the embryo begins with inductive signalling from epithelial and neural tissues, inducing the condensation of mesenchymal precursor cells. In the flat bones of the skull these cells then differentiate directly into osteoblasts; however, in

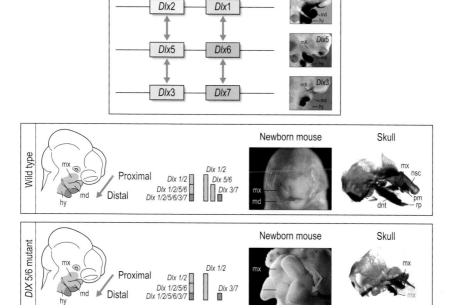

Figure 2.18 Patterning of the pharyngeal arches by Dlx genes. The pharyngeal arches have individual identity, which can be visualized along the proximal to distal axis in relation to the skeletal structures they give rise to. In addition, the first pharyngeal arch is itself subdivided into a proximal (maxillary) and distal (mandibular) process. It is thought that different combinations of Dlx gene expression in these arches generate specific skeletal structures accordingly. The six Dlx genes within the mammalian genome are arranged in pairs on three separate chromosomes. Each pair demonstrates an expression pattern that is progressively more restricted in a distal direction. Thus, in the maxillary and mandibular processes, *Dlx2/1* are expressed throughout, whilst *Dlx5/6* are expressed from the mandibular process back (distally) and *Dlx3/7* are expressed from the distal-most region of the mandibular process back (upper panel). By removing the function of both *Dlx5* and *Dlx6* in the mouse embryo, the mandibular process assumes the same code as the maxillary (the expression of *Dlx2/1* only) and there is a homeotic transformation. The maxilla is duplicated because in essence there are two maxillary processes. This maxillary duplication can be clearly seen in the newborn mice and the skeleton of their skulls (lower panels). Courtesy of Dr Michael Depew.

the remainder of the skeleton, these condensations differentiate into chondrocytes and form a cartilaginous intermediate of the developing bone, which becomes progressively ossified with the ingress of osteoblasts.

Endochondral ossification
During the process of endochondral ossification (Fig. 2.19):
- Chondrocytes differentiate from condensations of mesenchymal precursor cells to form a cartilaginous template of the future bone;

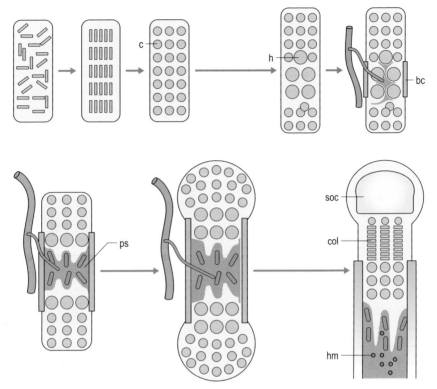

Figure 2.19 Endochondral ossification involves the differentiation of chrondrocytes and the formation of a cartilaginous template, which becomes vascularized and ossified via the ingress of osteoblasts. c, chondrocytes; h, hypertrophy; bc, bone collar; ps, primary spongiosum; col, proliferating chondrocytes; soc, secondary ossification; hm, haematopoetic marrow. Adapted from Kronenberg HM (2003), Developmental regulation of the growth plate. *Nature* 423: 332–336.

- This template increases in size through mesenchymal cell proliferation;
- Eventually, chondrocytes in the centre of this template stop proliferating; become hypertrophic and rapidly die;
- Blood vessels begin to invade the area to increase vascularization and osteoblasts differentiate from the local perichondrium to form a bony collar and matrix;
- In peripheral regions of the long bone, secondary ossification centres are established and between these regions of ossification, chondrocytes flatten and orientate themselves into proliferating columns, or growth plates along the long axis of the bone; and
- The rate of growth within the long bone represents the overall balance between chondrocyte proliferation and elongation or hypertrophy and ossification.

A number of transcription factors and signalling molecules have been identified as key regulators of endochondral bone formation. The SOX transcription factors are essential for chondrocyte differentiation. SOX9 is required for two crucial steps during this differentiation process:

- Formation of mesenchymal condensations; and
- Inhibition of maturation into the hypertrophic state;

whilst two other SOX transcription factors, L-SOX5 and SOX6, are required for the final step of chondrocyte differentiation.

Indian hedgehog (IHH) is a member of the Hedgehog family of signalling molecules and is a major regulator of:

- Chondrocyte proliferation and differentiation; and
- Osteoblast differentiation.

Ihh mutant mice have shortened long bones and a dwarf-like phenotype (St-Jacques et al, 1999). Ihh is also a powerful inducer of parathyroid hormone-related protein (PTHrP), which acts to maintain chondrocytes in the proliferative state and therefore encourage cartilaginous bone growth.

Fibroblast growth factor (FGF) signalling is also an important regulator of:

- Chondrocyte proliferation; and
- Chondrocyte differentiation.

Importantly, proliferation is inhibited through the FGF receptor FGFR3; *Fgfr3* mutant mice have excessive chondrocyte proliferation (Colvin et al, 1996; Deng et al, 1996) and constitutively active mutations in human *FGFR3* are the cause of achondroplasia or dwarfism (OMIM 100800) (Shiang et al, 1994).

Intramembranous ossification

Intramembranous ossification is dependent upon the direct proliferation of mesenchymal osteoprogenitor cells, which ultimately differentiate into osteoblasts. A key factor in the development of membrane bones within the skull is maintaining a correct balance between cellular proliferation and differentiation.

This process is directly influenced by activity of the MSX1 and MSX2 transcription factors (Ferguson, 2000). In particular, a lack of MSX2 activity in humans can lead to a reduction in calvarial ossification and a condition characterized by enlarged parietal foramina or bony defects in the skull vault (Wilkie et al, 2000). This condition is also seen in mice lacking Msx2 activity and interestingly, a lack of both Msx1 and Msx2 in the mouse leads to a lack of almost all membrane bone ossification in the skull, demonstrating the powerful combined effect of these proteins during development of the skull (Satokata et al, 2000). However, it is clear that the levels of MSX protein activity must be carefully controlled to coordinate normal skull development; mutations in the human *MSX2* gene that increase transcriptional activity of the protein can produce too much bone formation and premature fusion of the cranial sutures or craniosynostosis (Ma et al, 1996).

Osteoblast differentiation

A degree of commonality does exist between intramembranous and endochondral bones in that osteoblast differentiation, a pre-requisite of osteogenesis regardless of the embryonic origin of the bone, requires activity of the Runx2 transcription factor. Mice lacking the function of Runx2 have no osteoblasts and consequently no bone, either endochondral or intramembranous. In the growth plate, Runx2 also induces the differentiation of hypertrophic chondrocytes and therefore plays an additional role in cartilaginous ossification.

Further reading

COBOURNE MT (2000). Construction for the modern head: current concepts in craniofacial development. *J Orthod* 27:307–314.

SANTAGATI F AND RIJLI FM (2003). Cranial neural crest and the building of the vertebrate head. *Nat Rev Neurosci* 4:806–818.

MEIKLE MC (2002). *Craniofacial Development, Growth and Evolution* (Norfolk: Bateson).

LARSEN WJ (1998). *Essentials of Human Embryology* (Edinburgh: Churchill Livingstone).

References

BALDINI A (2005). Dissecting contiguous gene defects: TBX1. *Curr Opin Genet Dev* 15:279–284.

COLVIN JS, BOHNE BA, HARDING GW, ET AL (1996). Skeletal overgrowth and deafness in mice lacking fibroblast growth factor receptor 3. *Nat Genet* 12:390–397.

DENG C, WYNSHAW-BORIS A, ZHOU F, ET AL (1996). Fibroblast growth factor receptor 3 is a negative regulator of bone growth. *Cell* 84:911–921.

DEPEW MJ, LUFKIN T, AND RUBENSTEIN JL (2002). Specification of jaw subdivisions by Dlx genes. *Science* 298:381–385.

DUNCAN K, MCNAMARA C, IRELAND AJ ET AL (2008) Sucking habits in childhood and the effects on the primary dentition: findings of the Avon Longitudinal Study of Pregnancy and Childhood. *Int J Paed Dent* 18:178–188.

FERGUSON MW (2000). A hole in the head. *Nat Genet* 24:30–31.

FRANCIS-WEST PH, ROBSON L AND EVANS DJ (2003). Craniofacial development: the tissue and molecular interactions that control development of the head. *Adv Anat Embryol Cell Biol* 169(3–6):1–138.

GENDRON-MAGUIRE M, MALLO M, ZHANG M ET AL (1993). Hoxa-2 mutant mice exhibit homeotic transformation of skeletal elements derived from cranial neural crest. *Cell* 75:1317–1331.

GRAHAM A (2002). Jaw development: chinless wonders. *Curr Biol* 12:R810–R812.

GRAMMATOPOULOS GA, BELL E, TOOLE L, ET AL (2000). Homeotic transformation of branchial arch identity after Hoxa2 overexpression. *Development* 127:5355–5365.

HALL BK (1984). Developmental processes underlying the evolution of cartilage and bone. *Symposium, Zoological Society of London* 52:155–176.

HAMMOND P, HUTTON TJ, ALLANSON JE, ET AL (2005). Discriminating power of localized three-dimensional facial morphology. *Am J Hum Genet* 77:999–1010.

JAMES CT, OHAZAMA A, TUCKER AS, ET AL (2002). Tooth development is independent of a Hox patterning programme. *Dev Dyn* 225:332–335.

JIANG R, BUSH JO AND LIDRAL AC (2006). Development of the upper lip: Morphogenetic and molecular mechanisms. *Dev Dyn* 235:1152–1166.

LINDSAY EA, VITELLI F, SU H, ET AL (2001). Tbx1 haploinsufficieny in the DiGeorge syndrome region causes aortic arch defects in mice. *Nature* 410:97–101.

LUFKIN T, MARK M, HART CP, ET AL (1992). Homeotic transformation of the occipital bones of the skull by ectopic expression of a homeobox gene. *Nature* 359:835–841.

MA L, GOLDEN S, WU L, ET AL (1996). The molecular basis of Boston-type craniosynostosis: the Pro148–>His mutation in the *N*-terminal arm of the MSX2 homeodomain stabilizes DNA binding without altering nucleotide sequence preferences. *Hum Mol Genet* 5:1915–1920.

MUENKE M AND BEACHY PA (2000). Genetics of ventral forebrain development and holoprosencephaly. *Curr Opin Genet Dev* 10:262–269.

RIJLI FM., MARK M, LAKKARAJU S, ET AL (1993). A homeotic transformation is generated in the rostral branchial region of the head by disruption of Hoxa-2, which acts as a selector gene. *Cell* 75:1333–1349.

SATOKATA I, MA L, OHSHIMA H, ET AL (2000). Msx2 deficiency in mice causes pleiotropic defects in bone growth and ectodermal organ formation. *Nat Genet* 24:391–395.

SCAMBLER PJ (2000). The 22q11 deletion syndromes. *Hum Mol Genet* 9:2421–2426.

SCHILLING T (2003). Evolution and development. Making jaws. *Heredity* 90:3–5.

SCOTT MP (1992). Vertebrate homeobox gene nomenclature. *Cell* 71:551–553.

SHIANG R, THOMPSON LM, ZHU YZ, ET AL (1994). Mutations in the transmembrane domain of FGFR3 cause the most common genetic form of dwarfism, achondroplasia. *Cell* 78:335–342.

ST-JACQUES B, HAMMERSCHMIDT M AND MCMAHON AP (1999). Indian hedgehog signaling regulates proliferation and differentiation of chondrocytes and is essential for bone formation. *Genes Dev* 13:2072–2086.

WILKIE AO, TANG Z, ELANKO N, ET AL (2000). Functional haploinsufficiency of the human homeobox gene MSX2 causes defects in skull ossification. *Nat Genet* 24:387–390.

3 Postnatal growth of the craniofacial region

The adult skull is composed of twenty-eight individual bones and represents one of the most complex regions of the body. The skull bones either develop from a cartilaginous template, ossify directly from membrane, or are composite, being formed following contributions from both mechanisms (Fig. 3.1). Growth of this region therefore represents a combination of endochondral and periosteal modes of osteogenesis.

An understanding of the mechanisms underlying craniofacial growth is important for the orthodontist:

- Facial growth directly influences the skeletal relationship between the jaws and the occlusal position of the teeth;
- Orthodontic treatment is often carried out during a period when the craniofacial skeleton is growing and often attempts to alter or modify the pattern of jaw growth; and
- Previous patterns of facial growth can be useful for predicting future growth.

General growth of the body

A simple plot of height versus age (or height-distance curve) for either males or females reveals a relatively smooth and constant increase that occurs from birth to the late teenage years and results in an approximate threefold increase in height (Fig. 3.2). However, the height versus age curve does not demonstrate the dynamic changes in growth rate or velocity that occur from birth to adulthood. To do this, an incremental plot of height change, or a height–velocity curve is required, which shows three general phases in the growth curve (Fig. 3.3):

- A rapid rate of growth at birth, which progressively decelerates until around 3 years of age;
- A slowly decelerating phase, which persists until the adolescent growth spurt in the early teenage years and is interrupted by a brief juvenile growth spurt at around 6 to 8 years; and
- An adolescent growth spurt, which is followed by a progressive deceleration in growth velocity until adulthood.

Whilst the general trends associated with height change are similar in males and females, some fundamental differences do occur between the sexes. In particular, the adolescent growth spurt is greater and occurs later in males, giving them a longer overall period of growth, greater acceleration during adolescence and generally an increased overall height.

In contrast, other body tissues demonstrate quite different patterns of growth in comparison to height. For example, the central nervous system is well developed at birth and grows rapidly during the early years of life, being essentially complete by

Figure 3.1 Human fetus at around 20 weeks of embryonic development, stained with Alizarin red and cleared. With the exception of the clavicles, the axial and appendicular skeleton is characterized by endochondral ossification. The skull develops from a combination of endochondral and intramembranous ossification. Courtesy of the Gordon Museum, King's College London.

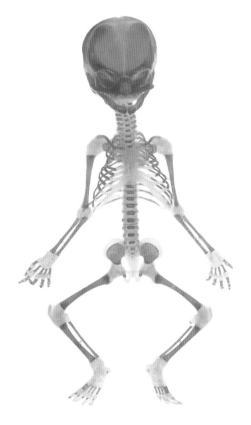

approximately 10 years of age; whilst the reproductive organs do not begin to increase in size until puberty (Fig. 3.4).

The skull at birth

One of the most striking features of a newborn child is the large size of the head in relation to the rest of the body (Fig. 3.5). This is because at birth, the cranial vault is approximately two-thirds of its final dimension, due to extensive prenatal growth and development of the brain. However, despite this large size the skull of the neonate differs significantly from that of an adult (Fig. 3.6):

- The face of the infant skull is disproportionately small because the nasal cavity, maxilla and mandible are all poorly developed. This reduced size is compounded by the relative enormity of the cranial vault and orbits.
- All of the individual bones within the neonatal skull are smaller than those in the adult, with the exception of the ear ossicles.
- Six fontanelles or fibrous membranes are present in the neonatal skull. These regions give a degree of flexibility to the skull as it passes down the birth canal and are all closed by 18 months of age (see Fig. 2.12).

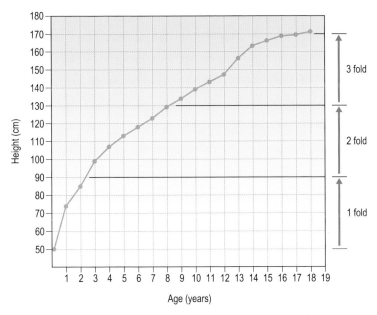

Figure 3.2 Height–distance curve for a male from birth to 18 years of age.

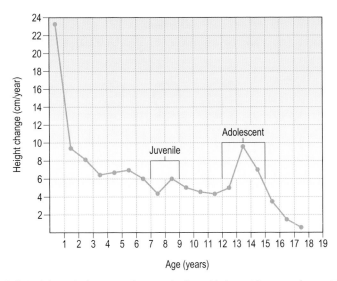

Figure 3.3 Height–velocity curve for a male from birth to 18 years of age. Note rapid deceleration of growth during the first three years and then a gradual deceleration, briefly interrupted by a juvenile growth spurt at 8 years and the more significant adolescent growth spurt at around 13 years of age.

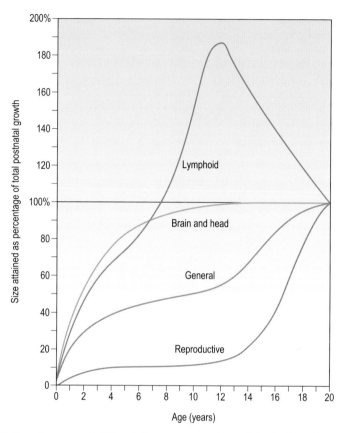

Figure 3.4 Growth curves of different tissue types, regions of the body and organ systems.

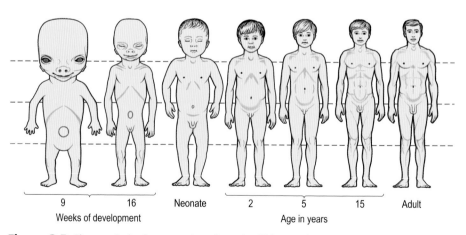

Figure 3.5 Changes in body proportions from the fifth month postconception to maturity. Note the large size of the head in relation to the rest of the body at birth. Redrawn from Medawar PB (1945), The shape of the human being as a function of time. *Proc R Soc Lond* 132:133–141.

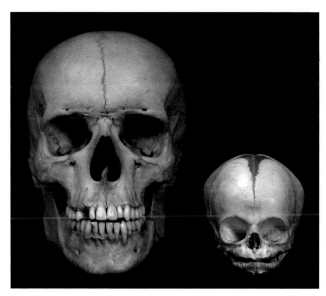

Figure 3.6 Comparison between adult and newborn skulls. The infant face is wide because of the precociously large cranium and orbits, but also short because of a lack of development within the nasal complex and jaws. The floor of the nasal cavity is sandwiched between the orbits and there is little vertical development of the maxilla and mandible in the neonate. The adult skull is characterized by a nasal cavity situated below the orbits and significant vertical elongation of the jaws.

- Additional sutures are present in the neonatal skull, including the metopic suture within the frontal bone (closes at 7 years) and symphyseal within the mandible (closes at 2 years).
- The spheno-occipital synchondrosis is a cartilaginous growth plate present between the basilar region of the occipital bone and the body of the sphenoid. This region is a significant growth centre, which persists until the end of the second decade.

Rapid growth of the cranial vault continues for the first year after birth, but this progressively decreases during the next two years and remains at a low level until adulthood (Fig. 3.7). However, by 5 years of age around 90% of the adult cranial dimension has been attained. Significantly, the dimensions of the cranium are not affected by the pubertal growth spurt.

In contrast to the cranial vault, the face is subject to a more significant change in postnatal dimension, which takes place over a longer period of time and does come under influence of the pubertal growth spurt. Facial growth results in anterior and vertical development of the nasal cavity and jaws relative to the cranial base and a significant change in overall proportions of the skull. By the mid-teenage years the cranial vault has attained adult dimensions, whilst the face is around 95% of its final size.

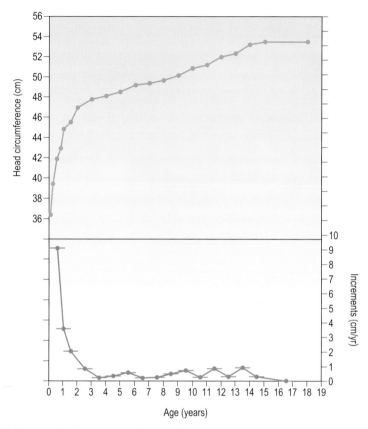

Figure 3.7 Growth in head circumference of a girl from birth until 18 years of age. The upper plot is the head circumference–distance curve, whilst the lower plot is the head circumference–velocity curve. It can be seen that growth in head circumference is most rapid during the first three years of life.

Mechanisms of craniofacial bone growth

It is clear from the direct comparison of different skull bones that postnatal growth of the craniofacial region does not result from a simple proportional enlargement of each individual bony element (Fig. 3.8). Endochondral bone growth occurs through cartilaginous replacement, whilst intramembranous bones grow as a result of periosteal remodelling. The complexity and diversity of the skull arises because the constituent bones enlarge differentially, in both a temporal and spatial manner (Fig. 3.9). The basic mechanisms underlying growth of the craniofacial region reflect this and produce:

- Relocation; and
- Displacement of individual bones.

The relocation of a bone takes place via differential changes in both size and shape, which are mediated by surface deposition and resorption. This remodelling occurs on both the outer (periosteal) and inner (endosteal) surfaces of each bone and the relocation, or cortical drift, will follow the direction of external bony deposition.

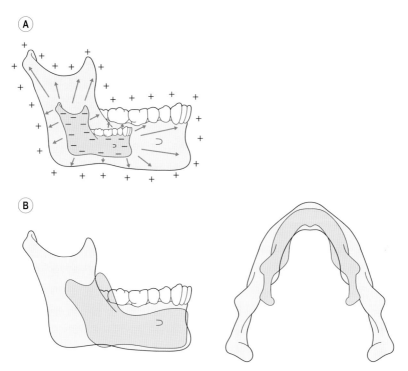

Figure 3.8 The mandible does not grow by a simple symmetrical enlargement (A); rather the condyle and ramus elongate in a posterior and superior direction, whilst the body of the mandible lengthens (B).

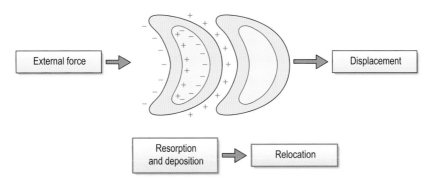

Figure 3.9 Periosteal resorption (–) and deposition (+) on the external and internal surfaces of a skull bone can produce differential changes in both size and shape, or relocation. This relocation will follow the overall direction of external bony deposition. Displacement of individual bones under the influence of external force also takes place, occurring as an independent process but often simultaneous with relocation. However, it should be remembered that relocation and displacement can occur in opposite directions.

The displacement of individual bones as single units also takes place, occurring as an independent process and often simultaneously with relocation. Displacement is mediated by the soft tissues, which apply external forces upon the bones, resulting in their displacement away from each other. Compensatory growth at the sutures maintains articulation of the bones as they move. The soft tissues include craniofacial muscles and connective tissues, primary and secondary cartilages and organs such as the brain and eyes. The relative importance and influence of these different forces upon craniofacial growth is controversial and they form the basis of several fundamental theories of growth control in this region.

Theories of craniofacial growth

Several theories that attempt to explain the mechanisms controlling postnatal growth of the craniofacial skeleton have been proposed. These theories have placed varying degrees of emphasis upon the role of genetic and environmental factors, or the significance of different tissues within this region; some being based upon experimental and biological observation and others having a more theoretical basis (Carlson, 2005).

The remodelling theory
The remodelling theory was presented by the anatomist James Couper Brash and represented the first attempt at a general theory explaining the fundamental mechanisms underlying craniofacial growth. This theory placed great emphasis upon remodelling as the primary mechanism by which all bones within the craniofacial complex grew. Thus, the cranial vault expanded via external deposition and internal resorption, whilst the facial bones grew downwards and forwards relative to the cranial vault by posterior resorption and anterior deposition.

The sutural theory
The sutural theory was largely the work of two anatomists, Joseph Weinmann and Harry Sicher, who suggested that primary growth of the craniofacial skeleton was genetically regulated, being controlled within the sutures and cartilages. Importantly, within this model, the sutures had an equivalent role to cartilage in being able to generate a tissue-separating force. For the cranial vault and maxillary complex, sutural growth was regarded as being the prime mediator of bony expansion and, in the case of the maxilla, downward and forward displacement relative to the anterior cranial base (Fig. 3.10).

The cartilaginous theory
In direct contrast to the sutural theory another anatomist, James Scott, suggested that sutures simply represented a continuation of the periosteum and endosteum of the craniofacial bones, in modified regions at their points of intersection. Growth in these regions should therefore be considered as periosteal in nature, being permissive rather than producing a tissue-separating force. Scott suggested that the bones abutting a suture could only be separated by the growth of an associated organ, such as the brain in the case of the cranial vault. Within this theory, great emphasis was placed upon the role of cartilage in producing the driving force of craniofacial growth: in particular, the nasal septal cartilage generating a downward and forward displacement of the maxillary complex, synchondroses elongating the cranial base and the condylar

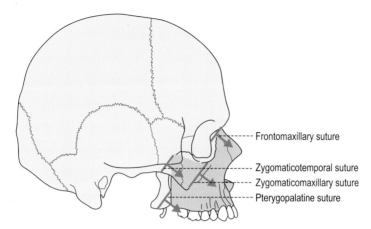

Figure 3.10 Downward and forward growth of the nasomaxillary complex as a result of sutural growth. The sutures are orientated parallel, downwards and forwards in relation to the anterior cranial base. Redrawn from Sicher H (1952), *Oral Anatomy* (St Louis: Mosby).

cartilage directing downward and forward growth of the mandible (Scott, 1953; 1954; 1956).

The functional matrix theory

The functional matrix theory of Melvin Moss describes bone growth within the craniofacial skeleton as being influenced primarily by function (Moss and Salentijn, 1969). In contrast to both the sutural and cartilaginous theories, this theory does not assume that growth of the skull is genetically determined. Indeed, this theory suggests that genes play no major role in determining postnatal growth of the craniofacial region.

Moss suggests that the head simply represents a region where a number of specific functions occur, each being carried out by a 'functional cranial component'. Functional cranial components consist of two elements:

- A functional matrix; and
- A skeletal unit.

The functional matrix represents all the tissues, organs and spaces that perform a given function, whilst skeletal units are the bones, cartilages and tendons that support this function. Two types of functional matrix exist:

- Periosteal matrices; and
- Capsular matrices.

The periosteal matrix consists of the soft tissues intimately related to a skeletal unit, such as muscles and tendons; whilst capsular matrices are the organs and tissue spaces associated with specific regions within the skull, such as the neurocranium, orbits and oropharynx.

Skeletal units are also further subdivided into:

- Microskeletal units; and
- Macroskeletal units.

Each skeletal unit does not necessarily represent an individual bone within the skull, some bones being composed of several microskeletal units or several bones uniting

Figure 3.11 The functional matrix hypothesis applied to the cranial vault. Primary growth of the brain or capsular matrix produces expansion of the flat bones and secondary growth at the sutures and synchondroses. This results in enlargement of the neurocranium or macroskeletal unit. During function, the temporalis muscle exerts pull on the periosteal matrix and bone growth of the temporal line (microskeletal unit). Redrawn from Carlson DS (2005), Theories of craniofacial growth in the postgenomic era. *Semin Orthod* 11:172–183.

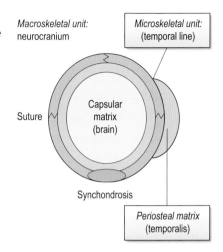

together to function as a single cranial component or macroskeletal unit. In general, the periosteal matrices primarily determine growth of microskeletal units, influencing the size and shape of bones; whilst macroskeletal growth is influenced more by the capsular matrices, producing displacement of cranial regions, such as the nasomaxillary complex or cranial vault (Fig. 3.11).

The servosystem theory

The primary cartilaginous skeleton of the craniofacial region is not influenced by the local and systemic environment to the extent that secondary cartilage of the mandibular condyle is. Based upon these observations, Alexandre Petrovic proposed that two principle factors determine growth of the craniofacial region:

- Genetically regulated growth of the primary cartilages within the cranial base and nasal septum determine growth of the midface and provide a constantly changing reference input, which is mediated via the dental occlusion; and
- The mandible is able to respond to this changing occlusal reference by muscular adaptation and locally induced condylar growth.

This theory provides a 'cybernetic' model of craniofacial growth (Fig. 3.12), which is based upon established biological principles concerning growth and function of primary and secondary cartilages, and the sutures. A strength of this theory is that it incorporates both genetic and environmental influences and assumes a role for both cartilaginous and periosteal tissues during growth of the head.

Growth of the cranial vault

The cranial vault is composed of the squamous parts of the frontal, temporal and occipital bones, and the paired parietal bones. Growth of the cranial vault is intimately linked with growth and expansion of the brain, which passively displaces the individual bones of the skull vault in a concentric manner. As this displacement takes place, the intramembranous bones of the cranium grow in two ways (Fig. 3.13):

- Compensatory bone growth at the sutures; and
- Surface periosteal and endosteal remodelling.

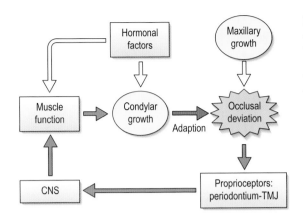

Figure 3.12 Servosystem theory of craniofacial growth as applied to the maxilla and mandible. Redrawn from Carlson DS (2005), Theories of craniofacial growth in the postgenomic era. *Semin Orthod* 11:172–183.

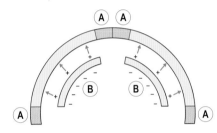

Figure 3.13 Bone growth in the cranial vault. As growth of the brain passively expands the flat bones, compensatory bone growth at the sutures maintains patency (A). Whilst external and internal surface remodelling reduces the curvature and adjusts their relationship as they are displaced radially (B).

Sutures are specialized fibrous joints situated between adjacent intramembranous bones and they mediate growth along the osteogenic fronts of these bones as they are displaced away from each other. Sutures are tension-adapted; they do not generate the forces underlying bone displacement, but respond to them, adding new bone in equilibrium with bony separation and therefore maintaining patency. This process must be closely regulated; too much bone formation can lead to the premature fusion of one or a number of sutures within the skull and prevent growth of these regions. This results in excess, compensatory growth within other regions of the skull and distortion as the soft tissues expand, a condition called craniosynostosis.

In addition to growth at the sutures, bones of the cranial vault also undergo remodelling along their external and internal surfaces to reduce their curvature and adjust their relationship as they are displaced radially.

Growth of the cranial base

The cranial base develops from a primary cartilagenous chondrocranium, which undergoes a programme of endochondral ossification that is well advanced at birth. A number of bones contribute to the cranial base, including the frontal, ethmoid, sphenoid and occipital. Postnatal growth of this region is achieved by the following mechanisms:

- Endochondral growth; and
- Surface remodelling.

Box 3.1   How much does the anterior cranial base grow?

The anterior cranial base is frequently used as a plane of reference for the superimposition and comparison of serial cephalometric radiographs. It is therefore important to know the amount and duration of growth that occurs within this region and in particular, when this growth is complete.

From the age of 5 through to 20 years, the distance from sella to nasion (see Chapter 6) will increase approximately 8-mm in females and 10-mm in males, with this growth being essentially complete by the age of 14 and 17 years, respectively. Interestingly, in comparison to growth of the anterior cranial base as a whole, the distance from sella to the foramen caecum (situated between the frontal and ethmoid bones) demonstrates proportionately very little growth (around 3-mm). In contrast, the distance from foramen caecum to nasion increases between 5 and 7-mm. Given that the total length of this dimension in the adult is only on the order of 10 to 12-mm, this is proportionately a huge amount of growth (Bhatia & Leighton, 1993). These differences reflect the fact that anatomically, the anterior cranial base is a relatively stable region for use in regional superimposition (Björk, 1968; Melsen, 1974), but care should be taken when using nasion, because growth of the frontal sinus and remodelling of the frontal bone can significantly influence the position of this landmark.

Isolated regions of cartilage, or synchondroses, persist within the cranial base for variable periods of time and make a significant contribution to postnatal growth of this region. They mediate pressure-adapted primary endochondral growth and act directly to increase the anteroposterior dimension of the skull base (Box 3.1). Once growth in the synchondroses has ceased, the cartilage is replaced by bone to form a synostosis.

- The sphenoethmoidal and sphenooccipital synchondroses make the most signifi-cant contributions to postnatal growth of the cranial base.
- The sphenoethmoidal synchondrosis is usually ossified at around 7 years of age.
- The sphenooccipital synchondrosis persists for longer. Direct histological examina-tion of autopsy material suggests that in females it closes around 13–15 years of age, whilst in males it remains patent until 15–17 years (Melsen, 1972).

Growth of the cranial base is not entirely endochondral in nature and considerable remodelling also occurs along its length. This is largely resorptive on the internal surface and depository externally, which contributes towards expansion and lateral relocation of the skull base. These patterns of remodelling activity within the cranial base have been mapped in some detail (Fig. 3.14) (Melsen, 1974). As the cranial base elongates and expands, via cartilagenous growth and surface remodelling, compensa-tory growth at the sutures maintains patency of the bony articulations within this region.

It is important to remember that coordinated growth of the cranial base does not occur in isolation within the skull and the influence of this region upon the face cannot be underestimated. The maxilla articulates with the anterior cranial base and the mandible is suspended beneath the middle cranial fossa, which is closely related to

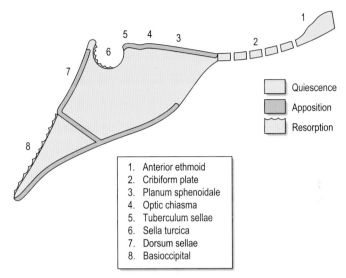

1. Anterior ethmoid
2. Cribiform plate
3. Planum sphenoidale
4. Optic chiasma
5. Tuberculum sellae
6. Sella turcica
7. Dorsum sellae
8. Basioccipital

Figure 3.14 Surface remodelling within the cranial base. The ethmoidal region is essentially stable after 4 years of age but bony apposition occurs along the planum sphenoidale (superior surface of the body of the sphenoid), optic chiasma and tuberculum sellae (anterior limit of the sella turcica) until the mid-teens. Within sella turcica, the anterior wall is stable from 5 years of age; however, the floor and posterior wall is resorptive until the late teens. Further posteriorly, the dorsum sellae is appositional, but the cerebral surface of the basioccipital bone is resorptive until around 17 years in females and 19 in males. Adapted from Melsen B (1974), The cranial base. *Acta Odontologica Scandinavica* 32:1–126.

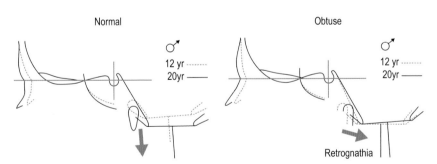

Figure 3.15 As the cranial base angle becomes more obtuse, the mandible becomes more retrognathic relative to the maxilla. Conversely, a more acute angle makes the mandible more prognathic. Redrawn from Björk A and Skieller V (1977), Growth of the maxilla in three dimensions as revealed radiographically by the implant method. *Br J Orthod* 4:53–64.

the posterior cranial base (Solow, 1980). Any degree of cranial base flexion between these two regions will directly affect the skeletal pattern of the jaws (Fig. 3.15). From the age of 12 there is very little change in this angle but individual variation in the size is high (Björk, 1955a).

Growth of the nasomaxillary complex

The nasomaxillary complex forms the middle part of the facial skeleton and is dominated by the orbits, nasal cavity, upper jaw and zygomatic processes. A number of bones make contributions to this region, including the frontal, sphenoid, zygomatic, lacrimal, nasal, maxillary, palatine, ethmoid and vomer.

The maxilla grows downwards and forwards in relation to the anterior cranial base, accompanied by the orbits and nasal cavity, with all three regions increasing in volume as they grow. The cheekbones and zygomatic arches also grow laterally and are relocated in a posterior direction within the face. A complex pattern of surface remodelling and sutural growth achieves these bony changes.

The maxillary arch is lengthened and widened by posterior and lateral deposition, with this depository activity giving way to anterior resorption below the zygomatic buttress. Growth of the maxilla has been extensively described in three dimensions using the implant method (Box 3.2) (Fig. 3.16) (Björk and Skieller, 1977):

- An increase in maxillary height occurs through sutural growth at the zygomatic and frontal articulations and deposition at the alveolar processes. This maxillary lowering is accompanied by resorption at the orbital and nasal floors, and deposition along the hard palate.

- An increase in maxillary width also occurs, achieved predominantly through growth at the midpalatal suture, with a smaller contribution from external remodelling. Growth of the midpalatal suture is greater posteriorly, which produces some transverse rotation between the two individual maxillary bones and a reduction in length along the sagittal plane.

- Downward and forward growth of the maxilla is often associated with a varying degree of vertical rotation. A forward rotation occurs when facial growth is greater

---

Box 3.2 The implant studies of Arne Björk

A great deal of information regarding postnatal craniofacial growth has been provided by a growth study carried out on children at the Royal Dental College in Copenhagen by Arne Björk. This landmark investigation began in the 1950s and combined the use of longitudinal cephalometric radiography with the placement of metallic implants into the jaws of around 100 children of each sex, covering an age period from 4 to 24 years (Björk, 1955b). The implants remained in position throughout the study and served as fixed reference points for radiographic superimposition. The stability of these implants meant that sites of growth and resorption could be identified within the individual jaws. This study highlighted many features of craniofacial growth that had not previously been recognized using cephalometric radiography alone. In particular were the findings that a significant amount of individual variation occurs in the pattern of facial growth when comparing subjects, that growth of the maxilla and mandible often contains a significant rotational component and that a number of naturally occurring and stable reference structures do exist within the craniofacial skeleton that can be used to compare serial cephalometric radiographs.

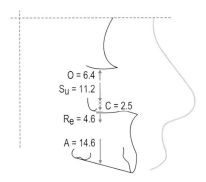

Figure 3.16 Average remodelling of the maxillary complex between 4 and 20 years of age in boys, as determined by the implant method. Su = sutural lowering; O = apposition along the orbital floor; Re = resorption of the nasal floor; A = apposition on the alveolar process; C = apposition at the infrazygomatic crest. Redrawn from Björk A and Skieller V (1977), Growth of the maxilla in three dimensions as revealed radiographically by the implant method. *Br J Orthod* 4:53–64.

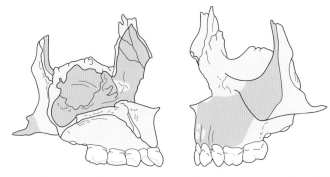

Figure 3.17 Maxillary remodelling. Resorptive surfaces are represented by dark shading and depository surfaces are unshaded.

posteriorly than anteriorly, whilst in a backward rotation the converse is true.

- The anterior surface of the zygomatic process is stable in the sagittal direction and can be regarded as a natural reference structure for maxillary growth analysis.
- The maxillary dentition is displaced anteriorly in relation to the maxillary bone as it grows.

These patterns of resorption and deposition occur over the surface of the maxilla (Fig. 3.17), as it is displaced downward and forward within the face. The origin of the displacing force has been a subject of some debate since the first studies on craniofacial growth were carried out. Indeed, the origin of the maxillary displacing force has formed a central theme for all of the major growth theories; be it periosteal growth at the sutures, cartilaginous growth at the nasal septum or the functional matrices associated with this bone.

Growth of the mandible

The mandible also grows downwards and forwards in relation to the cranial base and this is achieved by:

- Bony remodelling via subperiosteal resorption and deposition; and
- Cartilaginous growth at the condyle.

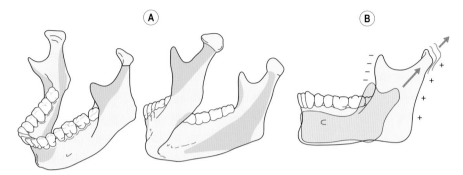

Figure 3.18 Mandibular growth. Surface remodelling (A) and elongation of the condyle (B). Resorptive surfaces are represented by dark shading and depository surfaces are unshaded.

The ramus is remodelled in posterior, superior and lateral directions by bony resorption and deposition. This elongation and posterior relocation of the ramus translates the body of the mandible downwards and forwards and increases the posterior arch length. The regions of bone remodelling are complex, but essentially involve bony deposition and resorption along the posterior and anterior margins of the ramus, supplemented by distinct patterns of resorption and deposition along lateral and lingual regions of the condyle, coronoid, ramus and angle (Fig. 3.18).

The condyle is also a major site of growth within the mandible, but controversy exists as to whether this contribution provides the primary force of mandibular displacement or whether this growth is more adaptive in nature.

Condylar cartilage

The condylar cartilage is a secondary cartilage that forms within the mandibular condyle at around 10 weeks of embryonic development. Initially, it forms a large carrot-shaped wedge within the whole of the condyle, but progressive ossification during early postnatal life results in a small cap of proliferating cartilage remaining beneath the fibrous articular surface of the condyle until around the end of the second decade.

- One view suggests that the condyle is a primary growth centre, generating a genetically predetermined increase in ramus height and mandibular length, and is the prime mover responsible for downward and forward mandibular growth.
- Alternatively, the condylar cartilage is regarded as being adaptive, maintaining articulation of the condyle within the glenoid fossa in response to downward and forward mandibular growth.

In reality, the condylar cartilage represents an essential adaptation of the mandible, allowing bone growth to occur at the condyle, which during function is in a field of compression. This adaptation is necessary because the mandible is an intramembranous bone, which in the skull grow via a periosteal mode of osteogenesis within fields of tension on the surface periosteum, endosteum and at sutures. Periosteal osteogenesis is not pressure-adapted and intramembranous bones are unable to grow within fields of compression. During function, the mandibular condyle undergoes compressive loading within the temporomandibular joint; therefore an adaptation is required within this region to allow bone growth to occur. Endochondral bones, such as the long bones of the axial skeleton, are able to grow under compression because they retain regions of cartilage at the epiphyses or growth plates. The cartilagenous growth plates have inherent growth potential and are able to produce skeletal growth under compressive force. The condylar cartilage is more adaptive, maintaining articulation of the condyle within the glenoid fossa as the mandible is translated downward and forward through regional growth (Box 3.3).

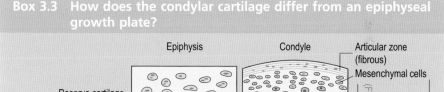

Box 3.3   How does the condylar cartilage differ from an epiphyseal growth plate?

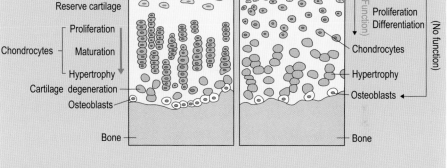

Superficially, the condylar cartilage resembles a primary growth plate such as an epiphysis or synchondrosis; however, considerable functional and anatomical differences exist between all of these structures.

The condylar cartilage is concerned with maintaining growth of an intramembranous bone (the mandible) within a field of multidirectional compression (the temporomandibular joint).

- The outer region of the condylar cartilage, or articular zone, is composed of a fibrous connective tissue layer, which is continuous with the fibrous layer of the mandibular periosteum.
- Below this, a zone of proliferating and undifferentiated mesenchymal cells is continuous with the osteogenic layer of the mandibular periosteum.
- These mesenchymal cells provide the key to function of the condylar cartilage because they are directly influenced by their local environment. During functional loading, they proliferate and grow, ultimately differentiating into chondrocytes, which secrete cartilage. Once differentiated, these condylar chondrocytes are unable to divide further, becoming randomly arranged within the cartilage, reflecting the multidirectional growth capacity of this region.

- In the absence of function the mesenchymal cells fail to proliferate and no growth occurs; instead, they differentiate directly into osteoblasts to form bone.
- Therefore, functional stimulation of mesenchymal cell proliferation provides the stimulus for cartilaginous growth. As cartilage is added superiorly, chondrocytes in the deeper layers eventually become hypertrophic and endochondral ossification takes place.

Epiphyseal growth plates are found within long bones and facilitate their elongation by endochondral ossification. Bone formation takes place within the peripheral calicified zone of the cartilage and growth is mediated by chondrocyte proliferation and cartilaginous replacement. An epiphyseal growth plate differs from the condyle in a number of respects:

- The outer region of the epiphysis is composed of a layer of hyaline cartilage, filled with small clusters of chondrocytes.
- Below this lies a region of proliferating chondrocytes, which form large elongated columns or palisades within the epiphysis. The ability of these cells to proliferate within a field of compression allows the epiphysis to grow, whilst the long bone supports the weight of the body.
- Deep to the proliferating zone lies a zone of maturation, where chondrocytes have ceased division and begun to increase in size, ultimately becoming hypertrophic. These hypertrophic chondrocytes degenerate to leave lacunae that become vascularized and populated by bone-forming osteoblasts.

Mandibular growth rotations

Growth in length of the mandibular ramus occurs essentially at the condyles, but this growth is variable in direction and often involves a component of rotation (Björk, 1955b; 1963). Large individual variation exists in the direction that is seen; with vertical, forward or backward growth taking place (Fig. 3.19). Three different types of mandibular growth rotation were originally described by Björk and Skieller, with the terminology associated with these different rotations being later simplified by Solow and Houston (Box 3.4) (Björk and Skieller, 1983; Solow and Houston, 1988):

- Total rotation represents a change in inclination of the body or corpus of the mandible relative to the anterior cranial base. The body is represented by a reference line constructed along the implants, or by natural reference structures present within this region.
- Matrix rotation represents a change in inclination of the soft tissue matrix of the mandible in relation to the anterior cranial base. A line drawn tangent to the lower border of the mandible represents the soft tissue matrix and the condyles lie at the centre of this rotation.

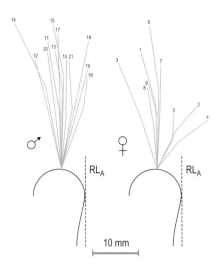

Figure 3.19 Variation in the direction of condylar growth direction. Adapted from Björk A and Skieller V (1972), Facial development and tooth eruption. An implant study at the age of puberty. *Am J Orthod* 62:339–383.

Box 3.4   The confusing nomenclature of mandibular growth rotations

Solow and Houston (1988) updated the original nomenclature proposed by Björk and Skieller (1983) in an attempt to simplify the subject of mandibular growth rotation.

- It was suggested that the term **true rotation** was used to represent a **total rotation**. The true rotation is the fundamental rotation that takes place between the mandible and cranial base.
- An **apparent rotation** of the mandible represented a **matrix rotation**. The apparent rotation is the result of true rotation and remodelling of the mandibular lower border and is the change apparent on a cephalometric radiograph in the absence of implants.
- **Angular remodelling** of the mandibular border represented an **intramatrix rotation**. The angular remodelling can only be visualized when the mandible is registered on implants or stable structures.

The sign convention for mandibular growth rotations was also clarified. With the head facing right, a forward or negative rotation is counterclockwise, whilst a backward or positive rotation is clockwise (Solow and Houston, 1988).

- Intramatrix rotation is the difference between the total and matrix rotations if the mandibular body rotates within the soft tissue matrix. This difference reflects bony remodelling that takes place along the lower border of the mandible and is defined by the change in inclination seen between an implant reference line and the mandibular lower border.

Figure 3.20 Mandibular growth rotations. (A) Forward rotator. (B) Backward rotator. Centres of rotation are marked (X).

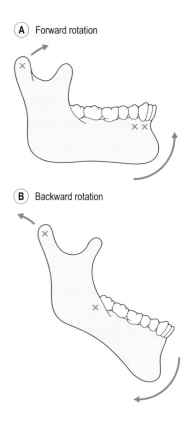

(A) Forward rotation

(B) Backward rotation

Mandibular growth rotations can take place in either a forward or backward direction, the total rotation representing the sum of the matrix and intramatrix rotations (Fig. 3.20). Forward rotations are the most common, associated with centres of rotation through the condyles, incisors or premolars; whilst backward rotations take place through centres in the condyles or the most distal-occluding molars (Björk, 1969). These different rotations all represent an imbalance in growth between anterior and posterior face height (Fig. 3.21). An excess of growth in the anterior face height will result in a total backward rotation of the mandible, whilst increased growth in posterior face height leads to a total forward rotation (Houston, 1988). In many cases of rotation, a normal occlusion is maintained because of dentoalveolar compensation; however, if the imbalance is severe, then a malocclusion such as anterior open bite or deep overbite may occur.

The presence, or likelihood of a mandibular growth rotation can have important consequences for orthodontic treatment. Extremes of rotation can influence the eruptive paths of the teeth and skeletal relationships of the jaws. It is therefore important to detect these types of mandibular growth rotation if at all possible. Unfortunately, orthodontists rarely have the benefit of fixed metallic implants to superimpose their radiographs on, and a total growth rotation cannot be evaluated by simply measuring the outer bony contours of the mandible because remodelling will mask it. A structural

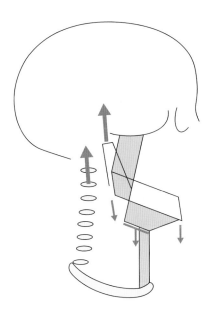

Figure 3.21 As the child grows, the cervical column increases in length and takes the head away from the shoulder girdle. This is associated with growth and stretch of a chain of muscle groups extending from the mandible to the base of the skull superiorly and from the mandible to the hyoid bone, and hyoid bone to shoulder girdle inferiorly. This produces a descent of the mandibular symphysis and hyoid bone relative to the cranial base and an increase in anterior face height. Posterior face height increases via growth of the middle cranial fossa and the condyle. Extremes of growth in these dimensions can lead to excessive anterior or posterior facial growth and rotations of the mandible. Redrawn from Houston WJ (1988), Mandibular growth rotations—their mechanisms and importance. *Eur J Orthod* 10:369–73.

method was therefore described, which was based upon identifying certain morphological features on a cephalometric radiograph that could be used to predict the presence and direction of a mandibular growth rotation (Björk, 1969). This method involves identifying and describing the following features (Fig. 3.22):

- Inclination of the condylar head;
- Curvature of the mandibular canal;
- Shape of the lower border of the mandible;
- Inclination of the mandibular symphysis;
- Interincisal angle;
- Interpremolar and intermolar angles; and
- Anterior lower face height.

There are conflicting results regarding the predictive ability of the structural method. An investigation using some of the more extreme cases from Björk's original sample demonstrated a high prognostic estimate of mandibular growth rotation using combined measures of mandibular inclination (Skieller et al, 1984). However, an alternative study tested the ability of five experienced clinicians to differentiate extreme backward rotators from forward using cephalometric radiographs and found this to be no better than chance (Baumrind et al, 1984).

Dentoalveolar compensation

A considerable amount of individual variation exists in the amount and direction of maxillary and mandibular growth that occurs during postnatal development. The dentoalveolar compensatory mechanism attempts to maintain a normal interarch occlusal relationship in the presence of variation in the skeletal pattern (Solow, 1980).

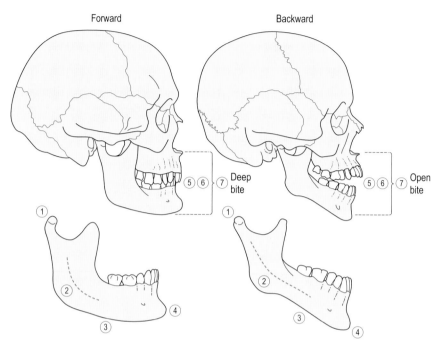

Figure 3.22 Structural signs of mandibular growth rotation. Björk identified seven structural signs within the mandible that could be associated with different growth rotations. Not all of these signs are found in each individual but the greater the number present, the more reliable the prediction of a forward or backward rotation. In the forward rotating mandible: (1) the condyle is inclined forward; (2) the mandibular canal has a curvature greater than the mandibular contour; (3) the lower border of the mandible is rounded anteriorly and concave at the angle, due to bony deposition along the anterior region and symphysis, and resorption below the angle; (4) the symphysis is inclined forward within the face and the chin is prominent; (5) the interincisor angle, (6) interpremolar and intermolar angles are all increased; (7) the anterior lower face height is reduced with a tendency towards an increased overbite. In contrast, the backward rotating mandible is associated with: (1) a backward inclination of the condyles; (2) a flat mandibular canal; (3) a lower border that is thinner anteriorly and convex, due to minimal remodelling along the lower border of the mandible and bony deposition at the posterior border of the ramus; (4) the symphysis is inclined backward within the face and the chin is receding; (5) the interincisor angle, (6) interpremolar and intermolar angles are all decreased; (7) the lower anterior face height is increased and there is an anterior open bite.

A number of different factors are responsible for dentoalveolar adaptation:
- Normal mechanisms of tooth eruption;
- Soft tissues forces; and
- Occlusal forces and mesial drift.

In the absence of adequate dentoalveolar compensation a malocclusion can therefore result. However, extremes of tooth position necessary to compensate for a jaw

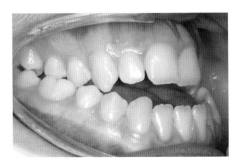

Figure 3.23 Incisor eruption has failed to compensate for a significantly increased anterior lower face height and class III skeletel base relationship. There is an anterior open bite and reverse overjet.

discrepancy might contribute towards crowding of the dental arches, exchanging one form of malocclusion for another. Alternatively, the size of the skeletal discrepancy might be such that successful compensation is not possible (Fig. 3.23). The amount of dentoalveolar compensation that has taken place in the presence of a skeletal discrepancy is an important factor when considering orthodontic treatment.

Adult craniofacial growth

Although most craniofacial growth is complete by the end of adolescence, longitudinal studies have demonstrated that a small amount continues during adult life. This tends to initially reflect the original growth pattern, especially when there is an underlying skeletal discrepancy; however, later in adult life, changes in the vertical dimension predominate. Rotational changes are also seen in the jaws, with males showing a greater tendency toward forward rotation of the mandible and females a backward rotation. It also appears that growth in females can re-accelerate in adulthood, especially during pregnancy. As well as these skeletal changes, considerable changes in the facial soft tissues take place with increasing age. In particular, the nose and chin tend to lengthen and the lips become more retrusive and less full with the passing of time.

Further reading

CAMERON N (2002). *Human Growth and Development*. (San Diego: Academic Press).
ENLOW DH (1990). *Facial Growth* (Philadelphia: WB Saunders).
ENLOW DH AND HANS MG (1996). *Essentials of Facial Growth*. (Philadelphia: WB Saunders).

References

BAUMRIND S, KORN EL AND WEST EE (1984). Prediction of mandibular rotation: an empirical test of clinician performance. *Am J Orthod* 86:371–385.
BHATIA SN AND LEIGHTON BC (1993). *A manual of facial growth. Oxford Medical Publications* (Oxford: Oxford University Press).
BJÖRK A (1955a). Cranial base development. *Am J Orthod* 41:198–225.
BJÖRK A (1955b). Facial growth in man, studied with the aid of metallic implants. *Acta Odontol Scand* 13:9–34.
BJÖRK A (1963). Variations in the growth pattern of the human mandible: longitudinal radiographic study by the implant method. *J Dent Res* 42(1)Pt 2:400–411.

BJÖRK A (1968). The use of metallic implants in the study of facial growth in children: method and application. *Am J Phys Anthropol* 29:243–254.

BJÖRK A (1969). Prediction of mandibular growth rotation. *Am J Orthod* 55:585–599.

BJÖRK A AND SKIELLER V (1977). Growth of the maxilla in three dimensions as revealed radiographically by the implant method. *Br J Orthod* 4:53–64.

BJÖRK A AND SKIELLER V (1983). Normal and abnormal growth of the mandible. A synthesis of longitudinal cephalometric implant studies over a period of 25 years. *Eur J Orthod* 5:1–46.

CARLSON DS (2005). Theories of craniofacial growth in the postgenomic era. *Semin Orthod* 11:172–183.

HOUSTON WJ (1988). Mandibular growth rotations—their mechanisms and importance. *Eur J Orthod* 10:369–373.

MELSEN B (1972). Time and mode of closure of the spheno-occipital synchrondrosis determined on human autopsy material. *Acta Anat (Basel)* 83:112–118.

MELSEN B (1974). The cranial base. *Acta Odontologica Scandinavica* 32:1–126.

MOSS ML AND SALENTIJN L (1969). The primary role of functional matrices in facial growth. *Am J Orthod* 55:566–577.

SCOTT JH (1953). The cartilage of the nasal septum. *Br Dent J* 95:37–43.

SCOTT JH (1954). The growth of the human face. *Proc R Soc Med* 47:91–100.

SCOTT JH (1956). Growth at the facial sutures. *Am J Orthod* 42:381–387.

SKIELLER V, BJÖRK A AND LINDE-HANSEN T (1984). Prediction of mandibular growth rotation evaluated from a longitudinal implant sample. *Am J Orthod* 86:359–370.

SOLOW B (1980). The dentoalveolar compensatory mechanism: background and clinical implications. *Br J Orthod* 7:145–161.

SOLOW B AND HOUSTON WJ (1988). Mandibular rotations: concepts and terminology. *Eur J Orthod* 10:177–179.

4 Development of the dentition

Humans have two dentitions, the deciduous (primary) and permanent (secondary). Each dentition is heterodont, meaning that it consists of teeth with different shapes and functions. The classes of human teeth are:

- Incisiform (incisor);
- Caniniform (canine); and
- Molariform (premolar and molar).

Deciduous teeth are progressively replaced by permanent teeth, with the addition of a molar dentition in the posterior region of the jaws.

Prenatal development of the dentition

Teeth form on the frontonasal process and on the paired maxillary and mandibular processes of the first pharyngeal arch. They are derived from two embryonic cell types:

- Oral epithelium, which gives rise to ameloblasts and enamel of the tooth crown; and
- Cranial neural crest, which contributes to formation of the dental papilla and follicle of the tooth germ and therefore, to the dentine, pulp and periodontal attachment of the fully formed tooth.

The anatomy of tooth development

In the human embryo, development of the deciduous dentition begins at around 6 weeks with the formation of a continuous horseshoe-shaped band of thickened epithelium around the lateral margins of the primitive oral cavity. The free margin of this band gives rise to two processes, which invaginate into the underlying mesenchyme:

- The outer process or vestibular lamina is initially continuous, but soon breaks down to form a vestibule that demarcates the cheeks and lips from the tooth-bearing regions.
- The inner process or dental lamina gives rise to the teeth themselves.

Discreet swellings of the dental lamina form the enamel organs of the future developing teeth. Epithelial cells of the enamel organ proliferate and progress through characteristic bud, cap and bell stages. Simultaneously, the dental papilla is formed by localized condensation of neural crest-derived ectomesenchymal cells around the epithelial invaginations. More peripherally, ectomesenchymal cells extend around the enamel organ to form the dental follicle. Together, these tissues constitute the tooth germ and will give rise to all structures that make up the mature tooth (Fig. 4.1).

The permanent dentition replaces the deciduous dentition and is composed of both successional and accessional teeth (Fig. 4.2):

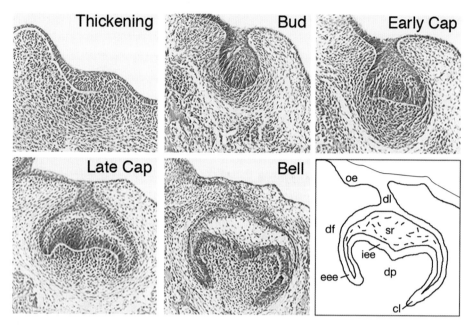

Figure 4.1 Early tooth development. Localized proliferation of the oral epithelium gives rise to a thickening, which invaginates into the underlying jaw mesenchyme to form the tooth bud. Simultaneously, neural crest cells condense around the bud and these two tissues form the tooth germ. At the cap stage, the tooth bud folds to demarcate the early morphology of the crown, which is modified by further folding at the bell stage. During the bell stage, the innermost layer of cells within the epithelial component of the tooth germ, the inner enamel epithelium, induce adjacent cells of the dental papilla to differentiate into odontoblasts, responsible for the formation and mineralization of dentine. Dentine formation is preceded by the formation of predentine. The first layer of predentine acts as a signal to the overlying inner enamel epithelial cells to differentiate into ameloblasts and begin secreting the enamel matrix. At the margins of the enamel organ, cells of the inner enamel epithelium are confluent with the outer enamel epithelial cells at the cervical loop. Growth of these cells in an apical direction forms a skirt-like sheet called Hertwig's epithelial root sheath, which maps out the future root morphology of the developing tooth and induces the further differentiation of root odontoblasts. Degeneration of this root sheath leads to exposure of the cells of the dental follicle to the newly formed root dentine and differentiation into cementoblasts, which begin to deposit cementum onto the root surface. Surrounding the enamel organ, the cells of the dental follicle produce the alveolar bone and collagen fibres of the periodontium. The developing tooth remains housed in this cavity of alveolar bone until the process of eruption begins. cl, cervical loop; dp, dental papilla; df, dental follicle; dl, dental lamina; eee, external enamel epithelium; iee, internal enamel epithelium; oe, oral epithelium; sr, stellate reticulum.

- Successional teeth have deciduous predecessors and consist of the incisors, canines and premolars. Formation begins between 20 weeks in utero and 10 months of age.
- Accessional teeth have no deciduous predecessors and consist of the three permanent molars. Formation begins between the fourteenth week in utero and 5 years of age.

The molecular control of tooth development

The histological basis of tooth development has been understood for some time, but in recent years progress has been made in understanding molecular mechanisms that underlie the process of odontogenesis using mouse models (Box 4.1). The generation of a tooth requires coordinated molecular signalling between epithelium of the early jaws and the underlying neural crest cells that migrate into these regions (Cobourne & Sharpe, 2003; Tucker & Sharpe, 2004).

Patterning the dentition: a molecular code for tooth shape

The mouse jaw is demarcated into future incisor and molar-forming regions on a molecular basis before any morphological evidence of tooth development has occurred. Fgf8 is a signalling molecule belonging to the fibroblast growth factor (Fgf) family, which localizes to the future molar regions of the jaw epithelium. In contrast, Bmp4, a signalling molecule of the bone morphogenetic protein (Bmp) family, localizes to the early incisor epithelium. These signalling molecules induce the expression of a number of homeobox-containing genes that encode transcription factor proteins in the tooth-forming neural crest-derived ectomesenchyme of the early jaws.

- Fgf8 induces expression of *Barx1* and *Dlx2* in the molar regions.
- Bmp4 induces expression of *Msx1* and *Msx2* in the incisor regions.

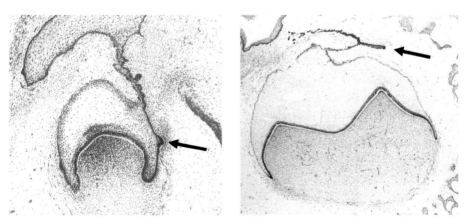

Figure 4.2 Successional teeth form as a result of localized proliferation within the dental lamina associated with each deciduous tooth germ (left, arrowed). In contrast, accessional teeth form as a result of backward extension of the dental lamina into the posterior region of the jaws (right, arrowed). Courtesy of Dr Barry Berkovitz.

Initially, signalling from the epithelium to neural crest cells that migrate into the jaws can induce expression of a range of genes. However, expression domains very rapidly become established and then independent of epithelial signalling. It has been suggested that the differing combinations of gene expression patterns act to specify tooth shape (Sharpe, 1995). The 'odontogenic homeobox code' predicts that for each tooth-forming region of the early maxilla and mandible, the morphology of the developing tooth is dictated by a specific combination of homeobox genes within the ectomesenchyme (Box 4.2). Thus, for the molar region of mouse jaws, an overlapping code of *Barx1* and *Dlx2* exists (Fig. 4.3). There are several important points to note with regard to the homeobox model (Sharpe, 2001):

- One specific gene is not responsible for each tooth shape;
- The absence of a gene is as important as the presence in terms of reading the code; and
- Because the code is overlapping it can specify a wide range of subtle differences in tooth shape.

This final point is important because the peripheral regions of overlap between teeth of different classes appear to be particularly vulnerable with regard to human hypodontia. In these cases, teeth at the end of a series (upper lateral incisors, lower second premolars, third molars) are those most commonly congenitally absent.

Initiation of tooth development

Once the ectomesenchyme within each mouse jaw has been regionalized into presumptive incisor and molar domains, tooth development is initiated within the jaw epithelium. A key player in this process is sonic hedgehog (Shh), a protein produced in localized regions of jaw epithelium where the teeth are going to form. Shh drives

Box 4.2 Transformation of tooth type by manipulation of homeobox genes

An incisor tooth germ has been converted into one demonstrating a molar crown shape by manipulating homeobox gene expression in the future incisor-forming region of the mouse jaw. *Barx1* is normally expressed in molar-forming mesenchyme of the jaws, this expression being established by Fgf8 signalling from the overlying epithelium. *Barx1* expression is restricted to the molar regions by antagonistic signalling from Bmp4, which is present in the incisor-forming epithelium and represses *Barx1* in the underlying mesenchyme. By artificially inhibiting Bmp4 activity in the incisor region of cultured jaws, the expression of *Barx1* can be extended into the incisor region. Moreover, Bmp4 normally induces *Msx1* in the incisor mesenchyme; therefore a loss of Bmp4 in this region also reduces expression of *Msx1*. The code of these early incisor regions is therefore altered into one resembling a molar region: a gain of *Barx1* and loss of *Msx1*. Transplantation of these early incisor regions into sites that allow tooth development to progress towards completion results in the formation of multicusped molar teeth rather than incisors. Thus, an experimental alteration of homeobox gene expression can re-specify the identity of developing teeth, which is powerful evidence in support of the 'odontogenic homeobox code' (Tucker et al, 1998).

proliferation of the dental lamina within these regions, resulting in formation of the tooth buds; if Shh signalling is lost in the early dental lamina, teeth fail to develop. Restriction of Shh production is therefore important in ensuring that teeth develop in the correct regions of the jaws and this is orchestrated by molecular compartmentalization of the jaw epithelium into tooth-forming and non-tooth-forming regions. Specifically, expression of the *Shh* gene is restricted to the tooth-forming regions because it is repressed throughout the non-dental epithelium by another signalling molecule called Wnt7b. Therefore, tooth formation in the correct regions of the jaws is established via reciprocal expression domains between two different signalling molecules within the jaw epithelium (Fig. 4.4).

Once the tooth bud has formed, a number of homeobox-encoding genes subsequently localize to the condensing dental papilla, including *Msx1* and *Pax9*. These genes play an important role in mediating later signalling between the underlying ectomesenchyme and the epithelial bud as tooth development progresses to the cap stage (Fig. 4.5). A loss of either gene leads to the arrest of tooth development at the bud stage in the mouse. Mutations associated with human *MSX1* and *PAX9* have also been implicated in hypodontia.

Progression to the cap stage: the production of shape
Formation of the tooth bud heralds an important transition for the tooth germ, from bud to cap stage. During the cap stage, the essential shape of the tooth crown is established by folding of the epithelial bud. Folding is mediated by a small group of

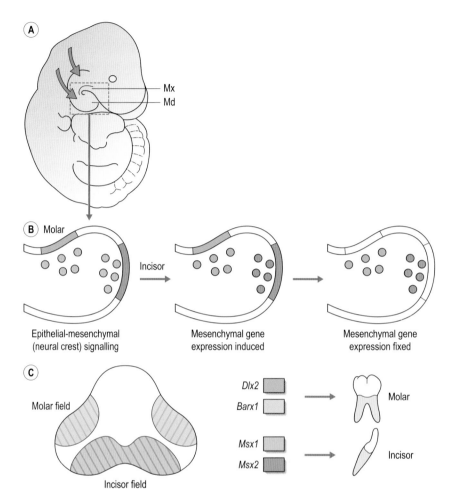

Figure 4.3 Establishing tooth pattern within the jaws. (A) In the early embryo, neural crest cells migrate into the tooth-forming regions of the primitive maxilla and mandible. (B) Highlight of cell signalling in the mandible. Signalling molecules are produced in the incisor and molar epithelium and these induce differential expression of homeobox genes in the underlying neural crest-derived mesenchyme. Initially, expression of these homeobox genes is dependent upon the presence of signals from the epithelium, but after a short space of time, these patterns of gene expression become independent and fixed. (C) Schematic and simplified representation of the odontogenic homeobox code. *Msx1* and *Msx2* code for incisors, whilst *Dlx2* and *Barx1* code for molars.

non-dividing cells within the epithelium of the tooth germ, called the primary enamel knot.

Cells of the enamel knot produce a wealth of signalling molecules and transcription factors, which influence differential growth of the epithelial cap and mediate changes in its shape. The primary enamel knot disappears during the late cap stage through

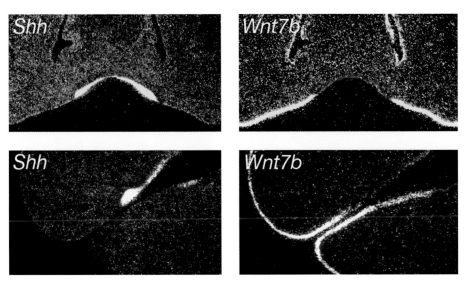

Figure 4.4 Expression of *Shh* and *Wnt7b* in the early maxilla (upper panel) and mandible (lower panel). Shh signalling is restricted to the early incisor and molar teeth, whilst *Wnt7b* is expressed in a reciprocal manner, in the regions of the jaw epithelium that will not form teeth.

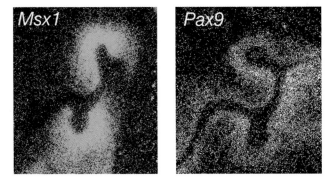

Figure 4.5 Expression of *Msx1* and *Pax9* in the dental mesenchyme surrounding bud stage molar teeth.

programmed cell death but in teeth with more complex crown structures, such as molars, a series of secondary enamel knots develop in the epithelium to sculpt more intricate cusp patterns (Fig. 4.6). Whilst the crown shape of a tooth is formed by cellular activity within the epithelial component of the tooth germ during the cap and bell stages, the molecular instructions for shape are established within the ectomesenchymal component much earlier in the developmental process.

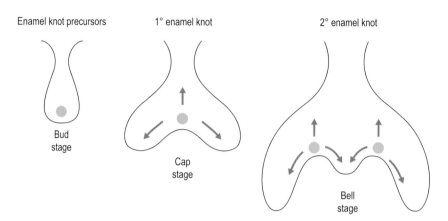

Figure 4.6 Signalling by the enamel knot is responsible for generating cusp shape.

Postnatal development of the dentition

When a child is born, mineralization of all the deciduous tooth crowns is well underway, with this process also beginning in the first permanent molars. The deciduous dentition will start to erupt in the first year of life and be completed by the end of the third. The permanent dentition is heralded by eruption of the first molars at around 6 years of age and completed in most cases by the appearance of third molars in the late teenage years.

The jaws at birth

At birth, the maxillary dental arch is characteristically horseshoe-shaped while the mandibular arch assumes a wider U-shape. The mucous membrane of both the maxilla and mandible is thickened in the newborn to produce gum pads, which cover the alveolar processes containing the developing deciduous teeth (Fig. 4.7). Formation of dentine and enamel begins in the deciduous tooth germs at around 4 to 6 months in utero and crown formation is completed during the first year of life. Each tooth is present within an individual segment of the gum pad, demarcated by characteristic transverse grooves within the mucous membrane. The grooves are particularly prominent distal to the deciduous canines in both arches and are known here as the lateral sulci.

The maxillary and mandibular gum pads have no fixed relationship during early life but the maxilla is usually positioned ahead of the mandible, resulting in a varying degree of increased 'overjet'. The gum pads rarely occlude but if they do this generally occurs in the molar region, leaving a prominent anterior space for the tongue to occupy, which facilitates suckling (Fig. 4.8). The variation in gum pad relationship at birth means it cannot be used to predict the future jaw relationship.

Occasionally a child is born with teeth already present or that undergo precocious eruption within the oral cavity (Fig. 4.9):

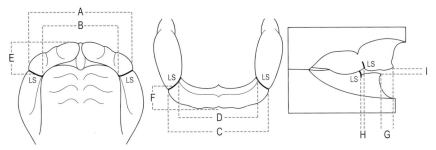

Figure 4.7 The maxillary (left) and mandibular (middle) gum pads in isolation and occlusion (right). Note the prominent lateral sulci (LS) present in both arches. A, C = external arch width; B, D = internal arch width; E, F = anterior arch length; G = overjet; H = anteroposterior relationship; I = overbite. Redrawn from Leighton BC (1977). Early recognition of normal occlusion. In: The Biology of Occlusal Development, Craniofacial Growth Series Monograph 7, University of Michigan. USA.

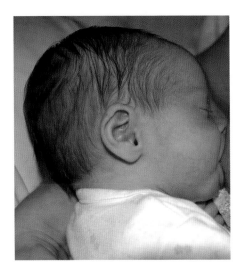

Figure 4.8 The primary role of the gum pads is to facilitate suckling in the newborn.

- Natal teeth are present at birth;
- Neonatal teeth erupt within the first month of life; and
- Pre-erupted teeth appear within the second and third months of life.

Natal and neonatal teeth occur in around 1:3000 children and are usually mandibular deciduous incisors, although rarely they can be supernumerary teeth (Leung & Robson, 2006). They are often poorly developed, mobile and can cause ulceration of the mouth and nipple during suckling. If these teeth give rise to problems they should be removed.

Figure 4.9 Natal teeth removed from a 6-week-old baby. Courtesy of Zahra Kordi.

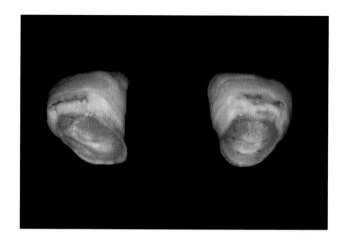

Figure 4.10 A sight for every proud parent, eruption of the first deciduous teeth. Courtesy of Miles Cobourne.

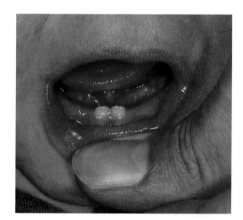

The deciduous dentition

The first year of life is characterized by rapid jaw growth in both the anteroposterior and transverse planes of space. This is particularly marked transversely during the first six months due to the presence of sutures within the midpalatal seam of the maxilla and mandibular symphysis. Thereafter, most dimensional change is the result of backward and outward extension of the alveolar processes (Box 4.3). This growth usually ensures that enough space is available in both jaws for the deciduous teeth to erupt without crowding, even though the deciduous tooth germs are often quite crowded within the jaws at birth. The early 'overjet' associated with the gum pads usually diminishes in the first six months as a result of rapid facial growth and increasing mandibular prognathism.

Eruption of the deciduous dentition begins at approximately 6 months of age (Fig. 4.10) and is complete by around $2\frac{1}{2}$ to 3 years (Fig. 4.11). The sequence can be variable (Fig. 4.12), but is characteristically:

Box 4.3 How much growth occurs in the dental arches during dental development?

The jaws grow considerably in size from birth to around 6 months of age (Clinch, 1934). After this time, very little increase in the dimensions of the tooth-bearing regions takes place in the deciduous dentition (Foster et al, 1972). During eruption of the permanent dentition, some transverse changes do occur in intercanine width, but the dimensions are small. A maximum increase of no more than 2 mm can be expected in the mandible and 4 mm in the maxilla, occurring up to the age of 12 years, with some of this increase being lost by the end of the second decade. This increase in the intercanine width is achieved largely through alveolar rather than skeletal change, during eruption of the permanent incisors and canines. In contrast to the maxilla, very little change occurs in the mandibular intercanine width once the incisor teeth have erupted, which is one of the reasons why mandibular incisor irregularity is so common. Some increase in the intermolar width is also seen in the mandibular and maxillary arches, and whilst this is also in the region of 2 and 4 mm respectively, this change differs from the intercanine width in that it occurs progressively from the age of 12 years through to 18 (Moyers et al, 1976). It should be remembered that wide individual variation is associated with all these dimensional changes, but generally there is more growth in boys than girls and the intermolar width will increase more than the intercanine width and over a longer period of time (Lee, 1999).

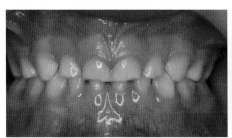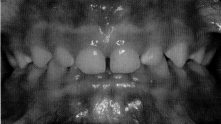

Figure 4.11 The complete deciduous dentition is usually present by around 3 years of age. Note the variation in overbite. Courtesy of Rupert Cobourne (left) and Isabelle George (right).

- Mandibular central incisors erupt first;
- Followed by the maxillary central incisors and soon after by the maxillary lateral incisors;
- Eruption of the mandibular lateral incisors completes the incisor dentition;
- First deciduous molars then erupt prior to the canines; and
- Mandibular and then maxillary second molars erupt.

The complete deciduous dentition is classically associated with a number of characteristic features:

- The arches are semi-circular in shape;
- The incisors are spaced, upright and associated with a positive overjet and overbite;
- Primate or anthropoid spaces are present, mesial to the maxillary deciduous canines and distal to the mandibular canines;
- The molar and canine relationship is class I; and
- The distal edges of the second deciduous molars are flush in the vertical plane.

However, these features are rarely all seen together and variation is very much the norm (Box 4.4).

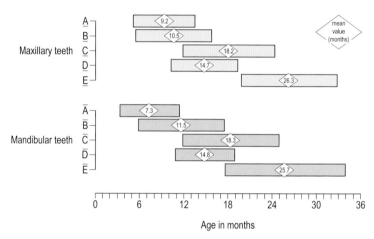

Figure 4.12 Eruption ages of deciduous teeth from a sample of indigenous British subjects. The mean value (in months) is indicated by the central diamond, whilst two standard deviations are shown by the horizontal bar. Redrawn from Leighton BC (1968). Eruption of deciduous teeth. *Dent Pract* 200:836–42.

Box 4.4 Does a normal deciduous dentition exist?

Foster and Hamilton studied the complete deciduous dentitions of 100 children aged between 2 ½ and 3 years. There was not a single child within this sample that had incisor spacing, primate spaces, upright incisors and flush terminal molars all present within the same dentition. Amongst these occlusal features, the presence of primate spaces was the most constant finding. Approximately one-third of the sample had spacing between all the incisor teeth, but the majority only had spacing between some of these teeth. Around half of the children had second deciduous molars that were flush in the terminal plane. The greatest variation was seen in the incisor relationship, with only a fifth of children having a normal overbite and almost three-quarters having some increase in the overjet (Foster & Hamilton, 1969).

Box 4.5 Can a future malocclusion be predicted from the deciduous dentition?

There is wide individual variation in occlusal development and predicting a malocclusion in the permanent dentition based upon an established deciduous dentition is difficult. Unilateral crossbite, anterior open bite and an increased overjet associated with a digit-sucking habit will usually spontaneously improve, if cessation of the habit occurs before the mixed dentition is established. However, in the absence of a digit-sucking habit, a markedly increased or reverse overjet will give a fairly accurate prognosis for the incisor relationship in the permanent dentition. Little predictive information regarding the potential for crowding in the permanent dentition is obtained from measuring the size of the deciduous teeth or the arch length. However, alignment of the incisor dentition can give a good indication of the potential for future crowding. If any incisor crowding exists in the deciduous dentition then this almost certainly means there will be crowding of the permanent teeth. Deciduous incisor teeth that are aligned but not spaced have approximately a 2 in 3 chance of crowding, whilst less than 3-mm of spacing gives a 1 in 2 chance. A total of 6-mm spacing is required in the deciduous incisor dentition to have little likelihood of crowding in the permanent dentition (Leighton, 1969).

Predicting a future malocclusion in the permanent dentition, based upon features of the deciduous dentition, is generally unreliable (Box 4.5). In addition, the deciduous dentition is not static and during the next two to three years, prior to eruption of the permanent teeth, a number of changes can occur:

- Occlusal wear of the teeth and more forward mandibular growth relative to the maxilla can produce an edge-to-edge incisor relationship and alteration of the molar relationship;
- Interproximal wear or premature loss of tooth substance due to caries can also produce an alteration of the molar relationship; and
- A prolonged digit or dummy sucking habit can induce an anterior open bite and posterior crossbites.

The mixed dentition

During the mixed dentition, both deciduous and permanent teeth are present. The permanent dentition is established in three phases:

- Eruption of first molars and incisors;
- Eruption of premolars, canines and second molars; and
- Eruption of third molars.

Eruption of first molars and incisors

Variations in the eruption sequence of the permanent teeth are common, but as a general rule the mandibular teeth erupt prior to the maxillary. Permanent teeth begin their eruption once crown formation is completed, taking between two and five years

Table 4.1 Chronology of permanent tooth development and eruption

	Crown completion	Eruption	Root completion
Maxillary teeth			
1	4.5	7.5	10
2	4.5	8.5	11
3	6.5	11.5	14
4	5.5	10.5	12.5
5	6.5	11.5	13
6	2.75	6.5	9.5
7	7.5	12.5	15
8	14	19	21
Mandibular teeth			
1	4.5	6.5	9
2	4.5	7.5	10
3	6.5	9.5	13
4	5.5	11	12.5
5	6.5	11.5	13.5
6	2.75	6.5	9.5
7	7.5	12.5	14.5
8	14	19	21.5

All dates in years. Adapted from Berkovitz, Holland and Moxham (2009), *Oral Anatomy Histology and Embryology* (St Louis: Mosby).

to reach the alveolar crest and a further one to two years to reach occlusion. Root development is usually completed within 2 years of eruption (Table 4.1).

The mixed dentition stage is heralded by eruption of the first permanent molars at around 6 years of age. This is generally followed by eruption of the first and then second permanent incisors between the ages of 7 and 8 years (Fig. 4.13), although in the mandible the first permanent incisors can erupt before or with the first molars.

During this phase of development the utilization of dental arch perimeter is crucial for establishing:

- Alignment of the permanent incisors; and
- Molar occlusion.

The collective mesiodistal dimensions of the permanent incisor tooth crowns are larger than their deciduous predecessors by approximately 5-mm in the mandible and 7-mm in the maxilla, a deficit known as the incisor liability. This increased space requirement for the permanent incisor teeth is gained from the following (Fig. 4.14):

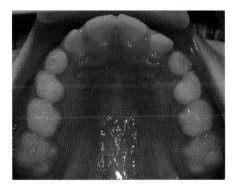

Figure 4.13 Early mixed dentition.
Courtesy of Wilf DiBiase.

- Residual spacing present between the deciduous incisors;
- Permanent incisors erupting into a more labial position (particularly in the maxilla) than their deciduous predecessors and therefore occupying a greater arch perimeter;
- Deciduous canines being moved distally as the incisors erupt; and
- Transverse increase in the intercanine arch width.

The initial occlusal relationship of the first permanent molars is directly influenced by the deciduous second molar position. If these teeth are flush in the terminal plane then the first permanent molars assume a cusp-to-cusp relationship when they erupt. In order to establish a class I molar relationship, some mesial movement of the mandibular first permanent molar will be required. This is achieved by two possible mechanisms (Fig. 4.14):

- Early mesial shift where the lower primate space (distal to the mandibular canine and therefore adjacent to the deciduous molar occlusion) is closed by forward movement of the mandibular molar dentition as the first permanent molar erupts; and
- Late mesial shift where the mandibular first molar only moves in a mesial direction after loss of the second deciduous molar; because the mesiodistal length of the mandibular second deciduous molar crown is greater than the maxillary, the loss of these teeth results in greater mesial movement of the mandibular first molar.

Occasionally, a mesial step occlusion of the deciduous molars might have been established prior to eruption of the permanent molars; in these cases they will tend to erupt directly into a class III occlusal relationship. Alternatively, there may be a distal step occlusion, in which case the first molars will erupt into a class II relationship. However, it should be remembered that all of these relationships affecting the deciduous molars and therefore establishment of the molar occlusion will be significantly influenced by the relative amounts of forward maxillary and mandibular growth that occur during this time.

During this period of the mixed dentition, a number of features associated with the maxillary incisor teeth can be present prior to establishing the early permanent dentition:

- Transient anterior open bite; and
- Physiological spacing (ugly duckling) stage.

A transient anterior open bite can be associated with eruption of the incisors as they approach the occlusal plane and this invariably improves with time. The maxillary

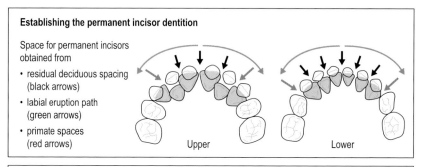

Establishing the permanent incisor dentition

Space for permanent incisors obtained from

- residual deciduous spacing (black arrows)
- labial eruption path (green arrows)
- primate spaces (red arrows)

Upper

Lower

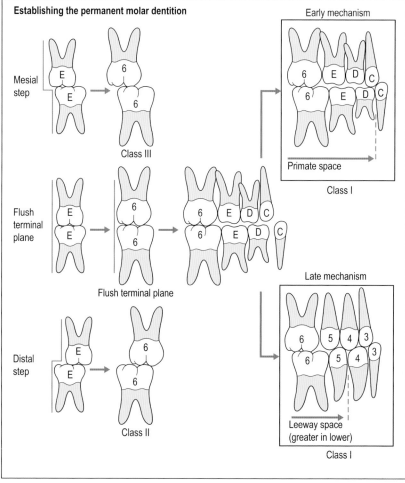

Establishing the permanent molar dentition

Early mechanism

Mesial step

Class III

Primate space

Class I

Flush terminal plane

Flush terminal plane

Late mechanism

Distal step

Class II

Leeway space (greater in lower)

Class I

Figure 4.14 Establishing the incisor and molar occlusions.

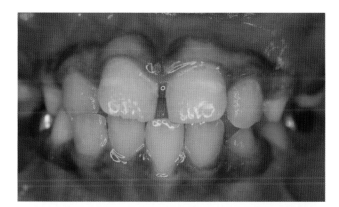

Figure 4.15
Physiological spacing or 'ugly duckling' stage.

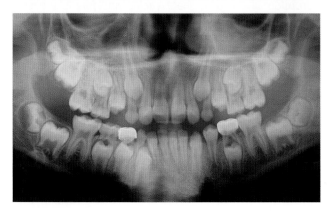

central incisors can also be quite distally inclined when they first erupt, which produces a midline diastema between them. This physiological spacing or 'ugly duckling' stage is thought to be due to the combined effect of the maxillary incisor apices being initially quite close together in the anterior maxilla as the incisors erupt and lateral pressure from the erupting maxillary lateral incisors and canines (Fig. 4.15). As these teeth erupt this pressure is transferred from the apical region of the maxillary incisors more coronally, improving their inclination and usually closing the diastema.

Eruption of premolars, canines and second molars
Further development of the dentition is characterized by eruption of the premolar and canine teeth, between the incisors at the front of the arch and the first molars at the back. Eruption of these teeth normally takes place between the ages of 9 and 12 years and as a general rule:

- In the mandible, the canine erupts ahead of the first premolar and this is followed by the second premolar; and
- In the maxilla, the first premolar usually erupts first, followed by the second premolar and then canine.

The consequences of these eruption patterns are that the mandibular second premolar and maxillary canine teeth are the most vulnerable for potential crowding (Fig. 4.16).

In contrast to the incisor dentition, the combined mesiodistal length of the deciduous canine and molar teeth is greater than that of the permanent canine and premolars, an excess known as the leeway space. In the maxilla, this is approximately 1.5-mm per quadrant, whilst in the mandible it is closer to 2.5-mm, because of the increased size of the lower second deciduous molar. However, successful alignment of the canine and premolar teeth within each quadrant relies upon a number of factors:

- The size of the leeway space;
- Previous encroachment by the incisors into the canine region; and
- The mechanism of molar relationship correction.

Clearly, the larger the leeway space present within each quadrant, the more potential space there will be for eruption of the permanent canine and premolar teeth. However, if earlier alignment of the permanent incisor dentition has utilized any space within the deciduous canine regions, this will now be at the expense of that available for the permanent canines. This can be particularly relevant in the maxillary arch, where the permanent canine has a long path of eruption and often appears after the premolar teeth. In addition, if substantial forward movement of the mandibular first permanent molar has occurred during establishment of the molar relationship or following the early loss of deciduous second molars, this will also leave less space for permanent canine and premolar teeth to erupt uncrowded. In this scenario it is often the mandibular second premolar that becomes crowded (Fig. 4.16).

The final part of this phase of dental development occurs with eruption of the second permanent molars, usually at around 12 years of age. Eruption of these teeth

Figure 4.16 Crowding of the maxillary canine and mandibular second premolar. The UR3 is buccally crowded due to timing of eruption, the LL5 is crowded due to early loss of the LLE.

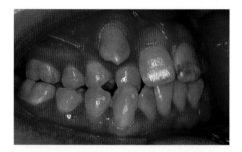

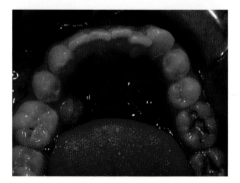

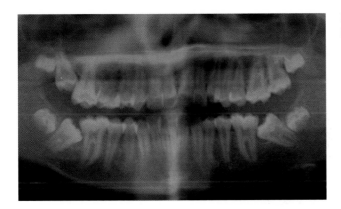

Figure 4.17 Impacted LL7, LR7 and UR7.

is often associated with some reduction in arch length, which manifests as increased crowding, particularly of the lower incisors (Lundy & Richardson, 1995). If the second permanent molars erupt precociously before the premolar dentition is established, in the lower jaw especially this can result in a considerable arch length reduction and crowding of the second premolar tooth. Occasionally, there is a lack of space in the posterior regions of the maxillary and mandibular dental arches and the second molars can become impacted (Fig. 4.17).

Third molar eruption

The appearance of the third molars is the final stage in establishing the permanent dentition. These teeth usually erupt between 17 and 21 years of age, but this is characteristically variable and in many cases they either remain unerupted or fail to develop completely. Controversy exists as to the effect of third molar impaction and eruption on mesial drift within the dental arches, particularly the mandibular, and the subsequent effect that this can have on the position of the incisors (Box 4.6). It is likely that third molar eruption, rather than impaction, does have an effect upon mandibular arch crowding often seen during the late teenage years, but this effect is one component of a multifactorial condition and prophylactic third molar extraction is unlikely to remove the problem (Richardson, 2002). The National Institute for Health and Clinical Excellence (NICE) in the UK has recommended that prophylactic removal of pathology-free impacted third molars, which includes removal to prevent occlusal changes in the incisor regions, be discontinued.

Occlusal changes in the permanent dentition

The dentition does not remain static throughout life as longitudinal studies on individuals who have not undergone orthodontic treatment have shown (Bishara et al, 1989; Moorrees et al, 1969; Sinclair & Little, 1983). Generally, the dental arches in males grow larger and for longer than in females during both the preadolescent and adolescent periods.

Apart from the effects of dental disease, which can result in major occlusal changes if teeth are lost, there is a gradual and progressive loss in arch length as age increases, particularly in the lower arch of females. The net effect of this is an increase

Box 4.6   Understanding the causes of late lower incisor crowding

Crowding of the mandibular incisors is one of the most common problems encountered in the permanent dentition and lower incisor alignment is one of the most likely things to relapse after orthodontic treatment. Studies of untreated subjects followed from the mixed dentition into adulthood have shown a tendency for the width and length of the mandibular arch to decrease and for crowding of the anterior teeth to increase (Sinclair & Little, 1985). Primary crowding refers to a discrepancy of tooth dimension and jaw size, mainly determined genetically. Secondary crowding is caused by environmental factors, including local space conditions in the dental arches and the position and function of the tongue, the lips and the buccal musculature. Tertiary crowding occurs during adolescence and post-adolescence with a predilection for the lower labial segment. Factors contributing to late lower incisor crowding may include:

- Mandibular growth rotations;
- Anterior component of occlusal force;
- Physiologic mesial drift;
- Soft tissue maturation;
- Degenerative periodontal changes allowing teeth to drift under light pressures;
- Change in diet and lack of interproximal wear;
- Tooth size and shape;
- Tooth loss and drifting leading to changes in occlusal function; and
- Mandibular third molars–presence and position.

In reality, all of these factors may contribute to the development of late lower incisor crowding but the contribution of developing third molars is regarded as being minimal as crowding can develop even in the absence of their development. The prophylactic removal of developing third molars is not recommended to prevent late lower incisor crowding.

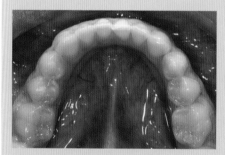 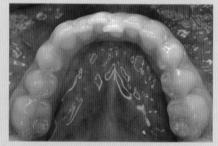

Late lower incisor crowding in an untreated mandibular arch.

in lower incisor crowding with age, although these changes are variable and difficult to predict. It is interesting to note that the changes found in untreated individuals in general are very similar in nature to those found in patients following orthodontic treatment.

Further reading

BURDI AR AND MOYERS RE (1998). Development of the dentition and occlusion. In: Moyers RE (ed). *A Handbook of Orthodontics*, 4th edn (Chicago: Mosby).
RICHARDSON A (2000). Interceptive Orthodontics, 4th Edition (British Dental Association: London)

References

BISHARA SE, JAKOBSEN JR, TREDER JE AND STASI MJ (1989). Changes in the maxillary and mandibular tooth size-arch length relationship from early adolescence to early adulthood. A longitudinal study. *Am J Orthod Dentofacial Orthop* 95:46–59.
CLINCH LM (1934). Variations in the mutual relationship of the maxillary and mandibular gum pads in the newborn child. *Int J Orthod* 20:359–372.
COBOURNE MT AND SHARPE PT (2003). Tooth and jaw: molecular mechanisms of patterning in the first branchial arch. *Arch Oral Biol* 48:1–14.
FOSTER TD, GRUND MC AND LAVELLE CL (1972). Changes in occlusion in the primary dentition between 2-and-one-half- and 5-and-one-half-years of age. *Trans Eur Orthod Soc* 75–84.
FOSTER TD AND HAMILTON MC (1969). Occlusion in the primary dentition. *Br Dent J* 126:76–79.
LEE RT (1999). Arch width and form: a review. *Am J Orthod Dentofacial Orthop* 115:305–313.
LEIGHTON BC (1968). Eruption of deciduous teeth. *Dent Pract* 200:836–842.
LEIGHTON BC (1969). The early signs of malocclusion. *Trans Eur Orth Soc* 353–368.
LEUNG AK AND ROBSON WL (2006). Natal teeth: a review. *J Natl Med Assoc* 98:226–228.
LUNDY HJ AND RICHARDSON ME (1995). Developmental changes in alignment of the lower labial segment. *Br J Orthod* 22:339–345.
MOORREES CF, GRON AM, LEBRET LM, ET AL (1969). Growth studies of the dentition: a review. *Am J Orthod* 55:600–616.
MOYERS RE, VAN DER LINDEN PGM, RIOLO ML ET AL (1976). *Standards of Human Occlusal Development*, Monograph 5, Craniofacial Growth Series. Ann Arbor, Michigan, Center for Human Growth and Development, University of Michigan.
RICHARDSON ME (2002). Late lower arch crowding: the aetiology reviewed. *Dent Update* 29:234–238.
SHARPE PT (1995). Homeobox genes and orofacial development. *Connect Tissue Res* 32:17–25.
SHARPE PT (2001). Neural crest and tooth morphogenesis. *Adv Dent Res* 15:4–7.
SINCLAIR PM AND LITTLE RM (1983). Maturation of untreated normal occlusions. *Am J Orthod* 83:114–123.
SINCLAIR PM AND LITTLE RM (1985). Dentofacial maturation of untreated normals. *Am J Orthod* 88:146–156.
TUCKER AS, MATTHEWS KL AND SHARPE PT (1998). Transformation of tooth type induced by inhibition of BMP signaling. *Science* 282:1136–1138.
TUCKER AS AND SHARPE P (2004). The cutting edge of mammalian development; how the embryo makes teeth. *Nat Rev Genet* 5:499–508.

5 Orthodontic tooth movement

If a force is applied to a tooth it will elicit a response within the periodontium, resulting in remodelling of the periodontal ligament and alveolar bone, and ultimately tooth movement. The physical and biological principles that underlie this process form the basis of orthodontic practice and are discussed in this chapter.

Biological basis of tooth movement

It was first noted in the nineteenth century that a mechanical stimulus applied to bone could lead to remodelling and this is the basic principle, which facilitates orthodontic tooth movement.

Physiology of bone

Bone is a hard tissue composed of a collagen matrix impregnated with mineral salts. As well as providing the foundation of the musculoskeletal system in most vertebrates, it serves as a storage site for many important elements, especially calcium. Bone consists of three principle components:

- An extracellular matrix, consisting predominantly of type I collagen and a variety of proteoglycans and bone-specific proteins;
- Inorganic mineral, which makes up approximately 67% of bone by weight and consists mainly of calcium and phosphate in the form of hydroxyapatite crystals; and
- Cells, which include osteoblasts responsible for laying down and mineralizing the bone matrix; osteocytes, which are osteoblasts that have become enveloped by bone as it mineralizes, and osteoclasts, which are large multinucleate cells derived from haematopoetic precursors within the circulation that resorb bone.

There is close intercellular communication between osteoblasts and osteocytes, the main function of this osteoblast–osteocyte complex being to maintain integrity of the bone matrix.

Bone remodelling

Bone is a dynamic tissue, with resorption and deposition continually occurring and being closely linked and regulated. This process produces remodelling of the skeleton, in simple terms by osteoblastic deposition and osteoclastic resorption. However, the situation is complex and in addition to their direct role in bony deposition, several osteoblastic responses have been identified that indirectly facilitate osteoclastic resorption:

Table 5.1 Factors affecting bone remodelling and maintenance of the periodontal space

Systemic factors	Local factors
Parathyroid hormone	Cytokines and growth factors
Vitamin D metabolites	Prostaglandins
Calcitonin	Leukotrienes

- Osteoblasts lining the bone represent a physical barrier to resorption and their retraction provides access for bone-resorbing osteoclasts;
- Osteoblasts remove unmineralized collagen or osteoid that lines the bone surface, which also acts as a physical barrier to osteoclasts; and
- Osteoblasts release a soluble activating factor, which has a direct action on osteoclasts.

Regulation of bony deposition and resorption is important for normal maintenance of the skeleton and when these mechanisms break down, pathological change can occur. Numerous systemic and local factors have been implicated in bone remodelling (Table 5.1).

Biomechanics of tooth movement

Early research into tooth movement investigated the histological response of tissues using animal models, whilst more recent work has focused on cellular activity following mechanical stimulation (Box 5.1).

Pressure–tension theory

Histological studies carried out independently by Carl Sandstedt and Albin Oppenheim at the turn of the past century provided the foundation for current understanding of orthodontic tooth movement. When a force is placed on a tooth, bone is laid down on the tension side of the periodontal ligament and resorbed on the pressure side (Fig. 5.1). On the pressure side, when the force is light, multinucleate cells resorb bone directly. However, if the forces are higher and exceed capillary blood pressure, cell death can occur and a cell-free area forms. This is described as hyalinization, due to the glass-like appearance of these regions when viewed with light microscopy resembling hyaline cartilage. Resorption of these areas proceeds at a much-reduced rate. This process is described as undermining resorption and will result in slower tooth movement and greater pain and discomfort for the patient. Later work showed that even forces as light as 30g will produce some areas of hyalinization, and this tends to occur more with tipping than bodily movement of teeth, presumably because the force is dissipated more evenly through the periodontal ligament during bodily movement (Reitan, 1964).

From histological and clinical studies there appears to be a range of force effective for tooth movement (Storey & Smith, 1952) although the optimum force magnitude for orthodontic tooth movement has yet to be described (Ren et al, 2003). Light continuous forces are thought to be more effective than heavy forces as these will increase the risk of hyalinization, with no increase in the desired tooth movement but with

Box 5.1   How has orthodontic tooth movement been investigated?

Early investigations into orthodontic tooth movement examined the histological effect within the periodontal ligament and alveolar bone of loading a tooth. Later experimental models were developed, both in vitro and in vivo, to study the effect that these forces had in greater detail. Numerous animal models have been used, including rats, cats and primates. Usually an orthodontic appliance is attached to the teeth and force applied over a given period of time, samples of cervicular fluid are collected for assay during the experimental period and then the animal is sacrificed for histological examination. Organ culture systems have also been used. As the periodontal ligament is similar to sutural joints, in both anatomy and function, one model involves placing mechanical stress across cranial sutures taken from newborn rabbits. Animal models tell us much about the histological and biochemical changes that occur during mechanical stress; however, the major drawback of such experiments is the difficulty in determining the individual cellular response. To examine this, a single cell type is cultured on a substrate that is mechanically deformed. Petri dishes with flexible bases are available, and these can be deformed by placing them over a convex template or applying a vacuum. Different cell types can be examined in this way and the size and periods of the deformation can be varied. Samples are taken periodically from the cell culture medium in which the cells are immersed for subsequent biochemical assay.

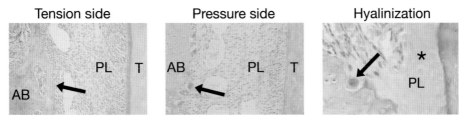

Tension side   Pressure side   Hyalinization

Figure 5.1 Histological appearance of the periodontium during orthodontic tooth movement. Osteoblastic bone deposition (arrowed) on the tension side. Osteoclastic frontal resorption (arrowed) on the pressure side. Hyalinization occurs in areas of excess pressure and is characterized by a glass-like appearance in regions of the periodontal ligament (*) and areas of undermining resorption (arrowed). AB, alveolar bone; PL, periodontal ligament; T, tooth. Courtesy of Professor Jonathan Sandy.

greater potential anchorage loss (Fig. 5.2). However, large variation does exist between individuals and more important than the absolute force is the stress generated in the periodontal ligament. Stress is force per unit area and depending on the type of tooth movement, stress distribution within the periodontium will vary. Therefore, different force levels are recommended for different types of tooth movement (Table 5.2). Tipping teeth requires less force than bodily movement, whilst intrusive forces need to be light as these are dissipated through the apices of the teeth, increasing the risk of root resorption.

Figure 5.2 Graph of force applied to the periodontal ligament and subsequent tooth movement. Up to a certain threshold, tooth movement increases with force. However, once this force exceeds a certain level, no additional movement is obtained. Indeed, extreme forces can even cause a reduction in movement.

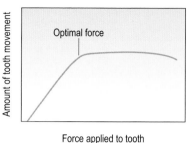

Table 5.2   Range of forces for different tooth movements

Tipping	30–60 g
Bodily movements	100–150 g
Rotational movements	50–75 g
Extrusion	50–75 g
Intrusion	15–25 g

Bone deflection and piezoelectricity

Orthodontic forces are transmitted within the periodontal ligament of the tooth and traditionally this has been thought to be via principle fibres of the periodontal ligament itself. However, when cross-linking of collagen is disrupted, the histological response of bone to orthodontic tooth movement appears normal (Heller & Nanda, 1979). Therefore, it has been proposed that the periodontal ligament represents a continuous hydrostatic system that distributes forces equally to all its regions (Baumrind, 1969). However, this would mean differential forces could not be distributed within the ligament, which is clearly not the case.

Teeth will displace a greater amount than the width of the periodontal ligament when force is initially applied to them, which implies that some deflection of alveolar bone also occurs. This might explain why differential forces can develop at the bone surfaces of the periodontal ligament. Bone deflection also produces stress-generated electrical potentials at the bone surface, which at one time were thought to be involved in bone remodelling. However, these are short-lived and very small and as such, unlikely to play an active role (McDonald, 1993).

Cellular shape change and signal transduction

When an external force is applied to a tooth, this stimulus generates an intracellular response, which ultimately leads to a change in function of affected and adjacent cells by production of local bone remodelling mediators.

A relationship appears to exist between cell shape and metabolic activity. Cell shape is controlled by the cytoskeleton, which terminates in specialized sites at the cell membrane, which form junctional complexes with the extracellular matrix. At these focal adhesion integrins, a family of proteins that span the cell membrane link the cytoskeleton to the extracellular matrix. They act as intracellular signalling receptors and are involved in numerous signalling pathways. Mechanical stress on cells within

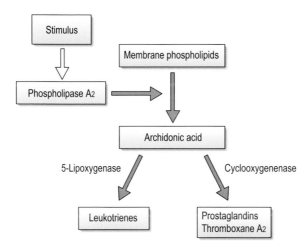

Figure 5.3 The arachidonic acid pathway producing prostaglandins, leukotrienes and thromboxanes.

the periodontal ligament initiates both the cyclic AMP and phosphoinositide pathways, which results in an increase in production of secondary messengers. This produces an increase in intracellular calcium levels, which mediates further cellular events, including a stimulation of DNA synthesis (Harell et al, 1977).

Production of arachidonic acid metabolites

Arachidonic acid is an unsaturated fatty acid produced from membrane phospholipids, which is metabolized into prostaglandins, leukotrienes and thromboxanes (Fig. 5.3). These molecules are potent mediators of inflammation and numerous in vitro and in vivo experiments have shown a relationship between mechanical stimulation and prostaglandin production in bone. Based on this work, prostaglandins have been used clinically via local administration in the gingivae to increase the efficiency of orthodontic tooth movement (Yamasaki et al, 1984). The other principle products of arachidonic acid metabolism, leukotrienes, have also been shown to increase around teeth moved orthodontically. This may explain the observation that on administration of a non-steroidal anti-inflammatory drug in an animal model, there is a decrease in osteoclast numbers, but not tooth movement (Sandy & Harris, 1984). This suggests some overlap between the pathways and a degree of redundancy within the system. Inhibition of leukotriene production itself results in inhibition of tooth movement (Mohammed et al, 1989).

Production of cytokines

Cytokines are low-molecular-weight proteins that regulate or modify the action of cells. These protein groups are diverse and complex, and include some potent stimulators of bone resorption. It appears that osteoclast activity is dependent on soluble factors produced by osteoblasts and stromal cells in the periodontal ligament, so-called osteoclast-stimulating factors. On mechanical stimulation, the initial response of bone is to inhibit the production of cytokines involved in osteoclast stimulation and hence promote osteogenesis.

Numerous cytokines are produced in the periodontal ligament when force is applied to teeth, including interleukins (ILs), tumour necrosis factors (TNFs) and epidermal growth factors (EGFs). Local production of these molecules by mechanically activated cells within the ligament may play an important role in mediating both the resorptive and formative phase of connective tissue remodeling.

Alteration in cellular function and remodelling

The ultimate effect of mechanical stimulation on cells within the periodontal ligament is an alteration in gene expression and cellular function; which allows remodelling to take place and teeth to be moved through alveolar bone. Initially there appears to be a reduction in DNA synthesis, followed by a gradual increase. In addition there is an increase in production of collagen and proteins associated with its breakdown, and that of components in the extracellular matrix, including metalloproteinases, collagenases and gelatinases. It appears that matrix degradation in the periodontal ligament is a prerequisite for cell proliferation, creating room to accommodate an increase in the cell population. On the compression side it is likely that enzymes produced by osteoblasts degrade the non-mineralized osteoid surface of the bone, while periodontal cells degrade the extracellular matrix of the periodontal ligament. There is an increase in recruitment and production of osteoclasts, mediated via factors released from cells in the periodontal ligament. Osteoclasts finally access the bone surface and degrade the mineralized matrix.

Mechanical basis of tooth movement

Orthodontic tooth movement is dictated by the force system delivered to the teeth and mediated through the orthodontic appliance and the biological response it evokes. The following are important concepts and definitions pertaining to orthodontic tooth movement and are relevant to its understanding:

- Force—a load applied to an object that has both magnitude and direction. Forces can be represented visually by vectors.
- Centre of resistance—the point at which bodily movement or translation of an object will result when a force is applied. In a free-floating body, the centre of resistance coincides with the centre of mass; however, teeth are fixed in bone and therefore, the centre of resistance is difficult to determine accurately. It is generally presumed to be located around one-third to halfway down the root of a healthy single-rooted tooth. The centre of resistance will move apically if bone support is lost due to periodontal disease (Fig. 5.4). For a multirooted tooth, the centre of resistance is between the roots, 1 to 2-mm apical to the furcation (Fig. 5.5).
- Moment—when a force is applied to a body at a distance from the centre of resistance a rotational effect or moment is created (Fig. 5.5). It is the product of the force and the distance from the centre of resistance, so the greater the distance the greater the rotation.
- Couple—this represents two equal and opposite forces. A couple exerts no net force to bodily move a tooth, as the forces are opposite in direction and cancel each other out. A couple acting alone on a tooth will produce a purely rotational

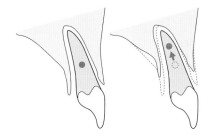

Figure 5.4 Centre of resistance of an incisor tooth in relation to the level of alveolar bone.

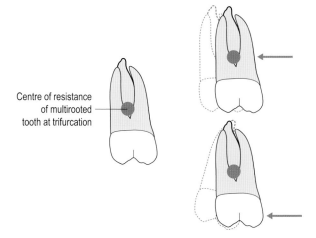

Centre of resistance of multirooted tooth at trifurcation

Figure 5.5 For bodily movement the force needs to pass through the centre of resistance of the tooth. If the force vector does not pass through the centre of resistance, a moment is created and rotation will occur.

movement (Fig. 5.6), whilst a couple combined with an additional force can produce bodily movement (see Fig. 5.8).

Tipping and bodily tooth movement

A significant problem with orthodontic tooth movement is that the centre of resistance of a tooth is not directly accessible to force application. Force must be applied to the tooth crown, which is at a distance from the centre of resistance and therefore, a moment and some rotational force is always produced.

Tipping movements are relatively easy to generate by point contact on the crown of a tooth and this is how the active components on a removable appliance work (Fig. 5.7).

Bodily movement is more difficult to produce and requires the combination of a force and a couple to control the rotational effect. This is essentially how the edgewise slot of a fixed appliance works. By placing a rectangular wire into the slot, a couple is created within the bracket slot, which will control root position and allow the tooth

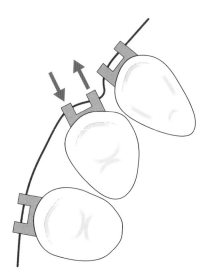

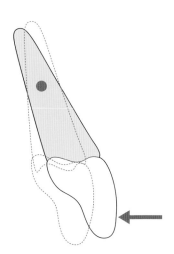

Figure 5.6 A couple is generated when a light archwire is engaged into the bracket slot of a rotated tooth.

Figure 5.7 Application of a single force to the crown of a tooth will result in tipping as a moment is created.

to move bodily in the direction of applied force (Fig. 5.8). The couple acts over the depth of the bracket slot and this will need to counter the moment created by a force applied at some distance from the centre of resistance of the tooth. Therefore, although the force applied to the tooth may be small, a large couple will need to be developed within the bracket to maintain bodily movement of the tooth. A small amount of space or 'slop' always exists between the archwire and bracket, so some tipping does occur. This can be countered by placing more torsion in the wire, or into the bracket base (Fig. 5.9). In reality, pure bodily movement or translation is an idealized impossibility. What happens is that the tooth or group of teeth will tip and then upright as they move along the archwire, giving the impression of bodily movement.

Force systems

In certain clinical situations the forces acting on the dentition and the resulting moments and couples can be readily determined. For example, with a cantilever spring acting on one tooth, the force system will consist of one force vector and the resulting couple and moment (Fig. 5.10). The movement of the tooth and the reactive forces are therefore fairly predictable. However, when using fixed appliances with continuous archwires numerous force vectors can be created and it becomes impossible to work out all the possible interactions. This is especially true in the initial alignment stage of treatment when numerous displaced teeth are often engaged with a flexible wire. Even so, all systems will follow the same basic physical laws, most notably Newton's third law of motion: 'For every action there is an equal and opposite reaction,' the sum of the forces and the sum of the moments for any appliance system equaling zero. Therefore care must be taken to elicit the planned tooth movements while limit-

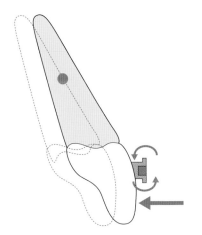

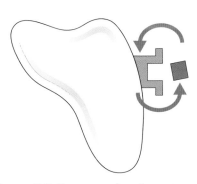

Figure 5.8 A force couple developed in an edgewise bracket slot with a rectangular wire will resist tipping and result in bodily tooth movement on application of an external force.

Figure 5.9 Placement of torsion or torque into the wire will counter the effect of tipping during bodily retraction.

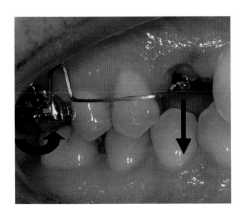

Figure 5.10 A simple cantilever spring to extrude a canine. This is described as a one-couple system because a couple is only generated at the site of full engagement in the molar tube. In this case this is resisted by the placement of a transpalatal arch.

ing the unwanted ones, as this can result in undesired treatment outcomes such as loss of anchorage.

Friction

Friction is the force that will resist the motion of two objects in contact with each other and acts tangentially to the two surfaces in contact. Friction affects tooth movement associated with all fixed appliances, but is particularly relevant for edgewise mechanics, which often rely upon sliding teeth along an archwire. Specifically, two types of friction need to be overcome:

- Static friction—the force that resists the motion of solid surfaces at rest with each other; and
- Kinetic friction—the force that resists the sliding motion of solid surfaces moving over each other at constant speed.

   Frictional resistance to sliding is proportional to the applied load and independent of the sliding surface area. In orthodontics, friction can result in binding between the archwire and bracket, leading to a reduction or failure of tooth movement, distortion of the archwires and loss of anchorage. Friction must be overcome before teeth will move and whilst frictional force can be measured in a laboratory, clinically the level is difficult to determine. In clinical practice with fixed appliances, friction is affected by a number of factors:

- The chemical and physical interaction of the archwire at the bracket–archwire interface—stainless steel exhibits the least friction, followed by nickel titanium. The greatest friction is shown by beta-titanium wire (Kapila et al, 1990). Archwire size, especially in the vertical dimension appears to have an effect on frictional resistance, with friction increasing as archwire thickness increases.
- The composition of the bracket itself—ceramic brackets exhibit higher levels of friction than those made of stainless steel. This is related to the surface hardness of ceramic materials and results in abrasive wear of the archwire surface and a build-up of debris during tooth movement. More recent ceramic bracket systems have tried to overcome this by incorporating a metal archwire slot.
- The angle of contact between archwire and bracket slot—teeth do not slide along brackets, but tip and then upright as the crowns are displaced initially a greater amount than the roots (Fig. 5.11). This results in an increase in the angle of contact between archwire and slot, which increases friction and binding between archwire and bracket. This is affected by the width of the bracket, with narrower brackets having been reported to result in greater friction—presumably as they allow greater tipping.
- The increase of frictional resistance with the force of ligation—elastomeric ligation and tightly secured steel ligatures will increase friction. Self-ligating brackets, which

Figure 5.11 Tooth moving along archwire showing as tooth tips. There is an increase in the contact angle between the wire and the bracket, resulting in an increase in friction.

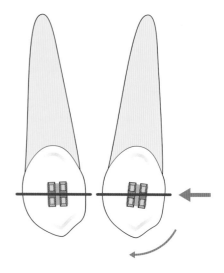

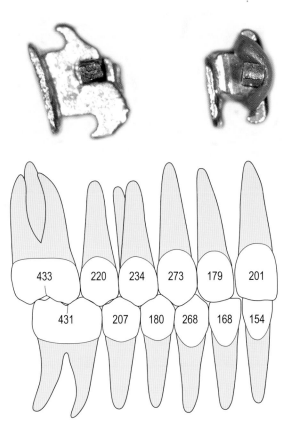

Figure 5.12 Self-ligating bracket (left) compared to conventionally ligated bracket (right), both with a rectangular steel archwire engaged in the slot.

Figure 5.13 Root surface area (mm²) of the permanent dentition, giving an indication of the relative anchorage value of each tooth (Jepsen, 1963).

secure the wire via a clip or gate, have been shown to reduce friction in laboratory studies (Fig. 5.12).

Anchorage

Anchorage is the resistance to unwanted tooth movement, or those sites that provide resistance to the reactive forces generated on activation of any orthodontic appliance. Anchorage needs to be carefully planned at the start of treatment to ensure the desired tooth movements are achieved. It maybe that equal movement of both the active and reactive units is desirable, such as expansion or closing a midline diastema, when anchorage is described as reciprocal. However, it is usual that to achieve the aims of treatment greater movement of the active than the reactive or anchorage unit is required. Depending how far the anchorage unit can move the anchorage requirements can be described as minimum or moderate. If no movement of the anchorage unit is permissible the requirement is described as maximum.

Sources of anchorage

- Root surface area—the more teeth present in the anchorage unit, the greater the combined root surface area and the less likely it is to move (Fig. 5.13).

Figure 5.14 Midline palatal implant providing anchorage via a palatal arch. Courtesy of David Tinsley.

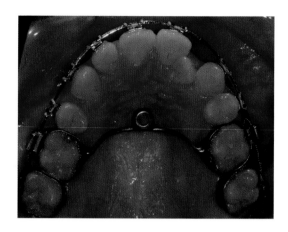

Figure 5.15 Mini screws placed in alveolar bone to provide anchorage during overjet reduction.

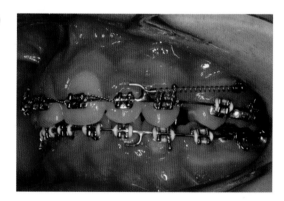

- Mucosa and bone—the palatal vault can be used as a source of anchorage via the acrylic base plate of removable appliance or acrylic button attached to palatal arches.
- Implants—absolute anchorage can be provided by implants which can be placed in any cancellous bone, but are routinely used in the palate. Implants require a period to osseointegrate and can be attached to the dentition by palatal arches to provide anchorage support (Fig. 5.14).
- Bone screws—developed more recently from those used for bony fixation during maxillofacial surgery, bone screws are much smaller than implants and do not osseointegrate. They can be placed in a variety of positions in both the maxilla and mandible, including interdentally and can be loaded immediately to provide anchorage (Fig. 5.15).

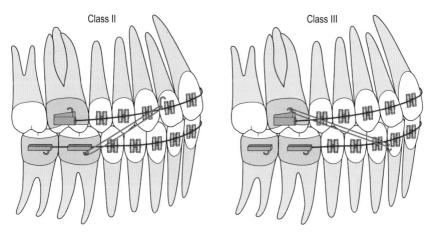

Figure 5.16 Intermaxillary elastics.

- Elastics—intermaxillary anchorage pits one dental arch against the other by using elastics. These elastics are defined as either class II or III, depending upon the direction of pull (Fig. 5.16). They must be changed at least daily and are therefore dependent upon good patient compliance. As well as the desired anteroposterior pull, they also have an extrusive and rotational effect. With class II elastics this can result in extrusion and mesial tipping of the lower molars, as well as lingual rolling as the elastics are usually run from the hook on the buccal aspect of the first molar band. Extrusion of the molars will result in reduction of the overbite, a desirable side effect in cases with reduce lower face height and an increased overbite. However, this is undesirable in those with increased lower face height and a reduced overbite to start with. Intermaxillary elastics will also tend to extrude and tip the incisors. So care must be taken when using class II elastics, particularly that the upper labial segment is not left excessively retroclined or the lower labial segment excessively proclined at the end of treatment.
- Extraoral anchorage—very useful and utilized for many years by orthodontists via the use of headgear. A force outside the mouth provided by elastics or springs attached to a head-cap or neck-strap is applied to the dentition using a Kloehn facebow (Fig. 5.17). The inner part of the bow can be attached to soldered tubes on removable appliances or directly to fixed appliances, via either tubes on molar bands or the archwire. One of the main problems encountered with the use of headgear is achieving the necessary compliance; wear can be difficult, associated with discomfort and socially disruptive, especially in older patients.

Headgear
Three factors should be considered when using headgear:
- Direction of force;
- Duration of force; and
- Level of force.

Figure 5.17 Components of headgear showing Kloehn facebow (KF), neck-strap (NS) and safety-release headgear springs (SR).

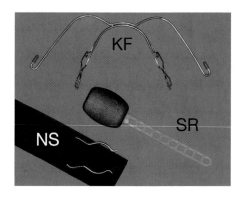

Occipital-pull   Cervical-pull   Combi-pull

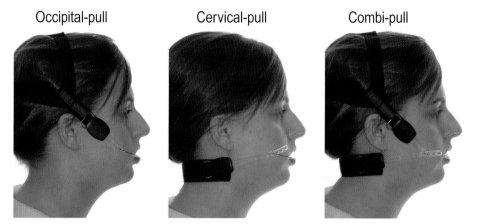

Figure 5.18 Occipital or high-pull, cervical or low-pull and combi- or straight-pull headgear.

Direction of force

The force direction can be defined as:

- High or occipital pull;
- Low or cervical pull; and
- Straight or combi pull.

Generally, high-pull headgear is used in cases with increased vertical proportions, which include high maxillary–mandibular plane angles and vertical maxillary excess, because it has an intrusive effect on the posterior dentition. Headgear force in this direction can help to avoid further bite opening and restrain vertical maxillary development during orthodontic treatment. Similarly, low-pull headgear is used in cases with reduced vertical proportion and will extrude the posterior dentition. In a growing individual this can be helpful in reducing a deep overbite. Straight or combi-pull headgear is generally used in the presence of normal vertical proportions and is useful for molar distalization (Fig. 5.18).

Duration of force

How long the patient is instructed to wear the headgear will depend on the aims of treatment. Not only is headgear effective at supporting anchorage it can also be used to distalize the buccal dentition and even restrict growth of the maxilla. To achieve these latter two objectives requires a greater duration of wear and a higher level of force magnitude. In general the duration of wear required is:

- Anchorage—10 to 12 hours per day; and
- Distalization or growth restriction—14 hours per day.

Level of force

The chosen force level will also depend upon the aims of treatment. A higher level of force is required for distalization and orthopaedic change:

- Anchorage—250 to 350g per side; and
- Distalization—450 to 500g per side.

Headgear and safety

The application of a removable extraoral force to an orthodontic appliance with headgear has led to injuries being reported in a small number of patients (Fig. 5.19). These are predominantly of two types (Samuels, 1996):

- Catapult injury—occurs when the facebow is disengaged from the tubes while still attached to the head or neck-strap, resulting in it springing back into the soft tissues of the mouth or face This type of injury can result from incorrect handling during the fitting and removal of headgear or inappropriate horseplay whilst the headgear is in place.

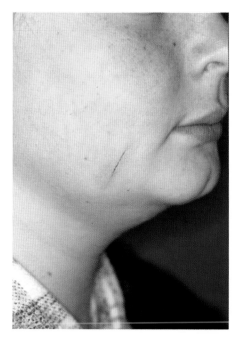

Figure 5.19 Facial laceration following accidental disengagement of a headgear facebow. Courtesy of Ricarda Kane.

Figure 5.20 NITOM locking facebow designed to prevent accidental disengagement.

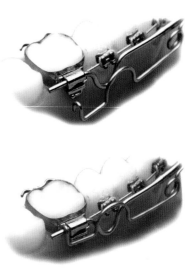

- Nocturnal disengagement—occurs when the facebow is unintentionally detached from the headgear during sleep and the inner bow causes intra- or extraoral injury.
    The most serious reported consequence of headgear injury is ocular damage, which can result in partial or total blindness in one or both eyes. Penetrating injuries of the eye can be relatively asymptomatic in the initial stages; however, oral microorganisms transmitted by the facebow can rapidly infect the eye because it acts as an excellent culture medium. These infections can be very difficult to treat and a sympathetic ophthalmitis can result, with the unaffected eye also becoming involved. Although the risk of this is small, because of the potentially devastating consequences, two independent safety devices are recommended when using headgear:
- Self-releasing head-cap or neck-strap—prevents catapult injury by detaching when a force exceeds a given amount (see Fig. 5.17); and
- Locking facebow—prevents disengagement at night by physically locking the facebow into the appliance (Fig. 5.20).

Anchorage loss
Anchorage loss is associated with undesirable tooth movement during orthodontic treatment. A common example is during overjet reduction, where teeth in the buccal segments move forward rather than those in the labial segments being retracted. If severe, too much space is lost and a residual overjet results. A number of factors can contribute to anchorage loss.

Heavy forces
Forces should be light enough to exceed the threshold for tooth movement where planned but below the threshold for movement of the anchorage unit. Heavy forces lead to unfavourable reactions in the periodontal ligament and tooth movement will plateau above a certain threshold. With greater force there is no increase in tooth movement. Assuming there are a greater number of teeth in the anchorage unit; by increasing forces, although there is no greater amount of tooth movement where it

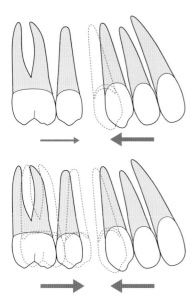

Figure 5.21 Forces should be kept light to reduce anchorage loss. All orthodontic force will produce some reciprocal force on the anchorage unit. If this is small, there will be minimal movement of these teeth. With heavier force there is a risk that the anchorage unit will move, with no additional desired tooth movement; in this case retraction of the maxillary canine.

is wanted, greater force is applied to the teeth in the anchorage unit and they are more likely to move (Fig. 5.21). Hence anchorage is lost with heavier forces. This is the differential force theory proposed by Begg and utilised in his treatment philosophy by pitching tipping of teeth, requiring very light forces against bodily movement of the teeth in the anchorage unit.

Maxillary arch
The maxillary arch is particularly susceptible to anchorage loss. This is probably due to a combination of factors, particularly the density of bone, width of the alveolus and more extensive tooth movement often required in the maxilla. Fortunately it is easier to support anchorage in the maxillary arch, primarily with the use of headgear.

Occlusal interferences
Interference between teeth or appliances in opposing arches can result in anchorage loss. This is seen commonly when correcting class II canines or when reducing an overjet prior to complete correction of an increased overbite.

Vertical growth pattern
Anchorage loss and space closure occurs more readily in patients with increased vertical proportion. This is possibly due to lower bite forces and less occlusal interference that occurs in cases with a reduced overbite.

Further reading

LINDAUER SJ (2001). The basics of orthodontic mechanics. *Sem Orthod* 7:2–15.
MEIKLE MC (2006). The tissue, cellular, and molecular regulation of orthodontic tooth movement: 100 years after Carl Sandstedt. *Eur J Orthod* 28:221–240.
QUINN RS AND YOSHIKAWA DK (1985). A reassessment of force magnitude in orthodontics. *Am J Orthod* 88:252–260.

References

BAUMRIND S (1969). A reconsideration of the propriety of the 'pressure-tension' hypothesis. *Am J Orthod* 55:12–22.

HARELL A, DEKEL S AND BINDERMAN I (1977). Biochemical effect of mechanical stress on cultured bone cells. *Calcif Tissue Res* 22 (Suppl):202–207.

HELLER IJ AND NANDA R (1979). Effect of metabolic alteration of periodontal fibers on orthodontic tooth movement. An experimental study. *Am J Orthod* 75:239–258.

JEPSEN A (1963). Root surface measurement and a method for X-ray determination of root surface area. *Acta Odontol Scand* 21:35–46.

KAPILA S, ANGOLKAR PV, DUNCANSON MG Jr, ET AL (1990). Evaluation of friction between edgewise stainless steel brackets and orthodontic wires of four alloys. *Am J Orthod Dentofacial Orthop* 98:117–126.

MCDONALD F (1993). Electrical effects at the bone surface. *Eur J Orthod* 15:175–183.

MOHAMMED AH, TATAKIS DN AND DZIAK R (1989). Leukotrienes in orthodontic tooth movement. *Am J Orthod Dentofacial Orthop* 95:231–237.

REITAN K (1964). Effects of force magnitude and direction of tooth movement on different alveolar types. *Angle Orthod* 34:244–255.

REN Y, MALTHA JC AND KUIJPERS-JAGTMAN AM (2003). Optimum force magnitude for orthodontic tooth movement: a systematic literature review. *Angle Orthod* 73:86–92.

SAMUELS RH (1996). A review of orthodontic face-bow injuries and safety equipment. *Am J Orthod Dentofacial Orthop* 110:269–272.

SANDY JR AND HARRIS M (1984). Prostaglandins and tooth movement. *Eur J Orthod* 6:175–182.

STOREY E AND SMITH R (1952). Force in orthodontics and its relation to tooth movement. *Aust J Dent* 56:11–18.

YAMASAKI K, SHIBATA Y, IMAI S, ET AL (1984). Clinical application of prostaglandin E1 (PGE1) upon orthodontic tooth movement. *Am J Orthod* 85:508–518.

6 The orthodontic patient: examination and diagnosis

Successful orthodontic treatment begins with the correct diagnosis, which involves patient interview, examination and the collection of appropriate records. At the end of this process, the orthodontist should have assimilated a comprehensive database for each patient, from which the appropriate treatment plan can be formulated. Examination and record collection are discussed in this chapter, whilst treatment planning is the subject of Chapter 7.

Patient's complaint and motivation

The demand for orthodontic treatment is primarily patient-driven and one of the most important components of an examination is the initial interview with the patient and their parent or guardian. It is important to ascertain what their main concerns are and the expectations of treatment. Over the past two decades there has been an increasing uptake in orthodontic treatment, with a greater awareness and demand for improved dental and facial aesthetics. Unfortunately this does not always accompany an appreciation of what orthodontic treatment involves (Tulloch et al, 1984). It can also be the case that the patient has no particular concerns regarding his/her dentition and it is the parent or dentist who has requested the consultation, which may make the acceptance of orthodontic treatment more difficult to obtain.

Dental history

Patients being considered for orthodontic treatment should be in good dental health and under the care of a general dental practitioner. It is important that the orthodontist and dental practitioner have a good working relationship because the orthodontist may often need to work closely with the dentist in a number of circumstances:

- Achieving a high enough standard of oral hygiene to allow orthodontic treatment;
- Treatment of any dental pathology as orthodontic appliance therapy should not be carried out in the presence of active dental disease;
- Facilitating elective tooth extraction;
- Requesting or coordinating any restorative work that may be required, either prior to or following orthodontic treatment (particularly in cases of hypodontia or trauma); and
- Assessing the occlusal impact of early tooth loss due to caries or trauma.

The general dental practitioner should be fully aware of the orthodontic treatment goals and good communication between the orthodontist, patient and dentist is therefore essential.

Medical history

A number of medical conditions may impact upon the provision of orthodontic treatment:

- Heart defects (with risk of endocarditis);
- Bleeding disorders;
- Childhood malignancies;
- Diabetes;
- Immunosuppression;
- Epilepsy;
- Asthma; and
- Allergies.

Infective endocarditis

Infective endocarditis (IE) is a serious condition characterized by colonization or invasion of the heart valves or mural endocardium by a microbiological agent, following a transient entry into the bloodstream (bacteraemia). A number of factors can put a patient at high risk of developing an endocarditis:

- Previous IE;
- Acquired valvular heart disease with stenosis or regurgitation;
- Heart valve replacement;
- Structural congenital heart disease, including surgically corrected structural conditions (but excluding isolated atrial-septal defect, fully repaired ventricular-septal defect and fully repaired patent ductus arteriosus); and
- Hypertrophic cardiomyopathy.

A number of invasive medical procedures have been causally associated with bacteraemia and endocarditis in susceptible patients and these include dental treatment. The British Society for Antimicrobial Chemotherapy previously recommended the use of antibiotic prophylaxis for any form of dentogingival manipulation in high-risk patients. These recommendations have now changed in the UK.

The National Institute of Health and Clinical Excellence (NICE) now advise that antibiotics to prevent IE should not be given to adults and children with structural cardiac defects at risk of IE who are undergoing dental interventional procedures and this includes orthodontic treatment. According to NICE, current evidence suggests that such antibiotic prophylaxis is not cost effective and may lead to a greater number of deaths through fatal anaphylactic reactions than from not using preventive antibiotics.

Bleeding disorders

Severe bleeding disorders such as haemophilia A do not contraindicate orthodontic treatment, but factor transfusion will be required to achieve haemostasis if dental extractions are necessary. Any risks of potential bleeding in the oral cavity during orthodontic treatment can be kept to a minimum by:

- Maintaining a high standard of oral hygiene; and
- Careful checking of appliances at each visit to ensure there are no wires or sharp surfaces traumatizing the soft tissues.

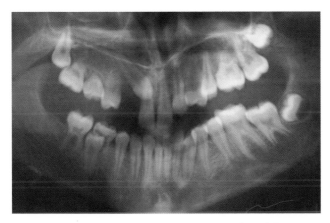

Figure 6.1 Localized root shortening in the upper right quadrant following cranial radiotherapy for treatment of a retinoblastoma.

These minor intraoral bleeds are an irritation to most patients, but can be a serious problem in this group. The orthodontist should also be aware of the increased risk of these patients being carriers for hepatitis or the human immunodeficiency virus (HIV).

Childhood malignancy
The commonest malignancies in childhood are the leukaemias, and amongst these, acute lymphoblastic leukaemia accounts for around 80% of cases. This condition mostly occurs in early childhood, before orthodontic treatment is routinely carried out. Treatment for a variety of malignances in children often involves the use of radiotherapy, which can affect the tooth-bearing tissues. This may result in tooth agenesis and root shortening (Fig. 6.1). Orthodontic treatment should be delayed for these patients until they are in a period of remission and if diagnosis occurs during orthodontic treatment it is usually advisable to suspend treatment and remove the appliances. For patients with severe root shortening orthodontic treatment is contraindicated.

Diabetes
Patients with insulin-dependent diabetes are more susceptible to periodontal disease and therefore excellent oral hygiene accompanied by regular periodontal maintenance is essential during orthodontic treatment.

Immunosuppression
Immunosuppressant drugs such as cyclosporin, which are routinely used in transplant patients to prevent rejection of the donor organ, can cause gingival hyperplasia, which can be exacerbated by orthodontic appliances. Excellent oral hygiene needs to be maintained during treatment and this can be reinforced with a chlorhexidine mouthwash. Gingivectomy of hyperplastic tissue may be necessary before or even during treatment.

Epilepsy
Removable orthodontic appliances should be avoided in the poorly controlled epileptic as there is a potential risk to the airway from displacement during seizures. These

patients can also be at risk from gingival hyperplasia due to the use of certain anti-convulsant drugs; therefore a high standard of oral hygiene must be maintained during treatment.

Asthma

The regular use of steroid-based inhalers can result in oral candida infections on the palate, which can be made worse by the use of palate-covering removable appliances. Patients with autoimmune and hyper-allergenic conditions can also be more prone to root resorption during orthodontic treatment.

Allergies

A patient may present with a reported history of allergic reaction. Although many materials used in orthodontics are capable of inducing an allergic response, the most relevant are natural rubber latex and nickel.

Allergy to latex was first recognized in the 1970s and its occurrence has increased in recent years, particularly amongst healthcare workers following the universal adoption of wearing protective gloves. Latex allergy has been reported in orthodontic practice in relation to gloves and orthodontic elastics. The most common allergic response is a type IV delayed hypersensitivity reaction triggered by the chemical accelerators used in the manufacture of latex. This causes a localized contact dermatitis, typically associated with a pruritic eczematous rash. The IgE-mediated type I reaction is less common but has more serious consequences, including anaphylaxis. Amongst the general public, type I sensitivity has been estimated to occur in around 6% of the population (Ownby et al, 1996). Investigation is via skin prick testing or immunoassay. Patients with a confirmed type I allergy should be treated in a 'latex-screened' environment where potential exposure to any allergens is minimized. Synthetic gloves composed of vinyl or nitrile are available as an alternative to latex gloves, whilst the use of orthodontic elastomeric auxiliaries containing natural rubber latex should be avoided. Latex-free silicone elastics are available but show greater force decay and as such, require more frequent replacement.

Orthodontic wires and brackets contain nickel and nickel allergy is thought to be present in approximately 10% of Western populations and more common in females. It is usually a type IV allergic reaction related to the wearing of jewellery or watches and body piercing. Fortunately, oral reactions are rare, although prolonged exposure to nickel-containing oral appliances may increase sensitivity to nickel (Bass et al, 1993). Intraoral signs are nonspecific and have been reported to include erythema, soreness at the side of the tongue and severe gingivitis, despite good oral hygiene. Definitive diagnosis is usually achieved via patch testing. Stainless steel wires and brackets contain a relatively low proportion of nickel and are considered safe to use in a patient with diagnosed nickel allergy although titanium or cobalt chromium nickel-free brackets are available. In contrast, nickel titanium archwires have a much higher content, and should be avoided in these patients.

Extraoral examination

Assessment of the patient should begin with an examination of the facial features because orthodontic treatment can impact on the soft tissues of the face. Although a number of absolute measurements can be taken, a comprehensive facial assessment

---

Box 6.1   Natural head posture

Natural head posture (NHP) is the position that the patient naturally carries their head and is therefore the most relevant for assessing skeletal relationships and facial deformity. It is determined physiologically rather than anatomically and varies between individuals; however, it is relatively constant for each individual (Moorrees & Keane, 1958). As such, NHP should be used whenever possible to assess the orthodontic patient. The patient is asked to sit upright and look straight ahead to a point at eye level in the middle distance. This can be a point on the wall in front of them, or a mirror so that they look into their own eyes. Ideally NHP should also be used when taking a lateral skull radiograph, allowing the clinical examination to be related more accurately to the cephalometric data.

---

involves looking at the balance and harmony between component parts of the face and noting any areas of disharmony. Extraoral examination should start as the patient enters the room and it is important to look at the face and soft tissues both passively and in an animated state. Once in the dental chair, the patient should be asked to sit and the face examined from the front and in profile, in a position of natural head posture (Box 6.1).

Frontal view

The frontal view of the face should be assessed vertically and transversely, with attention being paid to the presence of any asymmetry. In addition, the relationship of the lips within the face is examined in detail.

Vertical relationship

Vertically the face is split into thirds, with these dimensions being approximately equidistant. Any discrepancy in this rule of thirds will give an indication of disharmony within the facial proportions and where this lies. Of particular relevance is an increase or decrease in the lower face height. The lower third of the face can be further subdivided into thirds, with the upper lip falling into the upper third and the lower lip into the lower two-thirds (Fig. 6.2).

Lip relationship

The relationship of the lips should also be evaluated from the frontal view (Fig. 6.3):

- Competent lips are together at rest;
- Potentially competent lips are apart at rest, but this is due to a physical obstruction, such as the lower lip resting behind the upper incisors; and
- Incompetent lips are apart at rest and require excessive muscular activity to obtain a lip seal.

Lip incompetence is common in preadolescent children and competence increases with age due to vertical growth of the soft tissues, especially in males (Mamandras, 1988).

Incisor show at rest

In adolescents and young adults, 3 to 4-mm of the maxillary incisor should be displayed at rest (Fig. 6.4). In general, females tend to show more upper incisor than males, with

Figure 6.2 The face can be divided into thirds. The upper face extends from the hairline or top of forehead (trichion) to the base of the forehead between the eyebrows (glabellar). The midface extends from the base of the forehead to the base of the nose (subnasale). The lower face extends from the base of the nose to the bottom of the chin (menton). The lower third of the face can be further subdivided into thirds, with the upper lip in the upper one-third and the lower lip in the lower two-thirds.

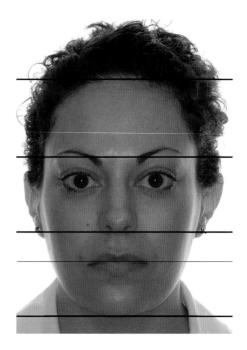

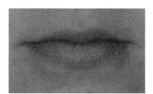 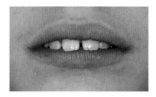 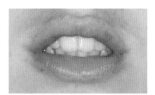

Figure 6.3 Competent (left), potentially competent (middle) and incompetent (right) lips.

the amount of incisor show reducing with age in both sexes. An increased incisor show is usually due to an increase in anterior maxillary dentoalveolar height or vertical maxillary excess. Occasionally it is due to a short upper lip. The average upper lip length is 22-mm in adult males and 20-mm in females.

Incisor show on smiling
Ideally 75 to 100% of the maxillary incisor should be shown when smiling (Fig. 6.4), but this also reduces with age. Some gingival display is acceptable, although excessive show or a 'gummy smile' is considered unattractive (Fig. 6.4).

Smile aesthetics is also an important component of orthodontic treatment planning and should be formally assessed (Box 6.2).

Transverse relationship and symmetry
The transverse proportions of the face should divide approximately into fifths (Fig. 6.5). No face is truly symmetrical; however, any significant facial asymmetry and the level at which it occurs should be noted. This can be done by assessing the patient from

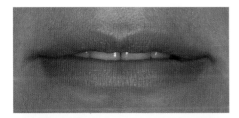

Figure 6.4 Normal upper incisor shown at rest (upper) and on smiling (middle). Increased upper incisor shown on smiling (lower panel).

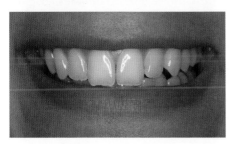

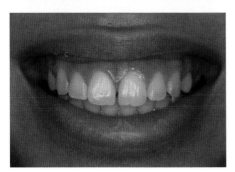

the front and also from behind and above, looking down the face (Fig. 6.6). The relative position of each dental midline to the relevant dental base should be recorded. Asymmetries of the lower face are particularly common in class III malocclusion with mandibular prognathism.

Mandibular asymmetry has been described as primarily of two types (Obwegeser & Makek, 1986):

- Hemimandibular hyperplasia—characterized by three-dimensional enlargement of the mandible, which terminates at the symphysis. There is an increase in height on the affected side, usually accompanied by a marked cant of the occlusal plane. This can be seen by asking the patient to bite onto a wooden tongue spatula.
- Hemimandibular elongation—characterized by a horizontal displacement of the mandible and chin-point towards the unaffected side. There is usually a marked centreline shift and a crossbite on the contralateral side, but no occlusal cant.

Profile view

The facial profile should be assessed anteroposteriorly and vertically.

Box 6.2 Aesthetics of the smile

During examination of an orthodontic patient the soft tissues should be assessed in animation and not just at rest. A key component of this is the smile. Smiling is an important part of communication and an unattractive smile can be a considerable social handicap, often providing a reason to seek treatment. Creating a pleasing smile is therefore a fundamental aim in orthodontics. Three principle characteristics of the smile need to be assessed (Sarver, 2001):

- Incisal and gingival show—the full height of the maxillary incisor crowns should be visible on smiling. Some gingival show is acceptable, but this should not be excessive. Generally, males show less tooth substance and gingiva then females on smiling, and in both groups this reduces with age; therefore, a full smile gives a youthful appearance. In addition, the gingival margins of the maxillary central incisors and canines should be level, with those of the maxillary lateral incisors being around 1-mm more incisal.
- Width—the lips should correctly frame the maxillary dentition with bilateral buccal corridors (the space between the buccal surface of the distal-most maxillary molar and the angle of the mouth on smiling) visible but not excessive. This relationship is affected by both the width of the dental arch and its anteroposterior position. However, excessive orthodontic expansion can result in complete elimination of the buccal corridors and an artifical denture-like smile.
- Relationship of the upper incisor edges with the lower lip—the upper incisor edges should be parallel to the curvature of the lower lip on smiling. This is known as the smile arc. Flattening of the smile arc will result in a less attractive smile, which can also be associated with premature aging.

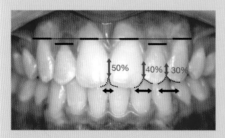 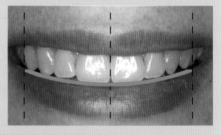

Pleasing gingival aesthetics. The gingival margin of the maxillary central incisors and canines are level, with the lateral incisor margin situated slightly below this. The embrasure spaces between the teeth (dotted lines) increase in size from the maxillary central incisors back. The connector areas (where the teeth appear to meet and indicated by red arrows) should be approximately 50, 40 and 30% of the maxillary central incisor crown length for the maxillary central incisors, central-lateral incisors and lateral incisors-canines, respectively (left panel). The maxillary incisor edges should also lie parallel to the curvature of the lower lip to produce a consonant smile arc (right panel) (Gill et al, 2007).

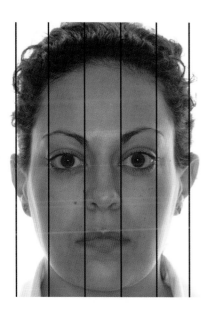

Figure 6.5 Transverse facial proportions should divide approximately into fifths (each one the width of the eye).

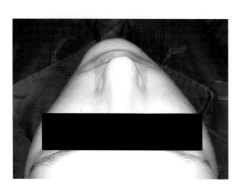

Figure 6.6 Facial asymmetry viewed from above and behind.

Anteroposterior relationship

An assessment should be made of the skeletal dental base relationship between the upper and lower jaws in the anteroposterior plane (Fig. 6.7). This can be achieved by mentally dropping a true vertical line down from the bridge of the nose (often called the zero meridian). The upper lip should rest on or slightly in front of this line and the chin slightly behind. Alternatively, the dental bases can be palpated labially.

- In a normal or skeletal class 1 relationship, the upper jaw should be approximately 2 to 4-mm in front of the lower;
- In a skeletal class 2 relationship the lower jaw is greater than 4-mm behind the upper; and
- In a skeletal class 3 relationship the lower jaw is less than 2-mm behind the upper.
  An assessment can also be made of the angle between the middle and lower third of the face (Fig. 6.7), with the profile being described as:

Class I   Class II   Class III

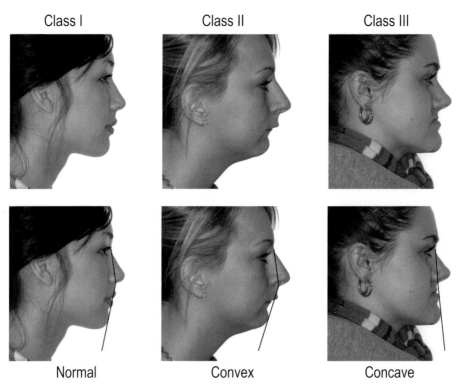

Normal   Convex   Concave

Figure 6.7 Skeletal class I (left), class II (middle) and class III (right) profiles. Facial convexity can also be described in relation to the angle between the upper and lower face.

- Normal or straight;
- Convex; or
- Concave.

Nasolabial angle and lip protrusion

The nasolabial angle is formed between the upper lip and base of the nose (columella) and should be between 90° and 110° (Fig. 6.8). It gives an indication of upper lip drape in relation to the upper incisor position. A high or obtuse nasolabial angle implies a retrusive upper lip, whilst a low or acute angle is associated with lip protrusion.

The lips should be slightly everted at their base, with several millimetres of vermillion show at rest, although they do tend to become more retrusive with age. Protrusion of the lips varies between ethnic groups, with patients of African origin being more protrusive than Caucasians. Lip protrusion is also relative to the size and shape of the chin. Generally, lips are considered too protrusive when both are prominent and incompetent.

Vertical relationship

The face can also be divided into thirds as described earlier and direct measurements made of the facial heights (Fig. 6.9).

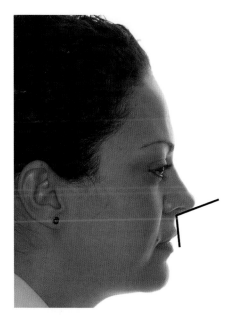

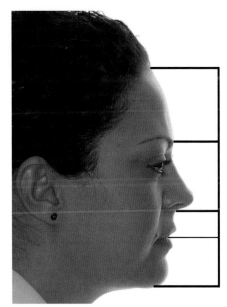

Figure 6.8 Normal nasolabial angle.

Figure 6.9 Facial profile divided into thirds.

The angle of the lower border of the mandible to the cranium should also be assessed. This can be done by placing an index finger along the lower border and approximating where this line points. If it points to the base of the skull around the occipital region, the angle is considered average. If it points below this, the angle is reduced, whilst above it the angle is increased (Fig. 6.10). This usually, but not always, correlates with measurements made of the anterior face height.

Intraoral examination

The intraoral examination is concerned primarily with the teeth in each dental arch, in both isolation and occlusion.

Dental health
The teeth present clinically should be noted and an assessment made of the general dental condition, including the presence of untreated caries, existing restorations and the standard of oral hygiene. Evidence of previous dentoalveolar trauma, such as chipped or discoloured incisor teeth, should also be recorded. Previous trauma will warrant further investigation in the form of vitality testing and radiographs. Other pathological signs, such as erosion or attrition, should also be noted.

Dental arches
Each dental arch is assessed independently, with the mandible usually described first. The following features should be recorded for both arches:

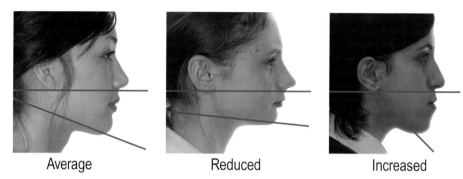

Average   Reduced   Increased

Figure 6.10 Clinical assessment of the vertical facial relationship.

Box 6.3   How is crowding measured?

Crowding represents a discrepancy between the size of the dental arch and the size of the teeth. It is important that the degree of crowding is assessed as accurately as possible. Ideally the mesiodistal widths of the teeth in each dental arch should be measured, added together and compared to the overall size of the arch. During the initial examination this can be done in the patient's mouth using a small metal ruler; however, a more detailed assessment can be made from the dental study casts during treatment planning. An important aspect of this process is deciding upon a suitable dental arch form. A number of ideal arch forms have been suggested in the orthodontic literature, but as a general rule the orthodontist should not attempt to change the existing arch form significantly. Generally it is best to decide on which of the incisors represents the ideal arch form for an individual patient and base the assessment of crowding upon this. It should also be borne in mind that rotations in the labial segments are a manifestation of crowding, whilst in the buccal segments they represent spacing. In general, crowding is usually described as mild (0 to 4-mm), moderate (5 to 8-mm) or severe (greater than 9-mm).

- Presence of crowding or spacing in the labial and buccal segments (Box 6.3) (Fig. 6.11);
- Tooth rotations, described in relation to the most displaced aspect of the coronal edge and the line of the dental arch;
- Tooth displacement in a labial or lingual direction in relation to the line of the arch;
- Position and inclination of the labial segment relative to the dental base. These are described as being average, proclined or retroclined. In the mandibular arch, the incisors should be approximately 90° to the lower border of the mandible. This can be assessed by retracting the lower lip in profile and visualizing the lower incisor inclination in relation to a finger or ruler placed along the lower border of the

Mild crowding   Moderate crowding   Severe crowding

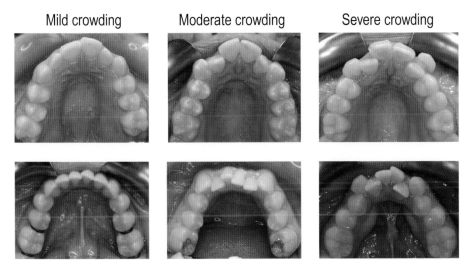

Figure 6.11 Upper and lower dental arch crowding.

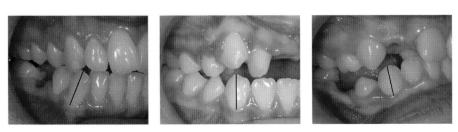

Figure 6.12 Mandibular canine angulation. Mesial (left); upright (middle); distal (right).

mandible. In the maxilla, the incisors should be approximately 110° to the maxillary plane, but this can be more difficult to assess clinically. Alternatively, the labial face of the maxillary incisors should be roughly parallel to the true vertical or zero meridian;

- Presence and position of the maxillary canines, which should be palpable buccally from the age of 10 years;
- Angulation of erupted canines, which should be recorded as mesial, upright or distal (Fig. 6.12); and
- Depth of the curve of Spee, which is described as normal, increased or decreased (Fig. 6.13). This will have a direct bearing on space requirements as an increased curve of Spee is a manifestation of crowding in the vertical plane and, as such, will require space to correct.

Static occlusion
When each dental arch has been assessed the patient is asked to occlude in intercuspal position (ICP) and the static occlusal relationship is recorded.

Figure 6.13 The normal occlusal plane of the maxillary and mandibular dental arches follows a curve in the anteroposterior plane, producing the curve of Spee. Any significant increase or decrease of the curve along either occlusal plane can influence the vertical dental relationship.

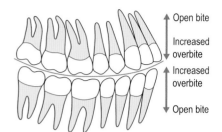

Open bite

Increased overbite

Increased overbite

Open bite

Incisor relationship

The incisor relationship is described using the British Standards Classification, but also needs to be supplemented with a description of the overjet and overbite.

Overjet

The overjet should be measured from the labial surface of the most prominent maxillary incisor to the labial surface of the mandibular incisors (Fig. 6.14). The normal range is 2 to 4-mm. If there is a reverse overjet, as can occur in a class III incisor relationship, this is also measured and given a negative value.

Overbite

The normal range is for the maxillary incisors to overlap the mandibular by 2 to 4-mm vertically, or one-third to one-half of their crown height (Fig. 6.15). Overbite is described as:

- Increased if the maxillary incisors overlap the mandibular incisor crowns vertically by greater than one-half of the lower incisor crown height;
- Decreased if the maxillary incisors overlap the mandibular incisors by less than one-third of the lower incisor crown height. If there is no vertical overlap between the anterior teeth, this is described as an anterior open bite and a measurement should be made of the incisor separation;
- Complete if there is contact between incisors, or the incisors and opposing mucosa; and
- Incomplete if there is no contact between incisors, or the incisors and opposing mucosa.

If the overbite is complete to the gingival tissues, it is described as traumatic if there is evidence of damage. This is most commonly seen on the palatal aspect of the upper incisors or labial aspect of the lower (Fig. 6.16).

Anterior crossbite

Teeth in anterior crossbite should also be noted along with the presence and size of any displacement of the mandible that may occur when closing in the retruded contact position (RCP) into the intercuspal position (ICP) (Fig. 6.17). An anterior crossbite with displacement can cause labial gingival recession associated with the lower incisors in traumatic occlusion, which if present, should be recorded.

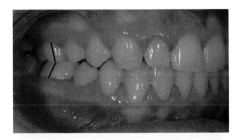

Figure 6.14 Occlusal variation. Class I occlusion; reduced overjet associated with a class II division 2 incisor relationship (the buccal segment relationship is half a unit class II); increased overjet associated with a class II division 1 incisor relationship (the buccal segment relationship is a full unit class II); reverse overjet associated with a class III incisor relationship.

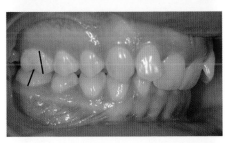

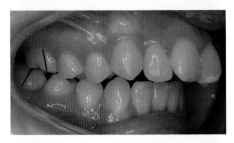

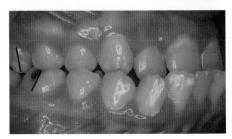

Centrelines

Maxillary and mandibular dental centrelines are assessed in relation to the facial midline and to each other. Displacement of a centreline can be due to:

- Asymmetric dental crowding (Fig. 6.18);
- Buccal crossbite with a mandibular displacement on closing (Fig. 6.19); and
- Skeletal asymmetry of the jaws (Fig. 6.20).

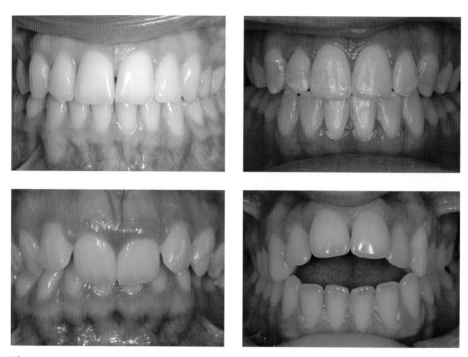

Figure 6.15 Variation in overbite. Normal (upper left), reduced (upper right), increased (lower left) and anterior open bite (lower right).

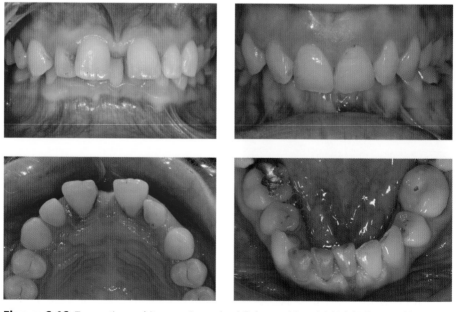

Figure 6.16 Traumatic overbites causing palatal (left panels) and labial (right panels) gingival trauma.

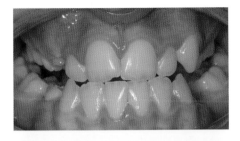

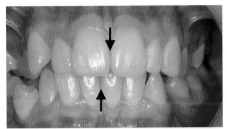

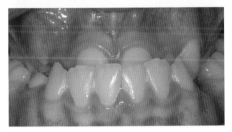

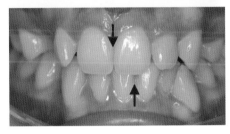

Figure 6.17 Anterior crossbite with a forward mandibular displacement on closing, which worsens the class III incisor relationship.

Figure 6.18 Centreline discrepancies due to asymmetric crowding.

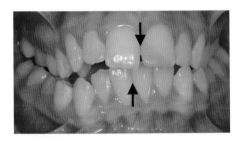

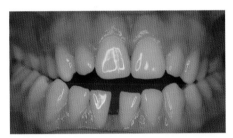

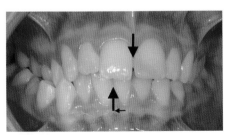

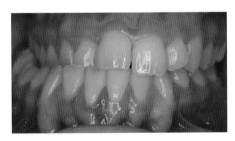

Figure 6.19 Lower-centreline displacement to the right, secondary to a mandibular buccal crossbite associated with a mandibular displacement to the right.

Figure 6.20 Skeletal asymmetries of the mandible producing centreline discrepancies to the right.

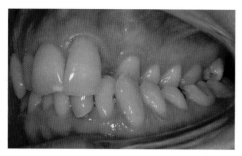

Figure 6.21 Mandibular buccal crossbite.

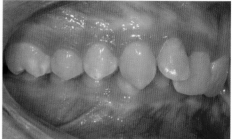

Figure 6.22 Mandibular lingual crossbite.

Buccal segments
The buccal segment relationship is described using the Angle classification (see Chapter 1). The molar and canine relationships should also be noted (see Fig. 6.14).

Posterior crossbite
The transverse relationship of the dental arches is described in occlusion. Crossbites are described in relation to the arch, whether they are localized or affect the whole segment of the dentition and if they occur uni- or bilaterally:
- A mandibular buccal crossbite exists when the buccal cusps of the mandibular dentition occlude buccally to the buccal cusps of the maxillary dentition (Fig. 6.21);
- A mandibular lingual crossbite exists when the buccal cusps of the mandibular dentition occlude lingually to the palatal cusps of the maxillary dentition (this can also be referred to as a scissors bite) (Fig. 6.22);
- A unilateral crossbite affects one side of the dental arch; and
- A bilateral crossbite affects both sides of the dental arch.

Teeth in crossbite should be recorded and any associated displacement of the mandible on closing from RCP to ICP. This can be achieved by ensuring the mandible is fully retruded by placing gentle pressure on the chin and asking the patient to put the tip of their tongue up towards the soft palate until initial occlusal contact is made on closing.

Functional occlusion
Any discrepancy between RCP and ICP should be recorded. The patient should also be asked to slide from ICP to the left and right, and the following should be detailed for each lateral excursion:
- Canine guidance or group function; and
- Non-working side interferences.

The patient should also be asked to slide the mandible forwards to check for disclusion of the posterior teeth.

Temporomandibular joint
The patient should be questioned about and examined for any signs and symptoms associated with both temporomandibular joints. These include:

- Clicking;
- Crepitus (a grinding noise or sensation within the joint);
- Pain (muscular and neurological); and
- Locking or limited opening.

Although some occlusal traits have a weak correlation with temporomandibular dysfunction, orthodontic treatment should be regarded as being neutral in relation to this condition. Treating a malocclusion is unlikely to have any long-term effect on symptoms, either positive or negative. However, a baseline record of temporomandibular joint health should be taken and any signs or symptoms should be recorded. If these represent the main complaint, they should be investigated further and managed before orthodontic treatment is considered.

Orthodontic records

Clinical orthodontic records are used primarily for diagnosis, monitoring of growth and development, and are a medico-legal requirement. They provide an accurate representation of the patient prior to orthodontic treatment, demonstrate treatment progress and allow communication between orthodontists, other healthcare professionals and the patient. Records also play an important role in research and clinical audit. It is essential that accurate clinical records are taken before commencing orthodontic treatment.

Study models
Impressions showing all the erupted teeth, full depth of the palate and good soft tissue extension are needed. These can be taken in alginate for study models and poured in dental stone (Fig. 6.23). A wax or polysiloxane bite should be taken with the teeth in ICP (Box 6.4). Orthodontic models should be trimmed with the occlusal plane parallel to the bases, so the teeth are in occlusion when the models are placed on their back. The bases are also trimmed symmetrically so the archform can be assessed and they are neat enough to be used for demonstration to the patient.

Box 6.4   Should articulated study models be used for orthodontic diagnosis?

The use of articulated study models has been advocated as a potential aid to orthodontic diagnosis and treatment planning. There is often a discrepancy between the occlusal relation in RCP and the full or habitual occlusion in ICP. Whilst a small shift is very common and not generally considered to be clinically important, larger shifts have been considered potentially damaging for both periodontal and temporomandibular joint health, although there is little substantial evidence for this. Small shifts can only be detected by articulating study models, but if these are unimportant, the value of articulation in most cases remains unproven (Ellis & Benson, 2003).

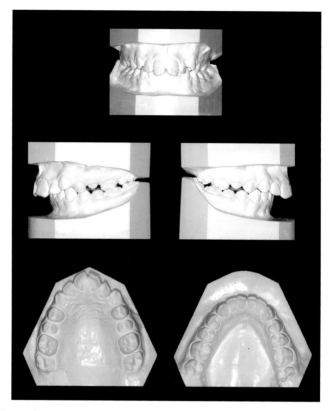

Figure 6.23 Angle trimmed cast stone orthodontic study models.

Accurate digital study casts are also now available, which have the advantages of occupying no physical storage space and having no deterioration over time, enabling indefinite storage (Fig. 6.24) (Santoro et al, 2003).

Clinical photographs

Good clinical photographs form an essential part of the clinical record. They provide a baseline record of the presenting malocclusion, are important in treatment planning especially in relation to facial and dental aesthetics, allow monitoring of treatment progress and are useful for teaching. The following views should be taken:

- Intraoral, taken with the occlusal plane horizontal:
  - Frontal occlusion;
  - Buccal occlusion (left and right);
  - Maxillary dentition; and
  - Mandibular dentition.
- Extraoral, taken against neutral background in natural head posture:
  - Full facial frontal;
  - Full facial frontal smiling;

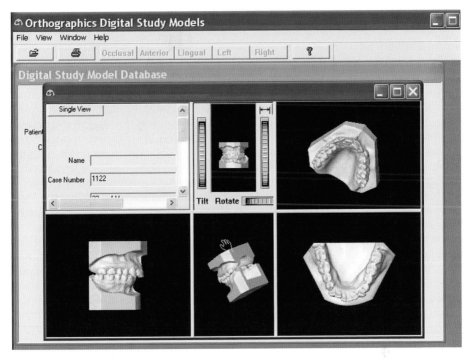

Figure 6.24 Digital orthodontic study models.

- Facial three-quarters; and
- Facial profile.

Radiographs

Radiographs are usually required prior to orthodontic treatment to assess:
- Presence or absence of permanent teeth;
- Root morphology of permanent teeth;
- Presence and extent of dental disease;
- Presence of supernumerary teeth;
- Position of ectopic teeth; and
- Relationship of the dentition to the dental bases and their relationship to the cranial base.

Radiation protection

Currently in the UK, the medical use of ionizing radiation is covered by two articles of legislation, which have been in force since 2000. The Ionising Radiation Regulations (1999) are concerned primarily with the safety of workers and members of the general public; whilst the Ionising Radiation (Medical Exposure) Regulations (2000) relate to the safety and protection of the patient. This legislation is based on the three basic principles of the International Commission for Radiological Protection (ICRP) that provide the foundation for all radiation protection measures:

- Justification;
- Optimization; and
- Limitation.

The dental practitioner is responsible for justifying the exposure of a patient to ionizing radiation and this should be based upon a defined clinical need. Once an exposure is clinically justified it should be optimized, keeping the dose as low as reasonably practicable (the ALARP principle) and maximizing the risk–benefit ratio to the patient. The main elements of this relate to the type of equipment and image receptor being used and to the use of selection criteria—the number, type and frequency of radiographs requested. Practical recommendations include using high kV equipment, fast speed film, rare earth intensifying screens or switching to digital radiography and collimating the size of the beam to the area of interest. Each view carries an estimated effective dose of radiation (Table 6.1). The effective dose for all diagnostic medical procedures is a converted whole body measurement, which takes into account the varying sensitivity of different organs and tissues to radiation and is usually measured using the Sievert (Sv) or micro-Sievert (µSv) subunit. The effective annual natural exposure to background radiation is approximately 2400 µSv and it is often easier to think of any further exposure in relation to this. To place the risks of dental radiographic exposure in context, a long haul flight to Singapore would result in an additional effective radiation dose of approximately 30 µSv, around 10 times that of a cephalometric lateral skull radiograph.

Comprehensive guidelines on how all these principles can be achieved in general dental and orthodontic practice have been published (Faculty of General Dental Practitioners UK, 2004; Isaacson et al, 2008). The fundamental principle, however, is that radiographs are only taken when clinically justified.

Table 6.1 Radiographs used in orthodontics and dose equivalence

Radiographic examination	Effective radiation dose (µSv)	Equivalent background radiation (days)	Risk of fatal cancer (per million)
DPT	3–30	0.5–5	0.2–1.9
Cephalometric lateral skull	2–3	0.3–0.45	0.34
Upper standard occlusal	8	1.2	0.4
Bitewing/periapical	1–10	0.15–0.27	0.02–0.6
CT scan (maxilla)	100–3000	15–455	8–242
CT scan (mandible)	350–1200	53–182	18–88
Chest	20	3	2

These figures are based upon Radiation Protection 136: European guidelines on radiation protection in dental radiology. The safe use of radiographs in dental practice (2004) European Commission. It should be emphasized that these only represent a guide and are regularly updated as new recommendations are made, particularly with regard to tissue weighting factors in the calculation of effective doses. CT = computerized tomography; DPT = dental panoramic tomograph.

Routine radiographs used in orthodontic assessment
A number of radiographic views are routinely used by the orthodontist:

Dental panoramic tomograph
Panoramic radiography or, more specifically, the dental panoramic tomograph (DPT) provides a useful screen for the presence or absence, position and general health of the teeth and their supporting structures with a relatively low-radiation dose. Because these radiographs are sectional in nature, they can be unclear in some regions, particularly the labial segments where variations in the depth of the anterior focal trough for different patients can influence clarity of the incisors.

Occlusal radiographs
Occlusal radiographs are taken with the film placed on the occlusal plane and can offer greater detail in the labial segments. They are particularly useful in the maxillary arch, for assessing root form of the incisors, the presence of midline supernumerary teeth and canine position, either alone or in combination with additional views using parallax.

Periapical radiographs
Periapical radiographs are also useful for the assessment of local pathology, root form and the presence or position of unerupted teeth. They can also be used for parallax, particularly in identifying the position of maxillary canine teeth. Either two periapicals are taken, incorporating a horizontal tube shift between them; or a single periapical is taken in conjunction with another radiographic view, such as an upper standard occlusal or DPT and a vertical tube shift utilized.

Bitewing radiographs
Bitewings are useful for the accurate detection of caries, the assessment of existing restorations and periodontal status.

Cephalometric lateral skull radiograph
A cephalometric lateral skull radiograph is a specialized view of the facial skeleton and cranial base from the lateral aspect, with the head position at a specific distance from the film. The uses and analysis of cephalometric radiographs are discussed in the next section.

When to take radiographs
The need for radiographic investigation will vary according to the age of the patient and their stage of dental development, in addition to the clinical presentation. Comprehensive guidelines regarding the need for orthodontic radiographic investigation are available (Isaacson et al, 2008).

Deciduous dentition
Radiographs are not routinely indicated in the preschool child. Indications include:
- Trauma to the upper labial segment for assessing potential risk to the permanent successors; and
- Dental caries for assessing both the extent and prognosis.

Mixed dentition

Radiographic investigation during the mixed dentition is indicated with evidence of dental disease or abnormal dental development. Specific orthodontic indications include:

- Asymmetric eruption pattern of the permanent dentition and significant retention of deciduous teeth. Failure of eruption associated with the maxillary incisors requires radiographic examination, as this can be due to the presence of supernumerary teeth. Similarly, maxillary canines should be palpable in the buccal sulcus by 10 years of age. If not, radiographic examination for detecting the presence of palatal impaction is indicated;
- Prior to any interceptive treatment, including extractions, particularly optimal timing for loss of first permanent molars with poor prognosis;
- Early treatment of class II malocclusion; and
- Early treatment of class III malocclusion.

Permanent dentition

Radiographic investigation is indicated prior to active orthodontic tooth movement for assessing dental health and root form. This will usually consist of a panoramic view supplemented with an anterior occlusal if the incisor region is unclear, or bimolar views plus an anterior occlusal. A cephalometric lateral skull radiograph is indicated as an aid to treatment planning in the presence of a skeletal discrepancy, or when treatment is being planned in both dental arches that involves extractions and bodily movement of incisors.

Three-dimensional imaging

Plain film and cephalometric radiography are invaluable for accurate diagnosis and treatment planning, but they only provide a two-dimensional image of a three-dimensional structure, with all the associated errors of projection, landmark identification, measurement and interpretation. A number of three-dimensional imaging techniques have been developed over the past decade, which help to overcome some of these shortcomings and give the orthodontist greater information for diagnosis, treatment planning and research (Box 6.5).

Imaging of the hard tissues composing the jaws and dentition using computed tomography (CT) had remained impractical until relatively recently, due to the high radiation dosage, lack of vertical resolution and cost. However, with the introduction of cone-beam computed tomography (CBCT), doses have been reduced and resolution increased, and although not yet used for routine orthodontic diagnosis, this technique is proving a very valuable tool in certain circumstances, particularly the diagnosis of impacted and ectopic teeth. It can also be very useful in airway analysis, assessment of alveolar bone height and volume prior to implant placement and imaging of temporomandibular joint morphology (Merrett et al, 2009).

Other less invasive techniques for generating three-dimensional images of the facial soft tissues have also been developed. Optical laser scanning utilizes a laser beam, which is captured by a video camera at a set distance from the laser and produces a three-dimensional image. Stereo photogrammetry involves taking two pictures of the facial region simultaneously, which creates a three-dimensional model image using

Box 6.5 Three-dimensional imaging in orthodontics

CBCT images of an impacted maxillary canine causing resorption of the central incisor (top). Soft tissue laser scan shows soft tissue facial changes following orthodontic treatment. Colours show areas of change from two superimposed scans (bottom).

The use of CBCT for exact localization of ectopic teeth, including maxillary canines has revealed much higher levels of root resorption associated with adjacent teeth than previously diagnosed from plain film radiography. Optical laser scanning offers the potential to image soft tissue changes in a safe, non-invasive and simple manner.

sophisticated stereo triangulation algorithms. These techniques have been used to study facial growth and soft tissue changes in normal populations and following orthodontic and surgical treatment.

Cephalometric radiography

Cephalometric radiography is a specialized radiographic technique concerned with imaging the craniofacial region in a standardized and reproducible manner. A cephalometric analysis identifies defined anatomical landmarks on the film and measures the angular and linear relationships between them. This numerical assessment can provide detailed information on the relationship of skeletal, dental and soft tissue elements within the craniofacial region.

Cephalometric analysis

Cephalometric analysis relies upon the production of a standardized lateral or (less commonly) posteroanterior head film. This is achieved by using a cephalostat, which holds the mid-sagittal plane of the head at a fixed distance from both the X-ray source and film, keeping the magnification constant for every radiograph (Fig. 6.25). For a cephalometric lateral skull radiograph, the mid-sagittal plane is orientated perpendicular to the X-ray beam and parallel to the film, whilst a posteroanterior film requires the mid-sagittal plane to be parallel to the X-ray beam and

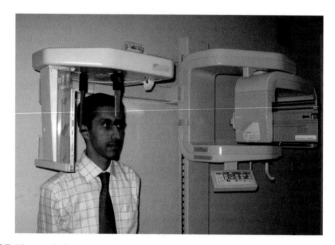

Figure 6.25 The cephalostat consists of ear rods to stabilize the position of the head, an aluminium wedge filter to reduce the intensity of X-rays that have passed through the soft tissues (and therefore improve their visibility on the film) and a film cassette holder. The X-ray source is at a fixed distance from the cephalostat and film. In addition, the beam is collimated to reduce irradiation by exposing only those structures of interest to the orthodontist, the cranial base, facial skeleton and jaws.

perpendicular to the film. Subjects are usually orientated in natural head posture or with the Frankfort plane horizontal and teeth in RCP. Because cephalometric films are reproducible, longitudinal views of the same subject or views of different subjects can be compared with one another. However, all machines produce some magnification of the image and this can vary. For accurate comparison of linear values between radiographs taken on different machines, the in-built magnification needs to be known.

Uses of cephalometrics
Cephalometric analysis can provide the orthodontist with much useful clinical information. Conventionally, this usually involves a lateral skull radiograph, but a posteroanterior film can also be useful, particularly in the diagnosis of facial asymmetry and in aiding visualization of impacted teeth. The taking of any cephalometric radiograph is not justified in all cases, particularly if only minor tooth movements are planned. A cephalometric analysis should supplement a thorough clinical examination and not attempt to replace it.

Diagnosis and treatment planning
Information on the relationship of the jaws and dentition in both the anteroposterior and vertical planes of space and their relationship with the soft tissue profile is an important factor in orthodontic diagnosis and treatment planning. A detailed analysis of the dentoskeletal relationship aids in treatment planning and determining the appropriate treatment approach.

Treatment decisions should be made with the use of a prognostic tracing; whereby planned tooth and jaw movements can be simulated on a radiograph and both the effects and feasibility of such movements studied in detail. A cephalometric radiograph can also provide information regarding:
- The position of unerupted and impacted teeth;
- The presence of pathology; and
- The size and morphology of the airway.

Monitoring treatment progress
A cephalometric radiograph taken during orthodontic therapy can provide information on how treatment is progressing. This allows the orthodontist to evaluate skeletal, dental and soft tissue relationships and assess what further changes will be required to produce an aesthetic and stable result. This is particularly useful for analysing the labiolingual position of the lower incisors. A cephalometric lateral skull radiograph is also essential prior to planning surgical movement of the jaws.

Research
The cephalometric analysis of head films derived from a number of human populations has provided normal average values (and standard deviations) for a variety of skeletal, dentoalveolar and soft tissue relationships, which are useful for orthodontic diagnosis and treatment planning (Table 6.2).

In addition, the serial comparison of films derived from both cross-sectional and longitudinal growth studies has produced important data on:
- The quantity and pattern of craniofacial growth in different populations; and
- Individual variation associated with human craniofacial growth.

Table 6.2 Cephalometric normal values for different racial groups

Cephalometric value	Caucasian[a]	African-American[b]	Arabic[c]	Japanese[d]
SNA	81 ± 3	87 ± 5	81 ± 4	82 ± 3
SNB	78 ± 3	82 ± 4	78 ± 3	79 ± 3
ANB	3 ± 2	5 ± 2	3 ± 2	3 ± 2
MMPA	27 ± 5	No value	25 ± 5	22 ± 4
UI Mx	109 ± 6	119 ± 8	111 ± 7	No value
LI Md	93 ± 6	99 ± 9	96 ± 5	95 ± 7

Values are given in degrees. SNA = angle SN (sella-nasion) to point A; SNB = angle SN to point B; ANB = difference between angles SNA and SNB; MMPA = maxillary–mandibular plane angle; UI Mx = upper incisor–maxillary plane angle; LI Md = lower incisor–mandibular plane angle.
[a] Ballard (1956).
[b] Beane et al (2003).
[c] Hamdan & Rock (2001).
[d] Mijajima et al (1996).

Cephalometric analysis also forms the basis of evaluating the effects of orthodontic treatment and is still the principle method for measuring treatment response in clinical studies.

Growth prediction

A number of workers have suggested that certain discreet features can be identified on a cephalometric lateral skull radiograph and used to predict the pattern of future jaw growth. There is little substantial evidence for this and the taking of such radiographs on the basis of growth prediction alone cannot be justified. A more accurate assessment of growth can be made from serial lateral skull radiographs taken approximately one year apart. These can be especially useful in those patients who present with a class III malocclusion; treatment decisions are delayed until the direction and extent of the growth discrepancy between the jaws can be determined.

Tracing a lateral skull cephalometric radiograph

A lateral skull radiograph should be hand-traced in a darkened room with suitable back illumination using a hard pencil and high-quality tracing paper attached to the radiograph. The peripheral regions of the radiograph should be masked to highlight the cranial base and facial complex. Bilateral structures should be traced independently and then averaged. Alternatively, the landmarks and tracing can be digitized directly into a computer using specialized software, which will instantly produce an analysis (see Fig. 12.11). A simple tracing and landmark identification is shown in Fig. 6.26.

Horizontal reference planes

A number of horizontal planes are commonly used as references in the construction of other measurements or they are related to each other within a cephalometric analysis (Fig. 6.27). In particular, they are used in the evaluation of skeletal relationships and the anteroposterior position of the dentition.

Frankfort horizontal plane

The Frankfort plane is a horizontal reference constructed as a line through porion to orbitale (Figs 6.27 and 6.28), which can be used both clinically and cephalometrically to orientate the head. It was first described at the Frankfort Congress of Anthropology in 1884 and was originally used for the orientation and comparison of dry skulls. The defining landmarks are easily located on a skull or subject in the clinic; however, several disadvantages are associated with the Frankfort horizontal as a cephalometric reference plane:

- Porion and orbitale are both difficult to locate on a cephalometric head film;
- Porion and orbitale are bilateral structures, which frequently do not coincide and therefore must be averaged; and
- The Frankfort horizontal does not lie in the mid-sagittal plane of the skull and can therefore be influenced significantly if the head is not correctly positioned in the cephalostat.

However, the Frankfort horizontal is one of the few reference planes that can be identified both clinically and on a radiograph, and it is used as the principle plane of reference in a number of cephalometric analyses.

Sella-nasion plane

The sella-nasion (SN) plane is constructed as a line extending from sella to nasion and represents the anteroposterior extent of the anterior cranial base (Fig. 6.27). It is commonly used as a reference plane because of its reliability:

- Sella and nasion are relatively easy to locate on a lateral skull radiograph; and
- Both these points lie in the mid-sagittal plane of the skull and are therefore under less influence of distortion if skull position deviates from the true vertical.

The SN reference plane is used principally:

- When relating the jaws to the anterior cranial base; and
- When superimposing serial lateral skull radiographs.

It should be remembered that nasion is not actually part of the anterior cranial base and can be subject to both vertical and horizontal growth changes, which can affect the accuracy of this plane (see Box 3.1).

Maxillary plane

The maxillary plane is constructed using a line connecting the anterior and posterior nasal spines, and serves as a horizontal reference for the maxilla (Fig. 6.27). It is useful for assessing:

- Vertical jaw relationship:
  - Maxilla to Frankfort plane;
  - Maxilla to SN plane; and
  - Maxilla to mandible.
- Inclination of the upper incisors to the maxillary skeletal base.

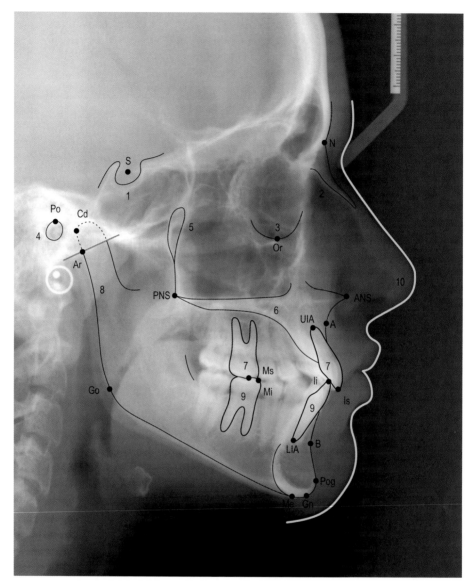

Figure 6.26 A simple cephalometric analysis can be achieved by identifying and tracing the following regions:

(1)   The pituitary fossa, extended to the anterior and posterior clinoid processes.
(2)   The external contour of the frontal bone past the frontonasal suture and down to include the nasal bone.
(3)   The lateral border and floor of the orbits.
(4)   The external auditory meatus.
(5)   The pterygomaxillary fissure, extending inferiorly to a point at the posterior nasal spine.

Figure 6.26 cont'd

(6)   From the posterior nasal spine, along the floor of the nasal cavity and then down along the anterior outline of the maxilla through the anterior nasal spine and down to the intersection of the alveolar crest with the most prominent maxillary incisor. This line is then continued along the outline of the palatal vault from the alveolar crest to the posterior nasal spine.

(7)   The outline of the most prominent maxillary incisor and the maxillary first molars.

(8)   The outline of the mandible, beginning from a point at the intersection of the alveolar crest with the most prominent mandibular incisor, moving down the anterior border of the symphysis and along the lower border, around the angle and up the ascending ramus to incorporate the condyle, notch and coronoid process, then moving down the ramus to the cervical margin of the most distal mandibular molar. In addition, the internal outline of the symphysis should also be traced.

(9)   The outline of the most prominent mandibular incisor and the mandibular first molars.

(10) The soft tissue profile, extending from the frontal region down around the nose, upper lip, lower lip, submental region and chin.

The following landmarks should also be identified:

Sella (S): the midpoint of the sella turcica (pituitary fossa).

Nasion (N): the most anterior point on the frontonasal suture in the midline.

Porion (Po): the upper- and outer-most point on the external auditory meatus.

Orbitale (Or): the most inferior and anterior point on the orbital margin.

Condylion (Cd): the most posterior and superior point on the mandibular condyle.

Articulare (Ar): the point of intersection of the posterior margin of the ascending mandibular ramus and the outer margin of the posterior cranial base.

Gnathion (Gn): the most anterior and inferior point on the bony chin.

Menton (Me): the most inferior point of the mandibular symphysis in the midline.

Pogonion (Pog): the most anterior point on the bony chin.

Gonion (Go): the most posterior and inferior point on the angle of the mandible.

Point A (Subspinale): The deepest point on the curved profile of the maxilla between the anterior nasal spine and alveolar crest.

Point B (Supramentale): the deepest point on the curved profile of the mandible between the chin and alveolar crest.

Anterior nasal spine (ANS): the tip of the bony anterior nasal spine in the midline.

Posterior nasal spine (PNS): the tip of the posterior nasal spine in the midline (located as a continuation of the base of the pterygopalatine fossa where it intersects with the nasal floor).

Incisor superius (Is): tip of the crown of the most anterior maxillary central incisor.

Upper incisor apex (UIA): root apex of the most anterior maxillary central incisor.

Incisor inferius (Ii): tip of the crown of the most anterior mandibular central incisor.

Lower incisor apex (LIA): root apex of the most anterior mandibular central incisor.

Molar superioris (Ms): the mesial cusp tip of the maxillary first molar.

Molar inferioris (Mi): the mesial cusp tip of the mandibular first molar.

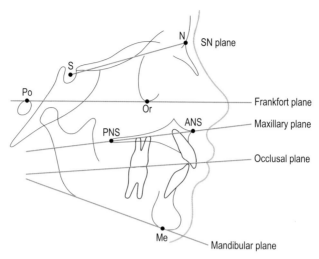

Figure 6.27 Horizontal reference planes.

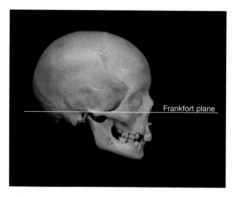

Figure 6.28 Frankfort plane.

Occlusal plane

- The occlusal plane is constructed using a line connecting the tip of the lower incisor edges to the midpoint between the upper and lower first permanent molar cusps (Fig. 6.27).
- The functional occlusal plane is a line constructed through the point of maximal cuspal interdigitation of the premolars or deciduous molars and first permanent molars.

A problem with both of these planes is the significant error associated with their construction.

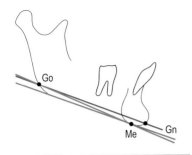

Figure 6.29 Methods of constructing the mandibular plane:
- As a line tangent to the lower border of the mandible and menton;
- As a line constructed from gonion to gnathion; and
- As a line constructed from gonion to menton.

(1) Tangent to lower border – Menton (red)
(2) Gonion – Gnathion (blue)
(3) Gonion – Menton (green)

Mandibular plane
The mandibular plane serves as a horizontal reference line for the mandible and can be constructed using several methods (Fig. 6.29). The mandibular plane is useful for assessing:
- Vertical jaw relationship:
  - Mandible to Frankfort plane;
  - Mandible to SN plane; and
  - Mandible to maxilla.
- Inclination of the lower incisors to the mandibular skeletal base.

Assessing the anteroposterior skeletal relationship
A number of methods for assessing the anteroposterior jaw relationship have been proposed.

The ANB angle
This method was first described as part of a cephalometric analysis proposed by Richard Riedel and relates the maxilla and mandible to the anterior cranial base (Riedel, 1952). The SN plane represents the anterior cranial base, whilst points A and B represent the anterior surfaces of the maxillary and mandibular apical bases, respectively (Fig. 6.30):
- The anteroposterior position of the maxilla is calculated by measuring the angle SN to point A (SNA) (81° ± 3°); and
- The anteroposterior position of the mandible is calculated by measuring the angle SN to point B (SNB) (78° ± 3°);
- The relative difference in the anteroposterior relationship of the maxilla and mandible is measured by the difference between the SNA and SNB angles, or ANB angle (3° ± 2°).

The ANB angle provides a relatively simple and commonly used assessment of anteroposterior jaw relations (Table 6.3). However, it is not beyond criticism:
- Both points A and B are used primarily because they are relatively easy to identify on a cephalometric radiograph. In reality they do not represent the true anterior

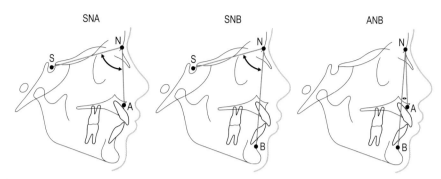

Figure 6.30 SNA, SNB and ANB angles.

Table 6.3 Classification of anteroposterior skeletal pattern using the ANB angle

Skeletal class	ANB angle
Class I	2–4°
Class II	> 4°
Class III	< 2°

extent of the skeletal bases and their positions can alter as a result of alveolar bone remodelling that occurs during orthodontic movement of the upper and lower incisor teeth.

● Variations in the position of the anterior cranial base can also affect interpretation of the jaw position using this method, a point discussed by Richard Mills as part of the Eastman cephalometric analysis.

Mills' Eastman correction
A potential problem of relating the maxilla and mandible to each other using the anterior cranial base is that any significant deviation in the position of this region within the skull will potentially affect interpretation of the jaw relationship (Fig. 6.31). Variation in the position of nasion can alter the SNA value. For example, the more anterior or superior the position of nasion, the lower the value of SNA, whilst a posterior or inferior position will produce a corresponding increase in SNA. Alterations in the value of SNA will, in turn, influence ANB and therefore estimation of the skeletal pattern. Mills introduced a correction for erroneous values of SNA (Mills, 1970):

● For every degree SNA is greater than 81 subtract 0.5 from the original ANB value; and

● For every degree SNA is less than 81 add 0.5 to the original ANB value.

The vertical position of sella will also influence orientation of the SN line, but unlike variations in the position of nasion, it affects SNA and SNB to the same extent and therefore does not alter ANB. In these circumstances, Mills' correction should not

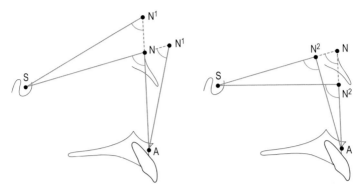

Figure 6.31 Anterior or superior positioning of Nasion (N¹) will reduce the SNA angle, whilst posterior or inferior positioning (N²) will increase the SNA angle. Both these changes will ultimately influence the ANB angle.

be applied. A simple check to ensure that sella is not in an erroneous position can be carried out by measuring the SN–maxillary plane angle, which should be 8° ± 3°.

Because of the problems associated with assessing the jaw relationship using the anterior cranial base, a number of alternative methods that assess the anteroposterior jaw position either in isolation or in relation to other regions of the skull have been described. It is useful to use at least one of these methods in addition to the angle ANB when assessing the skeletal pattern.

Wits appraisal
Alexander Jacobson described the Wits appraisal of jaw disharmony as a simple diagnostic aid that related the anteroposterior jaw relationship in isolation (Wits derives from an abbreviation for University of the Witwatersrand in South Africa where Jacobsen was employed) (Jacobson, 1975, 1976). The appraisal was based upon a sample of 21 adult males and 25 adult females selected on the basis of the excellence of their occlusion (Fig. 6.32).

By relating the maxilla and mandible to each other using the occlusal plane (which is common to both), this method avoids problems associated with relating them to the anterior cranial base, but gives no indication of the jaw position in relation to the face. Wits appraisal is useful as an additional measurement of the jaw relationship and should be used to supplement other methods of assessing the skeletal pattern. The most significant problem with this method is the potential error associated with localizing the occlusal plane.

Ballard's conversion tracing
Clifford Ballard described a simple method for assessing the anteroposterior jaw relationship by using the axial inclination of the incisor teeth (Ballard, 1951). This method removes any potential influence of the soft tissues and dentoalveolar compensation for a skeletal discrepancy by adjusting the inclination of the maxillary and mandibular incisors to their normal value relative to the maxillary and mandibular planes. By then measuring the overjet, a simple analysis of the skeletal pattern is achieved (Fig. 6.33):

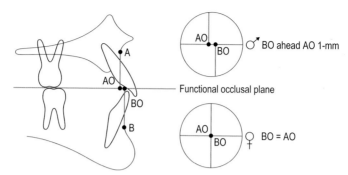

Figure 6.32 Wits method. Perpendicular lines are dropped from A and B points to the functional occlusal plane. For males BO should lie 1-mm ahead of AO, whilst for females AO and BO should coincide. In a skeletal class II AO lies ahead of BO, whilst in a class III discrepancy BO is significantly ahead of AO.

The validity of Ballard's method depends upon the premises that:
- The incisors bear a constant relationship to the jaw position;
- There is an average inclination of the incisors to the dental bases; and
- The incisors will always tip around a defined fulcrum.

As none of these premises are necessarily true, disagreement exists as to the validity of this technique (Bhatia & Akpabio, 1979; Houston, 1975).

Assessing the vertical skeletal relationship
The vertical jaw relationship can also be assessed in a number of ways (Fig. 6.34):

Maxillary–mandibular plane angle (MMPA)
The MMPA is a common method for evaluating the vertical jaw relationship, with horizontal reference planes that are easily located. The mean value is 27° ± 5°.

Frankfort–mandibular plane angle (FMPA)
The FMPA uses the Frankfort plane as a horizontal reference to the mandibular plane. This method ignores the maxillary plane, which if affected by a significant cant can give a misleading value to the vertical jaw relationship. It is useful to use this measurement in conjunction with the MMPA plane angle. The mean value is 27° ± 5°.

Anterior and posterior face heights
Anterior and posterior face heights are also used as a measure of vertical facial relationships (Fig. 6.35):
- Total anterior face height (TAFH) extends from nasion to menton, with both lines constructed perpendicular to the maxillary plane (mean 119-mm in an adult male). TAFH is further subdivided into:
  - Upper anterior face height (UAFH); nasion to maxillary plane (mean 54-mm);
  - Lower anterior face height (LAFH); maxillary plane to menton (mean 65-mm); and
  - The LAFH should be approximately 55% of the TAFH.

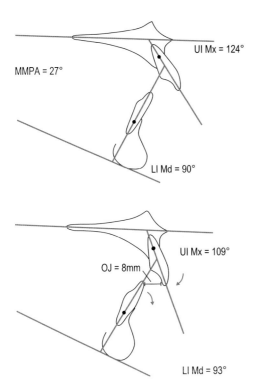

MMPA = 27°

UI Mx = 124°

LI Md = 90°

UI Mx = 109°

OJ = 8mm

LI Md = 93°

Figure 6.33 Ballard's conversion tracing. In the upper tracing, the UI to maxillary plane angle is 124°, whilst the LI to mandibular plane is 90°. The normal values should be 109° and 93°, respectively (the lower incisor to mandibular plane value is calculated by subtracting the MMPA from 120°). By adjusting these teeth to their normal values around a fulcrum approximately one-third of the root length from the apices, it can be seen that the overjet is still increased and therefore the skeletal pattern is class II.

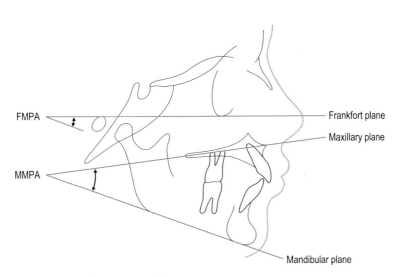

FMPA

MMPA

Frankfort plane

Maxillary plane

Mandibular plane

Figure 6.34 Vertical facial relationships.

Figure 6.35 Face heights.

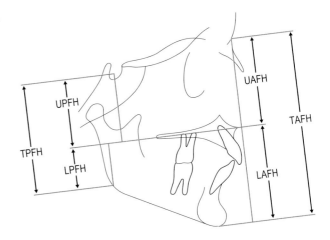

- Total posterior face height (TPFH) extends from sella to gonion, with both lines constructed perpendicular to the maxillary plane (mean 79-mm in an adult male). TPFH is therefore subdivided into:
  - Upper posterior face height (UPFH); sella to maxillary plane (mean 46-mm);
  - Lower posterior face height (LPFH); maxillary plane to gonion (mean 33-mm); and
  - The TPFH should be approximately 65% of the TAFH.

  It should be noted that the TPFH (unlike the TAFH) is influenced by a particularly superior or inferior position of sella and this will affect the TPFH/TAFH ratio. Referring to the SN–maxillary plane angle can check the relative position of sella within the cranium.

Assessing the dental relationship

Several methods of assessment are available for positioning the maxillary and mandibular dentition in relation to the jaws and face.

Maxillary incisor relationship

The inclination of the most prominent maxillary incisor is constructed using a line through UIA–Is and measured in relation to the maxillary plane (Fig. 6.36). The mean value is 109° ± 6°.

Mandibular incisor relationship

The inclination of the most prominent mandibular incisor is constructed using a line through LIA–Ii and measured in relation to the mandibular plane (Fig. 6.36). The mean value is 93° ± 6°; however, mandibular incisor inclination can be influenced by orientation of the mandibular plane. As the mandibular plane becomes steeper, the incisors will tend to retrocline. An alternative method of evaluating the correct mandibular incisor relationship is to subtract the MMPA from 120°.

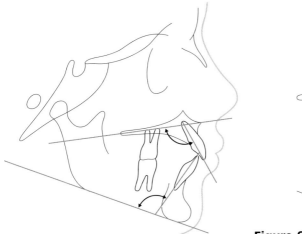

Figure 6.36 Incisor relationships.

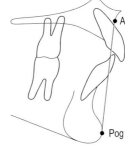

Figure 6.37 Lower incisor to A–Pogonion.

Mandibular incisor position within the face

The position of the mandibular incisors is so fundamental to orthodontic treatment planning that many individual analyses have been described for assessing position of these teeth.

Mandibular incisor to A–Pogonion

Relating the anteroposterior incisor position to a line drawn from point A to pogonion (A–Pog) was originally described in the Downs analysis for the upper incisors. However, it was Robert Ricketts who popularized the use of this line, for positioning the lower incisors within the face. He placed great emphasis on this measurement, suggesting that the lower incisor edge should be approximately 1-mm (±2) ahead of the A–Pog line for optimal facial aesthetics (Fig. 6.37) (Ricketts, 1960). This idea was further developed by Raleigh Williams, who emphasized the importance of this relationship for both aesthetics and long-term stability when planning treatment with the Begg fixed appliance (Williams, 1969). However, whilst this line provides a simple cephalometric assessment of lower incisor position in relation to the jaws, there is no evidence that deliberately positioning the lower incisor edges on the A–Pog line at the end of treatment will produce either improved aesthetics or stability (Park and Burstone, 1986; Houston and Edler, 1990).

Interincisal angle

The angle formed between the most prominent maxillary and mandibular incisors (Fig. 6.38). The mean value is 135° ± 10°.

Cephalometric analyses

The orthodontic literature contains many different cephalometric analyses that have been described by individual clinicians; each providing a detailed description of how

Figure 6.38 Interincisal angle.

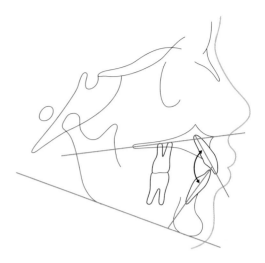

the facial skeleton and dentition should be positioned for maximal aesthetics. The scientific basis for many of these analyses is weak, with the quoted normal values often based upon very small sample sizes. In reality, very few are still used today in their entirety; however, individually they do contain many of the elements applied in modern analysis and it is useful to understand the origins of these measurements. A simple cephalometric analysis is shown in Table 6.4.

Downs analysis

William Downs was one of the first to propose a cephalometric analysis that attempted to describe the basis of facial skeletal pattern in the presence of normal occlusion (Fig. 6.39). His rationale was that if normal pattern and its range of variation could be described, then the abnormal could be judged by comparison (Downs, 1948, 1952, 1956).

Downs based his analysis on a study of 20 Caucasian boys and girls ranging in age from 12 to 17 years and selected on the basis of excellent occlusion and facial harmony. His analysis used the Frankfort plane as a horizontal reference and was subdivided into an assessment of the skeletal and dental patterns:

Skeletal pattern

- The facial angle represents the degree of recession or protrusion of the chin and is the inferior internal angle between the facial plane (N–Pog) and Frankfort plane;
- The angle of convexity is a measure of maxillary protrusion in relation to the total profile and is the angle formed between lines running from N–A to A–Pog. It can be positive or negative, depending on the amount of retrognathia or prognathia, respectively;
- The A–B plane in relation to the facial plane (N–Pog) relates the anterior limit of the dentition to the facial profile;
- FMPA is a measure of the angle between the Frankfort plane and the mandibular plane; and
- The y axis is a measure of the direction of facial growth and is formed by the angle between a line extending from S–Gn to the Frankfort plane.

Table 6.4 A simple cephalometric analysis

SNA	81° (± 3)°
SNB	78° (± 3)°
ANB	3° (± 2)°
SN Mx plane	8° (± 3)°
WITS	BO + 1 mm ahead AO (♂)
	BO = AO (♀)
MMPA	27° (± 5)°
UI Mx plane	109° (± 6)°
LI Md plane	93° (± 6)°
I/I	135° (± 10)°
LI APo	1 (± 2) mm
TAFH	Mean 119 mm
UAFH	Mean 54 mm
LAFH	Mean 65 mm
% LAFH	Mean 55%
NLA	100° (± 8)°
Lip relation to E-line	Upper –4 mm
	Lower –2 mm

SNA = angle SN (sella-nasion) to point A; SNB = angle SN to point B; ANB = difference between angles SNA and SNB; SN Mx plane = SN–maxillary plane angle; MMPA = maxillary–mandibular plane angle; UI Mx plane = upper incisor–maxillary plane angle; LI Md plane = lower incisor–mandibular plane angle; I/I = interincisal angle; LI APo = distance from lower incisor tip to A–Pog line; TAFH = total anterior face height; UAFH = upper anterior face height; LAFH = lower anterior face height; NLA = nasolabial angle.

Relationship of the dentition to the skeletal pattern
- Cant of the occlusal plane in relation to the Frankfort plane;
- Interincisal angle;
- Axial inclination of the mandibular incisors to the occlusal plane;
- Axial inclination of the mandibular incisors to the mandibular plane; and
- Maxillary incisor protrusion as measured by the distance of the maxillary central incisor edge to the A–Pog line.

Downs analysis was made simpler to interpret by plotting the results on a two-polygon graph or 'wiggleogram', one representing the skeletal pattern and one the denture pattern (Fig. 6.40) (Downs, 1956; Vorhies & Adams, 1951). Average values for each measurement were represented through the centre of the graph and the extremes of variation extended laterally, the best-balanced retrognathic faces to the left and prognathic faces to the right. By plotting the results of an analysis on such a graph, a very rapid quantitative and qualitative illustration of the facial type is generated.

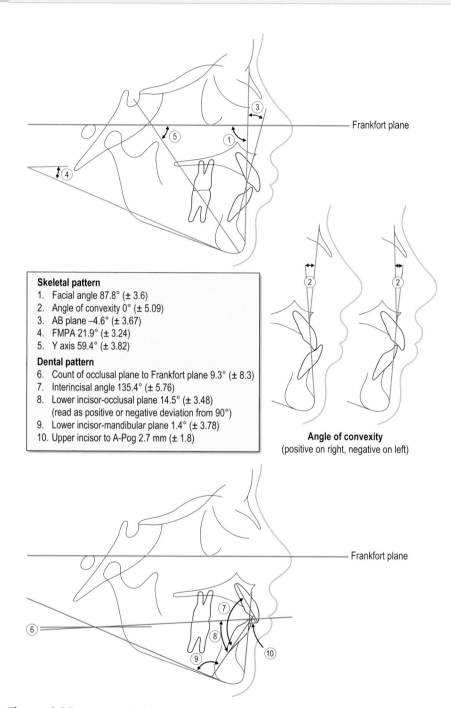

Frankfort plane

Skeletal pattern
1. Facial angle 87.8° (± 3.6)
2. Angle of convexity 0° (± 5.09)
3. AB plane –4.6° (± 3.67)
4. FMPA 21.9° (± 3.24)
5. Y axis 59.4° (± 3.82)

Dental pattern
6. Count of occlusal plane to Frankfort plane 9.3° (± 8.3)
7. Interincisal angle 135.4° (± 5.76)
8. Lower incisor-occlusal plane 14.5° (± 3.48) (read as positive or negative deviation from 90°)
9. Lower incisor-mandibular plane 1.4° (± 3.78)
10. Upper incisor to A-Pog 2.7 mm (± 1.8)

Angle of convexity
(positive on right, negative on left)

Frankfort plane

Figure 6.39 Downs analysis.

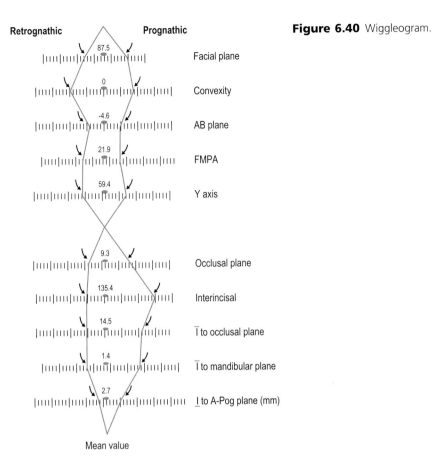

Figure 6.40 Wiggleogram.

Steiner analysis

The Steiner analysis was first described in 1953 by Cecil Steiner, an orthodontist in Beverly Hills, California (Steiner, 1953) and many elements of this analysis are still in popular use today (Fig. 6.41). Steiner utilized the SN plane as a point of horizontal reference, favouring it over the Frankfort horizontal for two main reasons:

- SN lies within the mid-sagittal plane of the skull and is therefore subject to minimal displacement by lateral movements of the head; and
- Both S and N points are readily identifiable on a profile radiograph.

Steiner compartmentalized his assessment into skeletal and dental components, later introducing a method of compromise for positioning the dentition in the presence of skeletal discrepancy.

Skeletal relationship

- The angle SNA represents the relationship of the maxilla to the anterior cranial base;
- The angle SNB represents the relationship of the mandible to the anterior cranial base;

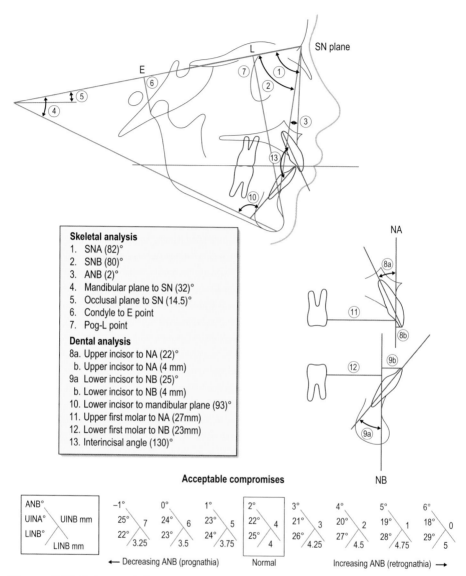

Figure 6.41 Steiner analysis.

- The angle ANB represents the relative position of the two jaws to one another;
- Mandibular plane (Go–Gn) to SN represents the vertical relationship of the mandible to the anterior cranial base; and
- The occlusal plane is also related to the SN plane.
  Further attention was placed upon locating the mandible and defining its relationship to other craniofacial structures:
- The mandible is located in space relative to the SN plane (via perpendicular lines from the distal-most point of the condyle and pogonion intersecting with SN (E and L points, respectively).

Dental relationship

- The upper central incisor is related to the line NA (the tip of the maxillary incisor crown should be 4-mm anterior to NA and the long axis at 22°);
- The lower central incisor is related to the line NB (the tip of the mandibular incisor crown should be 4-mm anterior to NB and the long axis at 25°);
- The lower central incisor inclination to the mandibular plane;
- Upper denture base length (most mesial point of the upper first molar crown to NA);
- Lower denture base length (most mesial point of the lower first molar crown to NB); and
- The interincisal angle.

Steiner recognized that not every individual would conform to a single set of cephalometric measurements and he further modified his analysis with the introduction of acceptable compromises for incisor position, if the values of ANB deviated from the ideal (Fig. 6.41) (Steiner, 1956).

McNamara analysis

James McNamara described his analysis as a method of evaluating the position of the dentition and jaws both to each other and to the cranial base for a more modern era, where the increasing use of functional appliances and orthognathic surgery was producing new possibilities in the treatment of skeletal discrepancies (Fig. 6.42) (McNamara, 1984). Normal values for the analysis were obtained by combining average values from three longitudinal cephalometric growth studies carried out in North America: Bolton, Burlington and Ann Arbor.

McNamara used the Frankfort plane as a horizontal reference and constructed a perpendicular line through nasion to provide a vertical reference. The analysis is subdivided into five principle sections defining the hard tissues, and an additional analysis of the airway:

- Relating the maxilla to the cranial base:
  - The distance from point A to the nasion perpendicular;
- Relating the mandible to the maxilla:
  - Effective lengths of the maxilla and mandible measured via lines from condylion to point A and gnathion, respectively;
  - Vertical dimension of the lower anterior face measured from the anterior nasal spine to menton;
  - Mandibular plane angle (Frankfort plane and mandibular plane); and
  - Ricketts facial axis;
- Relating the mandible to the cranial base:
  - The distance from pogonion to the nasion perpendicular;
- Relating the upper incisor to the maxilla:
  - A line is constructed through point A parallel to nasion perpendicular and the distance measured to the facial surface of the upper incisor;
- Relating the lower incisor to the mandible:
  - The distance from the facial surface of the lower incisor to a line drawn through point A and pogonion;

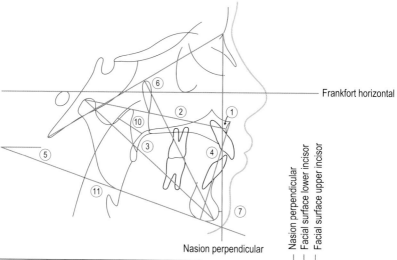

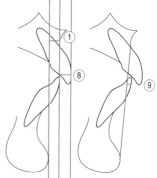

Maxilla to cranial base
1. A point to nasion perpendicular
   (mixed dentition 0 mm)
   (adult 1 mm)

Mandible to maxilla
2. Midfacial length (Co-A point)
3. Mandibular length (Co-Gn)
4. Lower anterior face height (ANS-Me)
5. FMPA
   (mixed dentition 25°)
   (adult 22°)
6. Facial axis (90°)

Mandible to cranial base
7. Pog to nasion perpendicular
   (mixed dentition –8 to –6 mm)
   (adult –2 to –4 mm)

Upper incisor to maxilla
8. Facial surface upper incisor to A point (4–6 mm)

Lower incisor to mandible
9. Facial surface lower incisor to A Pog (1–3 mm)

Airway analysis
10. Upper pharyngeal width (<5 mm)
11. Lower pharyngeal width (10–12 mm)

Composite norms		
Midfacial length	Mandibular length	LAFH
80	97–100	57–58
85	105–108	60–62
90	113–116	63–64
95	122–125	67–69
100	130–133	70–74
105	138–141	75–79

Bolton standards for midfacial and mandibular length					
	12 yrs		14 yrs		16 yrs	
	♂	♀	♂	♀	♂	♀
Midfacial length	98.6 (4.4)	98.6 (4.4)	98.6 (4.4)	98.6 (4.4)	98.6 (4.4)	98.6 (4.4)
Mandibular length	126.8 (4.7)	120.0 (3.4)	126.8 (4.7)	120.0 (3.4)	126.8 (4.7)	120.0 (3.4)

Figure 6.42 McNamara analysis.

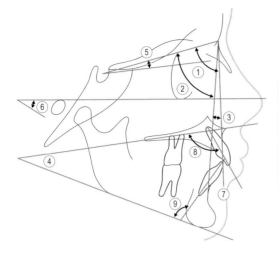

Skeletal analysis	
1. SNA	81 (± 3)°
2. SNB	78 (± 3)°
3. ANB	3 (± 2)°
4. MMPA	27 (± 5)°
5. SN Mx	8 (± 3)°
6. FMPA	27 (± 5)°
Dental analysis	
7. SN $\overline{\text{I}}$	= SNA
8. $\underline{\text{I}}$ Mx	109 (± 6)°
9. $\overline{\text{I}}$ Md	93 (± 6)°
SNA	>81°
	subtract 0.5°
	from ANB
SNA	<81°
	add 0.5° to ANB
[assuming SN Mx is from 5–11°]	

Figure 6.43 Eastman analysis.

- Airway analysis:
  - Both the upper and lower pharyngeal widths measured at the level of the soft palate and inferior border of the mandible.

Eastman analysis
The origin of this analysis is found in the work of Clifford Ballard who pioneered the use of cephalometric radiography in orthodontic diagnosis and treatment planning at the Eastman Dental Hospital in London. He based his standard values upon a random selection of 250 individuals gathered from a range of age groups (Ballard, 1956). The Eastman analysis was further developed by Richard Mills (Mills, 1982) and the core elements are still in popular use within the UK today, although usually supplemented with additional measurements. The original Eastman analysis was divided into skeletal and dental assessments (Fig. 6.43):

Skeletal relationship
- The anteroposterior jaw relationship:
  - SNA, SNB and ANB; and
  - Mills' correction (if applicable);

- The vertical jaw relationship:
  - MMPA;
  - SN–maxillary plane; and
  - FMPA;
- Dental relationship:
  - SN–I
  - UI–maxillary plane; and
  - LI–mandibular plane.

Soft tissue cephalometric analysis
The soft tissue profile can also be seen on a lateral skull cephalometric radiograph, and various methods for measuring this have been described.

Ricketts' E-line
Ricketts' E-line is a line drawn from tip of the nose to soft tissue pogonion. The upper lip should be 4-mm and the lower lip 2-mm behind this line. This line is age-related, as the lips tend to become more retrusive with age.

Nasolabial angle
The nasolabial angle can also be identified from the soft tissue profile on a cephalometric radiograph. The landmarks and mean values have been described previously (see Fig. 6.8).

Errors in cephalometric analysis
Cephalometrics is not an exact science and it should be recognized that a significant amount of error is associated with any cephalometric analysis (Houston, 1983).

It is important for the identification of a particular landmark to be reproducible, with successive measurements of the same dimension being identical. Reproducibility is influenced primarily by measurement error:

- There is a large difference in the reliability of identification between different landmarks.
- Every landmark has a characteristic non-circular envelope of error distribution in the x and y directions, explained by its anatomical position on the radiograph (Fig. 6.44) (Baumrind & Frantz, 1971a).
- Landmark error can also contribute to inaccuracy in both angular and linear measurements, depending upon the landmarks involved. In addition, the same landmarks are often used for the construction of different dimensions within an analysis and therefore error associated with these landmarks can be cumulative, resulting in artificial correlation between different measurements (Baumrind & Frantz, 1971b).
- The physical task of constructing, drawing and measuring lines on a cephalometric radiograph will also be associated with errors that affect reproducibility.

Another source of potential error is the validity of what is actually being measured. There is little merit in identifying landmarks and measuring particular dimensions to a high degree of accuracy if they do not represent what they are supposed to:

- Many landmarks are chosen because they are simple and convenient to locate rather than being anatomically accurate:
  - Points A and B represent the anterior limit of the jaw apical bases, but in reality no specific anatomical point exists. Both of these points are subject to remodelling as the incisor teeth move.

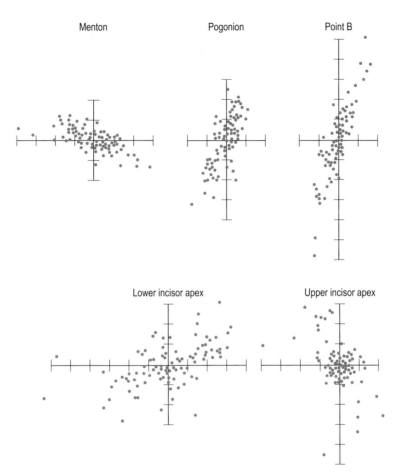

Figure 6.44 Envelope of error associated with cephalometric point identification. (Redrawn from Baumrind and Frantz, 1971a).

- Errors of projection also arise because a cephalometric radiograph represents the conversion of a complex three-dimensional object into a two-dimensional image:
  - Every cephalometric radiograph has an enlargement factor associated with it. In order for linear measurements to be compared from films taken on different machines, this enlargement must be known.
  - If the landmarks that contribute to an angle or linear value do not lie parallel to the film, this will also give rise to distortion, a fact often ignored because of the difficulty in calculating correction values.
  Methods to reduce cephalometric error include the following:
- The cephalometric radiograph should be of the highest quality:
  - Correct positioning of the subject in the cephalostat; and
  - Highest definition of skeletal and soft tissue structures.
- The cephalometric radiograph should be viewed under optimum conditions.

- Measurement error should be reduced as much as possible:
  - Hand-trace landmarks and then digitize using a computer;
  - Repeat measurements;
  - Magnification associated with the radiograph should be known; and
  - For large studies calibrate examiners.

Cephalometric superimposition

The comparison of longitudinal or cross-sectional cephalometric radiographs taken at different time points is a useful method for evaluating the effects of craniofacial growth, orthodontic treatment or both. Most commonly, superimposition is employed to evaluate:

- Changes in the facial skeleton;
- Maxillary growth and dentoalveolar change; and
- Mandibular growth and dentoalveolar change.

A prerequisite for accurate superimposition is that the anatomical structures used to superimpose one radiograph onto the other are stable over the period of observation between the films. In addition, for radiographs taken on different machines, the magnification must be taken into account.

Analysing changes in the facial skeleton

To accurately evaluate facial change, the region of superimposition not only needs to be stable, but must also be located outside the facial skeleton itself. The cranial base has completed much of its growth by 6 years of age and, therefore, is commonly used as a reference plane for this type of cephalometric superimposition. Several techniques have been described, but the most popular use the anterior cranial base:

Superimposition on anterior cranial base anatomy

Lucien de Coster described the basicranial line or anterior cranial base as a stable structure, which represented the axis of the skull base and was therefore suitable for the comparison of changes in the facial bones (Fig. 6.45) (de Coster, 1952). The de Coster line extends along the following landmarks:

- Anterior lip of sella turcica;
- Sphenoethmoid suture;
- Planum sphenoidale;
- Roof of the ethmoid; and
- Cranial side of the frontal bone.

Björk and Skieller subsequently modified this method of regional superimposition, further defining the precise anatomical landmarks along the anterior cranial base that should be utilized on the basis of stability (Fig. 6.46) (Björk & Skieller, 1983):

- Anterior wall of sella turcica and its intersection with the anterior clinoid process;
- Cribriform plate of the ethmoid;
- Frontoethmoidal crests; and
- Cerebral surface of the orbital roofs.

Superimposition on the SN plane, registered at S

The identification of anterior cranial base anatomy can be difficult because of a lack of radiographic clarity in this region and a degree of skill is required to carry out this

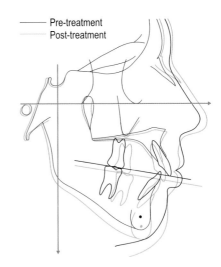

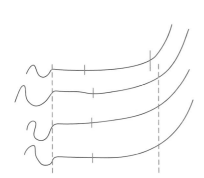

Figure 6.45 De Coster's line drawn from four members of the same family. Reproduced from de Coster (1952) with permission from Oxford University Press.

Figure 6.46 Structural superimposition of Björk at the cranial base. Reproduced from Männchen (2001), with kind permission from Roland Männchen and Oxford University Press.

procedure. An alternative method uses the SN plane, with registration at S. The clarity of sella and nasion, their relative stability and the position of SN in the mid-sagittal plane of the skull make this reference line an attractive and widely used alternative for cranial base superimposition. However, the position of nasion can change during growth of the frontonasal suture, and if this occurs in a vertical direction it can affect the accuracy of SN as a reference (see Box 3.1).

Studies comparing the accuracy of these different methods of anterior cranial base superimposition have demonstrated that all have appreciable levels of error and none are significantly more reliable (Baumrind et al, 1976; Ghafari et al, 1987).

Grid analysis
A number of grid-based analyses that attempt to differentiate between dental and skeletal changes that have occurred in the region of the jaws as a result of orthodontic treatment mechanics have been described. These analyses use cranial base superimposition and the construction of a vertical reference line to measure anteroposterior change.

- Pancherz analysis—Hans Pancherz devised this analysis to evaluate the interrelationship between skeletal and dental change within and between the maxilla and mandible (Pancherz, 1982). Skeletal and dental change is evaluated using a reference line constructed perpendicular to the occlusal plane with radiographs superimposed on the SN plane, registered at S.
- Pitchfork analysis—The Pitchfork analysis was described by Lysle Johnston as a simple method of analysing the effects of orthodontic treatment in the maxilla and mandible along the anteroposterior plane (Johnston, 1996). This analysis concen-

trates upon the relative contributions of skeletal and dental changes measured along the functional occlusal plane. The resulting 'pitchfork' diagram represents the combined numerical effects of skeletal change relative to the anterior cranial base and tooth movement (molar and incisor) relative to the basal bone of the jaws (Fig. 6.47).

Analysing changes in the maxilla and mandible
Superimposing on landmarks within or around the maxilla and mandible allows an analysis of the local growth and dentoalveolar change that has occurred in isolation from that produced by growth displacement. A number of techniques have been described for each jaw and they also rely on using stable or near-stable structures associated with each bone.

Analysing changes in the maxilla
A number of methods for analysing changes in the maxilla have been described:
- Superimposition on the maxillary plane (ANS–PNS), registered at ANS—this is one of the simplest methods of superimposition but it can result in an underestimation of anterior palatal development because of remodelling that occurs at ANS (Broadbent, 1937). An alternative method is to use the ANS–PNS plane but orientate to a best fit of the palatal surface of the maxilla, thereby removing the influence of ANS.
- Best fit on the superior and inferior surfaces of the hard palate—this method also eliminates any error associated with ANS by simply using the outline of the superior and inferior surfaces of the hard palate for orientation (Salzmann, 1960).
- The structural method of Björk (Fig. 6.48)—on the basis of extensive longitudinal growth studies using the implant method, Björk and Skieller found that the maxilla remodelled extensively during normal growth and that stable structures were not present within this bone. However, some regions surrounding the maxilla that

Figure 6.47 Pitchfork analysis.

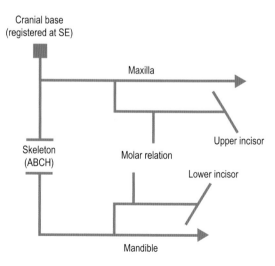

Cranial base
(registered at SE)

Maxilla

Upper incisor

Skeleton
(ABCH)

Molar relation

Lower incisor

Mandible

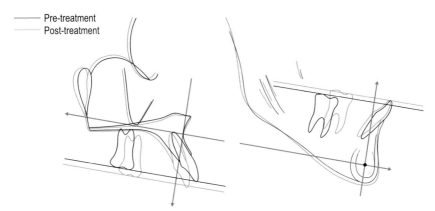

Figure 6.48 Regional superimposition of Björk for the maxilla (left) and mandible (right). Reproduced from Männchen (2001), with kind permission of Roland Männchen, Oxford University Press and the European Orthodontic Society.

underwent minimal remodelling and could be regarded as being stable and therefore used for maxillary superimposition were identified. It was recommended to superimpose on the anterior surface of the zygomatic process and then orientate the second radiograph so that resorptive lowering of the nasal floor is equal to apposition on the orbital floor (Björk & Skieller, 1977).

Analysing changes in the mandible

- Superimposition along the lower border and inner table of the symphysis—this method is relatively simple to carry out but is hampered by the extensive remodelling that occurs along the lower border, particularly at gonion, during growth and the variability associated with constructing the mandibular plane.
- The structural method of Björk (Fig. 6.48)—in contrast to the maxilla, Björk was able to identify stable natural reference structures within the mandible (Björk & Skieller, 1983). He described a list of mandibular structures that could be readily identified and then used to orientate longitudinal radiographs:
  - Anterior contour of the chin;
  - Inner contour of the cortical plate at the lower border of the symphysis;
  - Any distinct trabecular structure in the symphysis;
  - The contour of the mandibular canal; and
  - The lower contour of a mineralized molar tooth germ before root development has begun.

Further reading

BROWN M (1981). Eight methods of analysing a cephalogram to establish anteroposterior skeletal discrepancy. *Br J Orthod* 8:139–146.

FACULTY OF GENERAL DENTAL PRACTITIONERS UK (2004). *Selection Criteria for Dental Radiography*, 2nd edn. (London: Royal College of Surgeons of England).

MCDONALD F AND IRELAND AJ (1998). *Diagnosis of the Orthodontic Patient* (Oxford: Oxford University Press).

RADIATION PROTECTION 136: *European guidelines on radiation protection in dental radiology. The safe use of radiographs in dental practice* (2004) (Luxembourg: Office for Official Publications of the European Communities).

SARVER DM, PROFFIT WR AND ACKERMAN JL (2003). *Contemporary Treatment of Dentofacial Deformity* (St Louis: Mosby).

WHAITES, E (2007). *Essentials of Dental Radiography and Radiology*, 4th edn (Edinburgh: Churchill Livingstone Elsevier).

WILLIAMS P (1986). Lower incisor position in treatment planning. *Br J Orthod* 13:33–41.

References

BALLARD CF (1951). Recent work in North America as it affects orthodontic diagnosis and treatment. *Dental Record* 71:85–97.

BALLARD CF (1956). Morphology and treatment of class II division 2 occlusions. *Trans Eur Orth Soc* 44–55.

BASS JK, FINE H AND CISNEROS GJ (1993). Nickel hypersensitivity in the orthodontic patient. *Am J Orthod Dentofacial Orthop* 103:280–285.

BAUMRIND S AND FRANTZ RC (1971a). The reliability of head film measurements. 1. Landmark identification. *Am J Orthod* 60:111–127.

BAUMRIND S AND FRANTZ RC (1971b). The reliability of head film measurements. 2. Conventional angular and linear measures. *Am J Orthod* 60:505–517.

BAUMRIND S, MILLER D AND MOLTHEN R. (1976). The reliability of head film measurements. 3. Tracing superimposition. *Am J Orthod* 70:617–644.

BEANE RA, REIMANN G, PHILLIPS C ET AL (2003). A cepholometric comparison of black open-bite subjects and black normals. *Angle Orthod* 73:294–300.

BHATIA SN AND AKPABIO TA (1979). A correlation study of two methods of assessing skeletal pattern. *Br J Orthod* 6:187–193.

BJÖRK A AND SKIELLER V (1977). Roentgencephalometric growth analysis of the maxilla. *Trans Eur Orth Soc* 53:51–55.

BJÖRK A AND SKIELLER V (1983). Normal and abnormal growth of the mandible. A synthesis of longitudinal cephalometric implant studies over a period of 25 years. *Eur J Orthod* 5:1–46.

BROADBENT BH (1937). Bolton standards and technique in orthodontic practice. *Angle Orthod* 7: 209–233.

DE COSTER L (1952). The familial line, studied by a new line of reference. *Trans Eur Orth Soc* 50–55.

DOWNS WB (1948). Variations in facial relationships: their significance in treatment and prognosis. *Am J Orthod* 34:812–840.

DOWNS WB (1952). The role of cephalometrics in orthodontic case analysis and diagnosis. *Am J Orthod* 38:162–182.

DOWNS WB (1956). Analysis of the dentofacial profile. *Angle Orthod* 26:191–212.

ELLIS PE AND BENSON PE (2003). Does articulating study casts make a difference to treatment planning? *J Orthod* 30:45–49; discussion 22–23.

GHAFARI J, ENGEL FE AND LASTER LL (1987). Cephalometric superimposition on the cranial base: a review and a comparison of four methods. *Am J Orthod Dentofacial Orthop* 91:403–413.

GILL DS, NAINI FB AND TREDWIN CJ (2007). Smile aesthetics. *Dent Update* 34:152–158.

HAMDAM AM AND ROCK WP (2001). Cepholometric norms in an arabic population. *J Orthod* 28:297–300.

HOUSTON WJ (1983). The analysis of errors in orthodontic measurements. *Am J Orthod* 83:382–390.

HOUSTON WJ AND EDLER R (1990). Long-term stability of the lower labial segment relative to the A-Pog line. *Eur J Orthod* 12:302–310.

HOUSTON WJB (1975). Assessment of the skeletal pattern from the occlusion of the incisor teeth: a critical review. *Br J Orthod* 2:167–169.

ISAACSON KG, THOM AR, HORNER K ET AL (2008). Orthodontic radiographs. *British Orthodontic Society*.

JACOBSON A (1975). The 'Wits' appraisal of jaw disharmony. *Am J Orthod* 67:125–138.

JACOBSON A (1976). Application of the 'Wits' appraisal. *Am J Orthod* 70:179–189.

JOHNSTON LE Jr (1996). Balancing the books on orthodontic treatment: an integrated analysis of change. *Br J Orthod* 23:93–102.

MAMANDRAS AH (1988). Linear changes of the maxillary and mandibular lips. *Am J Orthod Dentofacial Orthop* 94:405–410.

MCNAMARA JA Jr (1984). A method of cephalometric evaluation. *Am J Orthod* 86:449–469.

MERRETT SJ, DRAGE NA, DURNING P (2009). Cone beam computed tomography: a useful tool in orthodontic diagnosis and treatment planning. *J Orthod* 36:202–210.

MIJAMIMA K, MCNAMARA JA, KIMURA T ET AL (1996). Craniofacial structure of Japanese and European-American adults with normal occlusions and well-balanced faces. *Am J Orthod Dentofacial Orthop* 110:431–438.

MILLS JRE (1970). The application and importance of cephalometry in orthodontic treatment. *The Orthodontist* 2:32–47.

MILLS JRE (1982). *Principles and Practice of Orthodontics* (Edinburgh: Churchill Livingstone).

MOORREES CFA AND KEANE MR (1958). Natural head position, a basic consideration in the interpretation of cephalometric radiographs. *Am J Phys Anthropol* 16:213–234.

OBWEGESER HL AND MAKEK MS (1986). Hemimandibular hyperplasia–hemimandibular elongation. *J Maxillofac Surg* 14:183–208.

OWNBY DR, OWNBY HE, MCCULLOUGH J ET AL (1996). The prevalence of anti-latex IgE antibodies in 1000 volunteer blood donors. *J Allergy Clin Immunol* 97:1188–1192.

PANCHERZ H (1982). The mechanism of Class II correction in Herbst appliance treatment. A cephalometric investigation. *Am J Orthod* 82:104–113.

PARK YC AND BURSTONE CJ (1986). Soft-tissue profile–fallacies of hard-tissue standards in treatment planning. *Am J Orthod Dentofacial Orthop* 90:52–62.

RICKETTS RM (1960). A foundation for cephalometric communication. *Am J Orthod* 46:330–357.

RIEDEL RA (1952). The relation of maxillary structures to cranium in malocclusion and in normal occlusion. *Angle Orthod* 22:142–145.

SALZMANN JA (1960). The research workshop on cephalometrics. *Am J Orthod* 46:834–847.

SANTORO M, GALKIN S, TEREDESAI M, ET AL (2003). Comparison of measurements made on digital and plaster models. *Am J Orthod Dentofacial Orthop* 124:101–105.

SARVER DM (2001). The importance of incisor positioning in the esthetic smile: the smile arc. *Am J Orthod Dentofacial Orthop* 120:98–111.

STEINER C (1953). Cephalometrics for you and me. *Am J Orthod* 39:729–755.

STEINER C (1956). Cephalometrics in clinical practice. *Angle Orthod* 29:8–29.

TULLOCH JF, SHAW WC, UNDERHILL C ET AL (1984). A comparison of attitudes toward orthodontic treatment in British and American communities. *Am J Orthod* 85:253–259.

VORHIES JM AND ADAMS JW (1951). Polygonic interpretation of cephalometric findings. *Angle Orthod* 21:194–197.

WILLIAMS R (1969). The diagnostic line. *Am J Orthod* 55:458–476.

7 The orthodontic patient: treatment planning

One of the most difficult, but important aspects of orthodontic management is treatment planning. With the advent of modern fixed appliance systems it is deceptively easy to straighten teeth. The skill of the orthodontist lies in placing the dentition in the optimal position and achieving the correct aesthetic and occlusal result for each patient. This process starts with clinical examination, record collection and diagnosis. The next stage is treatment planning, which should ideally be carried out in a formal manner and away from the patient, using the clinical data and collected records. It is a two-stage process, initially defining the treatment aims and then deciding how these are to be achieved. In this chapter, treatment aims and the general principles of treatment planning are discussed. The specifics of treatment for different types of malocclusion are covered in Chapters 10 and 11.

Timing of treatment

Many traits of a malocclusion can manifest in the early mixed dentition and there is often a temptation to begin treatment at this stage. In particular, both 'arch development' (or expansion) to relieve crowding and growth modification to correct a skeletal discrepancy have been proposed by some to benefit from an early approach.

Advocates of these early treatment strategies suggest that they maximize growth potential, compliance and orthopedic change in the young patient, reduce the risk of trauma when maxillary incisors are prominent, simplify any further treatment that may be required in the permanent dentition, reduce the need for extractions and ultimately establish a more stable result. They can also have a psychological benefit, promoting self-esteem by correcting potentially socially debilitating malocclusions early.

However, there are disadvantages associated with starting treatment too soon. The overall duration will be extended, because almost inevitably a second phase of treatment will be required in the permanent dentition and this can lead to problems with compliance over the longer term. The original arch form and growth patterns will tend to reimpose themselves following the first phase of early treatment and a prolonged retention period may be required to maintain any correction during the transition from mixed to permanent dentition. Finally, there is a growing body of evidence to suggest that the treatment result for growth modification will be the same whether carried out in the early mixed or permanent dentition, the only difference being the increased duration if started early (Harrison et al, 2007). In the case of arch development in the early mixed dentition, the long-term results are poor, particularly with regard to the stability of tooth alignment (Little et al, 1990).

The most appropriate time to start treatment aimed at growth modification is usually the late mixed dentition, essentially just before loss of the second deciduous molars. This results in the shortest treatment time, whilst still utilizing growth potential and is least demanding upon compliance. The majority of routine orthodontic treatment with fixed appliances is carried out in the early permanent dentition and this is generally the best time to address problems of crowding. However, there are exceptions and some malocclusions will benefit from earlier treatment:

- Class III cases associated with maxillary hypoplasia can benefit from interceptive treatment to move the maxilla forward with protraction headgear. This appears to be more effective if carried out in the early mixed dentition (see Figs 10.45 and 10.46) (Kim et al, 1999).
- Treatment to correct a class II skeletal base relationship is most effective during the adolescent growth spurt. In females, this will generally occur earlier than in males and is poorly correlated with dental age. Therefore, this type of treatment should often be started earlier in females than males.
- Certain malocclusions, especially an increased overjet, can be a source of teasing and bullying, which can be very distressing. In these circumstances, early treatment may be indicated.
- An increased overjet increases the risk of dentoalveolar trauma, especially before the age of ten. Early treatment to reduce the overjet is indicated in those individuals where little protection is provided by the lips, due to gross lip incompetence and marked maxillary protrusion.
- Early treatment of a posterior crossbite associated with a displacement can prevent perpetuation into the permanent dentition (Harrison & Ashby, 2001). An anterior crossbite can result in mucogingival problems associated with the lower incisors (see Fig. 10.42). Both these forms of malocclusion are amendable to simple removable appliance treatment in the early mixed dentition.

Aims of treatment

The principle aims of orthodontic treatment relate to aesthetics and function:
- Positioning the dentition within the skeletal and soft tissue environment for optimal facial and dental aesthetics; and
- Achieving a stable and ideal static, and functional occlusion.

The extent to which these aims need to be considered will vary between patients and depend upon the diagnosis. The treatment required to achieve them may range from simple occlusal change to complex multidisciplinary intervention.

Facial aims

There is a greater awareness amongst orthodontists of the importance associated with facial and soft tissue aesthetics in treatment planning (Box 7.1). Obtaining a class I incisor and canine relationship is usually a fundamental aim of treatment, but this must not be achieved at the expense of the soft tissue profile. Reconciling the facial and occlusal aims of treatment can be difficult and will depend in part on the underlying skeletal relationship:

- In the absence of any significant discrepancy in the skeletal pattern, treatment planning will be concerned primarily with obtaining the correct occlusal relationship (Fig. 7.1).

Box 7.1   Planning treatment around the face

Orthodontic treatment planning should begin with the position of the dentition, particularly the upper incisors, within the face. This represents something of a shift in emphasis from planning based around the lower incisor position and treating to isolated static occlusal goals.

In the infancy of orthodontics it was assumed that if all the teeth were aligned and the occlusal goals achieved, each individual would have ideal facial aesthetics. However, it soon become apparent that this was not the case, resulting in extreme protrusion of the dentition in some cases and extensive relapse in others. With the advent of cephalometric analysis, it was argued that facial growth was genetically determined and that orthodontic treatment could have little influence on the facial skeleton. Treatment became based around arbitrary hard tissue cephalometric standards, especially in relation to lower incisor position, even though these bear little relation to the soft tissues and facial profile (Park & Burstone, 1986). Since then, conventional thinking has shifted again, with the soft tissues defining the limits of orthodontic treatment in each individual (Ackerman & Proffit, 1997). The main reasons for this are a resurgence of interest in functional appliance therapy, advances in orthognathic surgical techniques, a greater understanding of orthodontic relapse and the acceptance of long-term retention strategies. There is also an appreciation of how the face ages and therefore how treatment carried out in the teenage years will impact on facial appearance many years into the future.

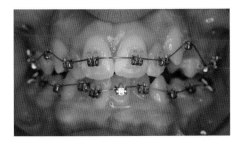
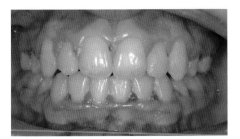

Figure 7.1 Occlusal correction of a crowded class I case using fixed appliances following the extraction of four first premolar teeth.

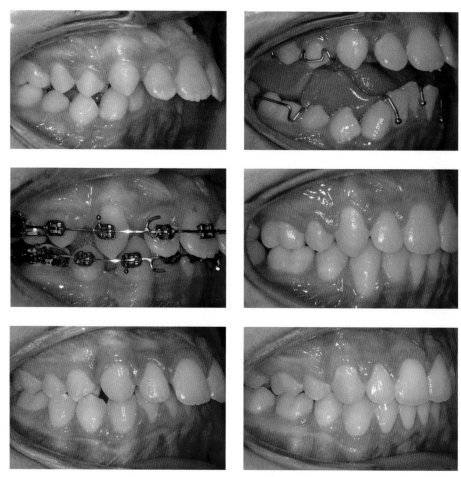

Figure 7.2 Correction of class II division 1 malocclusion. A case with a moderate class II skeletal base relationship treated initially with a functional appliance to correct the anteroposterior discrepancy. This was followed by the extraction of four premolars to alleviate crowding and fixed appliances to detail the occlusion (upper four panels). A case with a milder skeletal discrepancy treated with orthodontic camouflage involving premolar extraction and fixed appliances (lower two panels).

- If there is a mild to moderate skeletal discrepancy, appliances aimed at growth modification can be used in an attempt to improve the skeletal relationship. These appliances tend to rely on good patient compliance combined with favourable facial growth, results can be variable and they are much more effective at correcting class II discrepancies than class III. Alternatively, orthodontic camouflage may be appropriate, accepting the skeletal pattern and planning the necessary occlusal changes to correct the malocclusion (Fig. 7.2) (Box 7.2).

Box 7.2   Camouflage treatment

In a young patient with a class II skeletal discrepancy, utilizing growth with a functional appliance can facilitate treatment, which is not possible in an older patient or adult, where growth potential either is poor or has disappeared. In these cases there are two treatment options: surgically repositioning the jaws or moving the teeth to mask the skeletal discrepancy. The latter is known as camouflage treatment and can be very successful in mild to moderately severe skeletal class II cases. One of the main limiting factors in this type of treatment is the soft tissue profile, as treatment will involve retraction of the upper incisors and with them, the upper lip. If the upper lip is protrusive, some retraction will be beneficial to the profile. However, if the lip profile is retrusive and the nasolabial angle obtuse, any further retraction will increase prominence of the nose and worsen aesthetics. Similarly, over-retraction of the lower incisors to camouflage a class III skeletal discrepancy can result in unacceptable prominence of the chin. Therefore, when planning camouflage treatment, although it may be possible to achieve a good occlusal result, it should not be done at the expense of facial aesthetics. Generally the more severe the skeletal discrepancy, the harder it is to achieve camouflage with tooth movement alone.

- If the skeletal discrepancy is severe and the patient is growing, growth modification should certainly be considered, but success will be less predictable. However, orthodontic camouflage in these cases can be more problematic, particularly in terms of achieving good facial aesthetics. Surgical repositioning of the jaws is a definitive method of changing a more severe skeletal pattern, but this is only carried out once facial growth is complete. Attempts have been made to define the relative limits of orthodontic and surgical tooth movement for the correction of malocclusion, but these can only ever represent a guide (Fig. 7.3).

Occlusal aims

The occlusal aims of treatment are defined in terms of dental aesthetics and both static and functional occlusion (Table 7.1) and are generally listed in the order in which they will be corrected. Whilst these will vary between cases, in practical terms occlusal correction will usually require some or all of the following:
- Creating space to relieve crowding;
- Levelling and aligning the dental arches;
- Correcting the buccal segment relationship; and
- Correcting the incisor relationship.

A further consideration related to the occlusion is health of the temporomandibular joints, but this is a contentious area. Despite evidence showing orthodontic treatment having little impact on temporomandibular dysfunction (Luther, 2007a, b), much conjecture exists regarding the ideal position for the condyle at the end of treatment and the need to treat to an ideal functional occlusion. However, orthodontics is one area in dentistry where treatment can result in significant occlusal change. Therefore it would seem sensible practice to aim for an ideal static and functional occlusion wherever possible.

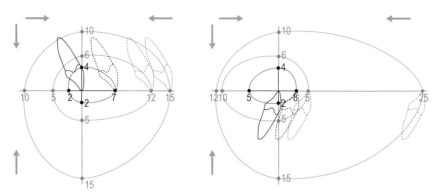

Figure 7.3 The envelope of discrepancy showing the tooth movements theoretically possible for correcting a malocclusion. With the ideal position shown at the origin of the *x* and *y* axes, the movement possible with orthodontics alone (inner black envelope), growth modification (middle red envelope) and surgery (outer red envelope) are shown. Redrawn from Proffit WR, White RP Jr and Sarver DM (2003). *Contemporary Treatment of Facial Deformity* (St Louis: Mosby).

Table 7.1   Occlusal aims of orthodontic treatment

- Andrews six keys;
- Canine guidance or group function;
- No non-working side interferences;
- Anterior guidance; and
- RCP and ICP coincident.

Table 7.2   Positioning the upper incisors within the face

- Vertically around 3–4 mm of the upper central incisors should be shown at rest;
- The labial face should be parallel to the true vertical and adequately support the upper lip;
- Curvature of the incisal edges should be parallel with the lower lip on smiling; and
- The dental centreline should be coincident with the facial midline.

Planning to achieve the facial aims of treatment

Treatment planning should begin with some consideration regarding the upper incisor position and whether this needs to be changed (Table 7.2). Achieving an ideal position for these teeth will be more difficult in the presence of a skeletal discrepancy and in some cases may not be possible with orthodontic treatment alone.

Anteroposterior position of the upper incisors
The upper incisors can be positioned too far forward within the face as a result of maxillary skeletal excess or simple dentoalveolar disproportion. The skeletal and soft tissue morphology will influence the resulting incisor relationship:

- The overjet can be increased, resulting in a class II division 1 relationship. The upper incisors are normally inclined or proclined. If they are proclined this is often due to the position of the lower lip or a digit sucking habit.
- The upper incisors can be retroclined, resulting in a class II division 2 relationship with an increased overbite, which is usually due to a high lower lip position (see Fig. 1.8).

In a growing child with skeletal maxillary excess, restraint of maxillary growth can be achieved with extraoral force, although the use of a functional appliance can also provide some maxillary restraint, particularly when used in combination with headgear. Any associated mandibular retrognathia is indicative of the need for a functional appliance.

Alternatively, the position of the maxilla can be accepted and orthodontic camouflage carried out to retract the upper incisors into a class I occlusion, by either tipping or bodily movement, depending upon their position. In many cases, space will be required to facilitate this movement and this can be achieved by retraction of the buccal segments using headgear or by extractions.

Conversely, the upper incisors can be positioned too far back within the face, resulting in a class III relationship. This can again be associated with dentoalveolar disproportion but is more commonly due to skeletal maxillary deficiency. A patient in the mixed dentition with marked maxillary deficiency may be a candidate for attempted growth modification to improve the maxillary position. This will require extraoral force to the maxilla provided by a facemask and reverse headgear. A rapid improvement in the incisor relationship can be achieved using this type of treatment; however, it requires excellent cooperation and the subsequent pattern of facial growth will significantly influence long-term stability of any change achieved (see Figs 10.45 and 10.46).

A class III incisor relationship can also be associated with mandibular excess, either alone or in combination with maxillary deficiency. These cases are even less amenable to growth modification and likely to worsen with age. Definitive treatment will almost always require surgical intervention, which should be delayed until facial growth is complete.

Vertical position of the upper incisors
Any significant vertical excess in the upper incisor position, particularly when associated with a gummy smile, can be difficult to correct with orthodontic intrusion and ideally will require either growth modification or surgery for correction. As the face ages there is a tendency to show less upper incisor and it is important that these teeth are not overintruded during treatment; otherwise, the smile can become prematurely aged. In a growing child, a full-coverage maxillary intrusion splint in combination with high-pull headgear can be used to restrict vertical maxillary growth and reduce upper incisor show. However, treatment of this type is difficult, requiring excellent compliance and favourable growth to be successful. In an adult, excess incisor show in the vertical plane will require surgical impaction of the maxilla for definitive correction.

Lower incisor position
The planned upper incisor position will also need to be decided in relation to the lower incisors to achieve a class I relationship—a fundamental aim of treatment in most cases. Longitudinal studies have demonstrated that any labial movement of the lower incisors with an orthodontic appliance is inherently prone to relapse in the long-term (Mills, 1966, 1968). Therefore, as a general rule it is advisable to avoid proclining these teeth to any significant extent during treatment, although some exceptions to this do exist (Table 7.3).

Table 7.3   Clinical situations where lower incisor proclination may be acceptable

- Mild lower incisor crowding;
- Class II division 2 cases with retroclined lower incisors;
- Lower incisors retroclined by an active lower lip; and
- Decompensation prior to orthognathic surgery.

Class I malocclusion

If the incisor relationship is initially class I, the anteroposterior position will not require correction during treatment and labiolingual movement of the lower incisors to any great extent can be easily avoided. An exception to this is a class I incisor relationship with significant bimaxillary proclination. If a goal of treatment is the correction of this position, some retraction of the lower incisors will be required and this will usually mean extractions to provide the necessary space.

Class II malocclusion

The lower incisors can be set back within the face in association with mandibular retrognathia, which will also give rise to a class II relationship. In common with class II cases associated with maxillary excess, more severe mandibular deficiency and habitual positioning of the lower lip behind the upper incisors tends to result in an increased overjet and class II division 1 incisor relationship; whilst class II division 2 cases are more commonly seen with milder skeletal discrepancies, reduced vertical proportions and a high lower lip line.

A class II incisor relationship will require some change in the position of these teeth to obtain the goal of a class I occlusion. How this is achieved will depend upon the underlying skeletal and soft tissue relationships and it should be remembered that wide variation is seen in the extent and combinations of skeletal patterns that occur.

For class II cases associated with a normal or only mild skeletal discrepancy and an acceptable profile, the existing lower incisor position will generally be accepted and a class I incisor relationship achieved by changing the upper incisor position. The necessary tooth movement is often relatively minor and rarely has any negative consequences for the facial profile.

In moderate class II malocclusions, it may be possible to achieve a class I incisor relationship with orthodontic tooth movement alone. Camouflage treatment of this kind will usually involve mid-arch premolar extractions, maxillary incisor retraction and maintenance of lower incisor position (although some class II division 2 cases can be very demanding to treat in this manner without some lower incisor proclination). More severe class II cases, particularly those associated with mandibular retrognathia, may require significant upper incisor retraction to achieve camouflage, which can worsen a retrusive soft tissue profile as the lips move back with the teeth. There is not a simple relationship between incisor retraction and lip movement, and how far the lips can be acceptably retracted depends upon many factors, including their thickness and competence, the original incisor position and the underlying skeletal anatomy (Handelman, 1996; Ramos et al, 2005). However, care must be taken not to over-retract incisors, particularly in the more severe cases that already have a retrusive soft tissue profile.

In a growing child with a moderate or severe class II skeletal pattern associated with mandibular deficiency, treatment with a functional appliance aimed at modifying growth should always be considered in an attempt to improve the incisor relationship.

> **Box 7.3   Lower incisor position and the functional appliance**
>
> A general principle of orthodontic treatment planning is to avoid proclination of the lower incisors. However, an optimal solution in class II cases with mandibular retrognathia is to encourage forward movement of these teeth as a result of mandibular growth, facilitated by a functional appliance. This can be difficult to achieve and care must be taken with these appliances not to simply tip the lower incisors forward. In addition, any forward growth of the mandible should ideally occur in the absence of any increase in lower facial proportions; otherwise, the anterior direction of incisor movement can be lost as the mandible rotates downwards and backwards due to an increase in the lower anterior face height.

In successful cases this will improve the lower incisor position through advantageous jaw growth and dentoalveolar change prior to a second phase of treatment aimed at achieving the final occlusal aims (Box 7.3).

In patients with increased vertical proportions or maxillary excess in combination with mandibular retrognathia, some attempt should be made at restraining maxillary development with headgear, which will aid forward development of the mandible.

In adults, and those patients who have responded poorly to growth modification either due to poor compliance or an adverse growth pattern, a decision has to be made whether to accept the underlying skeletal base relationship and correct the malocclusion with orthodontic camouflage, or wait until facial growth has ceased and definitively correct the skeletal base relationship and malocclusion with a combination of orthodontics and orthognathic surgery.

Class III malocclusion
When there is a class III incisor relationship with a mild skeletal discrepancy, a class I position can be achieved with orthodontic camouflage, usually involving a combination of upper incisor proclination and lower incisor retroclination. Fortunately, the lower incisor position is often stable following retraction in class III cases, particularly in the presence of a positive overbite, and in these milder cases, this will be the treatment of choice.

The management of class III cases associated with a more severe skeletal discrepancy can be problematic (Box 7.4). In the presence of maxillary deficiency, some attempt can be made to encourage forward movement, but this will require a young child, extraoral force, excellent cooperation and some improvement in the pattern of facial growth for long-term success. In cases with marked mandibular prognathia, there is a limit how far the lower incisors can be retracted and surgery will often be required. In adolescent patients the decision as to whether a class III malocclusion can be treated orthodontically will depend on several factors (Table 7.4).

Planning to achieve the occlusal aims of treatment

Once the facial aims have been planned, the occlusal aims need to be considered. These are not mutually exclusive and often can both be achieved with orthodontic tooth movement alone. Planning involves initially visualizing the tooth movements needed and assessing what space is required to bring them about. If done formally, this is

Box 7.4   The problem of managing a class III malocclusion

Although a class III incisor relationship only represents a small percentage of malocclusions, they can be some of the most difficult to manage. The main reason for this is the uncertainty surrounding facial growth. In class III cases with a significant skeletal component, the mandible will tend to grow more and later than in class I individuals (Baccetti et al, 2007). Unlike class II malocclusions, where any forward mandibular growth is generally favourable, in class III cases this is not the case. There is a significant risk that a patient who has had orthodontic camouflage to correct a class III incisor relationship in the presence of an underlying skeletal III base will outgrow this treatment if there is further mandibular growth. This is a potential problem because the orthodontic tooth movements aimed at camouflaging a class III malocclusion and those required prior to surgical correction of the skeletal base relationship are essentially opposite in nature. Orthodontic camouflage will maximize dentoalveolar compensation already present, whilst presurgical orthodontics will remove it to optimize the surgical change possible. Treatment decisions should be delayed until the direction and extent of growth is known. Accurate individualized growth prediction from a single cephalometric image is not possible. However, by taking serial lateral cephalograms and study models a better picture of facial growth will be formed. The stability of class III correction not only depends on growth, but also achieving a positive overbite and overjet at the end of treatment. Patients with reduced overbites at the start of treatment, especially in the absence of an anterior displacement, are often not suitable for orthodontic correction alone.

Table 7.4   Prognostic indicators for treatment of class III malocclusion

Indications for orthodontic treatment of class III malocclusion:
- Class I or mild class III skeletal base relationship;
- Average or reduced lower face height;
- Average or increased overbite;
- Proclined lower incisors;
- Upright or retroclined upper incisors; and
- Anterior displacement on closing from RCP into ICP.

Contraindications for orthodontic treatment of class III malocclusion:
- Moderate to severe class III skeletal base relationship;
- Increased lower face height;
- Reduced overbite;
- Retroclined lower incisors;
- Proclined upper incisors;
- No anterior displacement on closing from RCP into ICP; and
- A significant class III molar relationship.

known as a space analysis and can greatly assist in the process of treatment planning because it provides a numerical value for the space required within each dental arch. This can aid in deciding whether teeth need to be extracted and how the mechanics and anchorage are managed to ensure the treatment aims are achieved (Box 7.5).

Space creation

Space may be required in the dental arches to achieve a number of treatment aims relating to the malocclusion:

- Relief of dental crowding (Fig. 7.4);
- Arch levelling and overbite reduction (Fig. 7.5);

Box 7.5   Space analysis

Whether done formally or informally, a space analysis or visualized treatment objective is an essential part of orthodontic treatment planning. The concept of space analysis in orthodontics is not new and numerous analyses have been described; however, one of the most practical and comprehensive is provided by the Royal London space planning exercise (Kirschen et al, 2000a, b). In essence it will give a measurement of the space required to achieve the orthodontic treatment aims. However, it should not be prescriptive. It is carried out in two phases using the patient records including dental study casts, photographs and a cephalometric analysis. The first assesses space requirements in each dental arch. The second is an assessment of how space will be created and used in treatment. This includes planning buccal segment movements required for occlusal correction and the effect future growth will have. If the analysis has been correctly done and the treatment aims accounted for, the balance of space required and how this is created and used should equal zero. If not, the treatment aims should be reviewed and modified appropriately. The advantages of such a space analysis is that it leads to a disciplined approach to treatment planning, realistic treatment aims, a greater anticipation of anchorage requirements and better information for patients. This is very helpful, especially for less experienced operators and those in training.

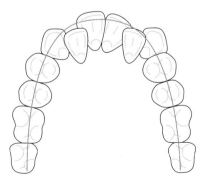

Figure 7.4 Crowding should be measured to the arch form that reflects the majority of the teeth.

Figure 7.5 An increased curve of Spee represents slipped contact points vertically and to level it requires space to avoid lengthening the arch.

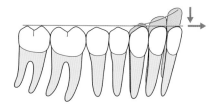

Figure 7.6 Teeth angulated (bottom) occupy more space in the arch than those upright (top).

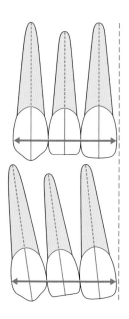

- Correction of tooth angulation (Fig. 7.6);
- Overjet reduction (Fig. 7.7); and
- Correction of tooth inclination or torque (Fig. 7.8).
  There are essentially four methods available to the orthodontist for the creation of space within the dental arches:
- Extraction of teeth;
- Transverse expansion of the dental arch;
- Anteroposterior lengthening of the dental arch; and
- Reduction in tooth width.

Extraction of teeth
One of the most effective ways to create space is by the extraction of teeth. There has been a long history of debate in orthodontics regarding the merits of extraction-based treatment (Box. 7.6); however, the decision to extract and the choice of teeth will depend upon a number of factors.

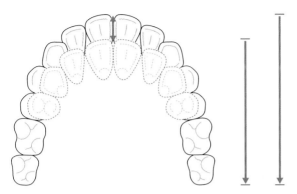

Figure 7.7 To reduce an overjet requires space. If this is created by mid-arch extractions, arch length will shorten.

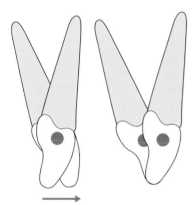

Figure 7.8 Correcting the inclination of a retroclined upper labial segment will require space to prevent an increase in the overjet.

Degree and site of crowding

Dental crowding most commonly manifests in the incisor regions but it is not routine practice to remove these teeth, particularly in the maxillary arch, because they are integral to both dental and smile aesthetics. If the degree of crowding is severe enough to require extraction, teeth are usually removed from the buccal segments. However, the further a tooth is situated from the site of crowding, the less space will be available for tooth alignment. It is also mechanically simpler to extract teeth closer to the site of the crowding.

For the alignment of incisors where moderate to severe crowding exists, first premolar teeth are often the first choice for extraction. Indeed, if correctly timed, the extraction of first premolars can allow for much spontaneous relief of dental arch crowding in a growing child, particularly if the mandibular canines are mesially angulated and the maxillary canines buccally displaced. Inappropriate extraction of first premolars in cases with mild crowding can lead to excessive space and over-retraction of the labial segments following space closure with fixed appliances. Therefore, if dental crowding is mild, consideration should be given to extraction of second premolars, or non-extraction treatment if possible. General guidelines for extraction in the lower arch are given in Table 7.5.

Box 7.6 The great extraction debate

The debate regarding the merits of extractions in orthodontics is as old as the specialty itself and has at times been both emotive and vitriolic. Edward Angle was vehemently opposed to extractions, because he felt that achieving ideal aesthetics and stability necessitated having an intact dentition. To achieve his goals the dental arches were invariably expanded and any overjet corrected with heavy elastic wear. Bone had been shown to remodel under stress in the peripheral skeleton and Angle assumed he was growing alveolar bone with his appliances. Unfortunately, ideal aesthetics and stability were not necessarily achieved in many cases, but despite the protestations of a few, the influence of Angle was so great that non-extraction treatment was the norm in America until the 1940s.

Following the death of Angle, one of his former pupils, Charles Tweed, presented cases that he had re-treated following relapse with the extraction of four premolar units, which showed greater stability and less protrusion of the dentition and soft tissues. Another former student of Angle, Raymond Begg, also concluded that premolar extraction was justified in many cases. Treatment became based around camouflaging skeletal discrepancies and to achieve this, extractions were often necessary.

However, the pendulum soon swung again. From longitudinal studies over several decades, it became apparent that extracting teeth provided no guarantee for long-term stability. Facially, the current desire is for a fuller, more youthful profile, which is aided by non-extraction treatment. There is also a fear of litigation in some quarters following successful claims alleging temporomandibular dysfunction associated with retraction-based orthodontics following extraction. With modern appliances expansion is easy, and many patients can be treated without extraction. However, despite re-branding this as arch development, expansion of the lower arch is still inherently unstable and should be avoided.

One of greatest criticisms leveled at mid-arch premolar extraction as part of orthodontic treatment is that it can lead to flattening or a dishing-in of the facial profile and a loss of face height. These claims are often supported by the use of anecdotal case reports; however, the current body of evidence would suggest that they are not true. Certainly, after extractions the soft tissues are often slightly more retrusive at the end of treatment, but the differences between extraction and non-extraction cases are minimal and difficult to judge (Rushing et al, 1995). Even in borderline cases, both extraction and non-extraction patients have been perceived to benefit in terms of the soft tissue profile from orthodontic treatment (Paquette et al, 1992). In fact, lip retraction must be considerable before the profile is regarded as unattractive by dental professionals and the general public (Bowman & Johnston, 2000). How the soft tissues of the lower face respond to movement of the incisors is complex and difficult to predict, and there is wide individual variation.

Table 7.5 Guidelines for extraction in the lower arch

Amount of crowding	Extraction choice
Mild (1–4 mm)	Non-extraction or second premolars
Moderate (5–8 mm)	First or second premolars
Severe (9+ mm)	First premolars

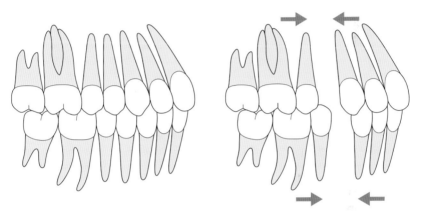

Figure 7.9 If the buccal segment is class I, extracting the same tooth in both arches will help maintain it.

Crowding in the buccal segments is often a consequence of early loss of deciduous molars. Although this can be relieved by the loss of a premolar it can result in excessive space. The loss of second molars can provide a small amount of space, particularly in the lower buccal segment for the relief of crowding. However, this benefit must be tempered with the difficulty associated with extracting these teeth in a young child, the problematic nature of achieving a good eruptive position of the third molar and the fact that little space will be available for relief of crowding in the labial segment (Richardson & Richardson, 1993; Thomas & Sandy, 1995). In the upper arch, second molar extraction provides little mesial space, but does facilitate distalization of the buccal segments with headgear and is associated with more reliable third molar eruption.

Type of malocclusion
In a class I malocclusion requiring premolar extraction to relieve crowding in the mandibular arch, the corresponding premolar teeth are usually extracted from the maxillary arch. This helps maintain the buccal segment relationship as class I (Fig. 7.9).

In a class II malocclusion, one of the aims of treatment will be to correct the incisor relationship and as such, space requirements are often larger in the maxillary arch. Again, if premolar extractions are required to treat crowding in the mandibular arch, it is usual practice to extract at least as far forward in the maxilla. A

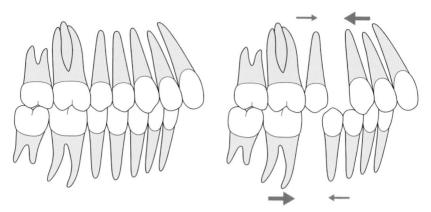

Figure 7.10 If the buccal segment is class II, extracting further distally in the lower arch will help correction.

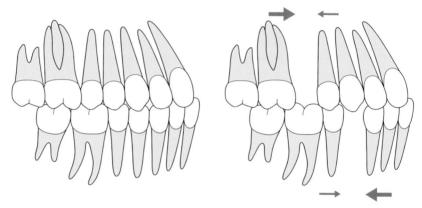

Figure 7.11 If the buccal segment is class III, extracting more mesially in the lower arch will help correction.

common extraction pattern for class II cases involves lower second premolars and upper first premolars, which aids both molar and incisor correction, but this will depend upon the space requirements in the mandibular arch (Fig. 7.10). If they are great, it may be necessary to extract first premolars; if space requirements are minimal in the mandibular arch, a decision may be taken to extract in the upper arch only, correcting the malocclusion and finishing to a class II molar relationship.

Conversely, in class III malocclusions, the mandibular incisors may need to be moved lingually, which will increase the space requirement in the lower arch. If premolar extractions are needed, it is usual practice to extract further forward in the lower arch than in the upper. In these circumstances, extraction of lower first premolars and upper second premolars is a common choice (Fig. 7.11). If the upper arch is well aligned, an alternative is the extraction of lower premolars only, finishing with a class III molar relationship after incisor retraction; or even a single lower incisor to allow retroclination of the remaining lower incisors to correct the class III incisor relationship

(Fig. 7.12). However, any extractions in the lower arch of a class III case should be planned with care (see Box 7.4).

Presence and position of teeth

In cases of hypodontia, upper lateral incisors and lower second premolars are often absent. If one upper lateral incisor is congenitally missing, loss of the remaining upper lateral incisor is often a viable option to maintain arch symmetry, especially if it is diminutive in form. This may also involve modifying the shape of the maxillary canine crowns to more resemble lateral incisors (Fig. 7.13). In addition, when the upper lateral incisors are palatally crowded, their extraction can simplify and shorten treatment considerably.

Maxillary canines are commonly associated with impaction; although not usually a choice for extraction, if the malocclusion requires space provision in the maxillary arch and one or both canines are in a poor position, consideration can be given to their removal (Fig. 7.14).

Dental health of teeth

Heavily restored, carious or hypoplastic teeth should always be considered for elective extraction in the developing dentition, particularly if arch space is required. Similarly, during planning for orthodontic extractions, a potentially compromised tooth should always be removed in preference to a healthy one. First permanent molars with a poor long-term prognosis are often encountered and these teeth are not usually a routine

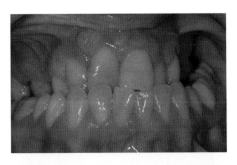

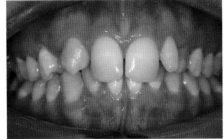

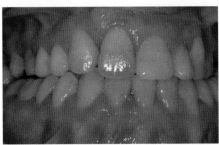

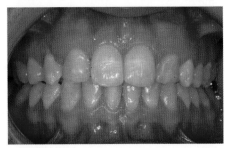

Figure 7.12 Extraction of a lower incisor to correct a class III incisor relationship.

Figure 7.13 Extraction of a diminutive UL2 to balance a congenitally absent contralateral tooth. Courtesy of Padhraig Fleming.

choice for orthodontic extraction as the space created is distant from the site of crowding. However, with the use of fixed appliances and careful anchorage management, the extraction of first molars can be considered as a treatment option in cases where their prognosis is poor (Fig. 7.15).

Upper central incisors are the teeth most commonly affected by trauma. Their importance for dental aesthetics means that they are not usually electively extracted; however, if the prognosis is such that extraction is required, whether an acceptable

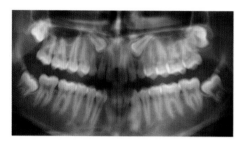
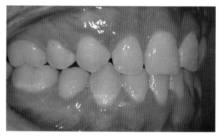

Figure 7.14 Poorly positioned maxillary canines electively extracted as part of an orthodontic treatment plan. The maxillary first premolar makes a good substitute for the canine. Courtesy of Padhraig Fleming.

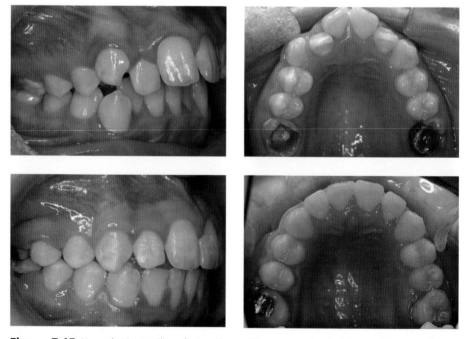

Figure 7.15 Hypoplastic maxillary first molars, which were extracted to provide space for the relief of crowding and reduce the overjet.

result can be achieved with space closure depends on the form and shape of the lateral incisors (Fig. 7.16).

Transverse arch expansion

Increasing dental arch dimensions, in both the anteroposterior and transverse planes can create space. Problems with this strategy can arise because the teeth occupy a zone of equilibrium between the soft tissue forces of the tongue on one side and the lips and cheeks on the other. If the teeth are moved excessively in either buccal or labial directions, they will move outside this zone of stability and potentially be subject to unbalanced forces that will tend to return them to their previous position. In particular, there are significant restrictions on how far the position of the teeth can be changed in the lower arch, especially the intercanine width. This dimension is established early during development of the dentition and any subsequent expansion is inherently unstable (Fig. 7.17). Expansion of the lower arch to relieve labial segment crowding should therefore be avoided.

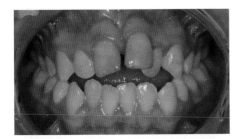

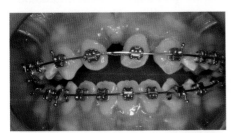

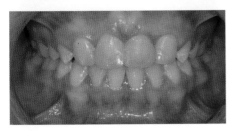

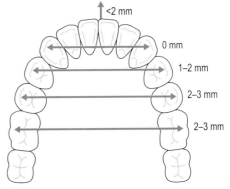

Figure 7.16 Upper central incisors with a history of trauma that became ankylosed were extracted and replaced by the lateral incisors, which were subsequently built up with composite. Courtesy of Padhraig Fleming.

Figure 7.17 Limits of expansion in the lower arch. Redrawn from Ackerman JL and Proffit WR (1997). Soft tissue limitations in orthodontics: treatment planning guidelines. *Angle Orthod* 67:327–336.

In contrast, some expansion of the maxillary arch is appropriate in the presence of a buccal crossbite, especially when there is an associated displacement. This can be achieved with either fixed or removable appliances, but the space created within an arch is equal to only approximately half the amount of expansion (O'Higgins & Lee, 2000). In addition, regardless of the method, any maxillary arch expansion will be associated with some relapse in the long-term.

Anteroposterior arch lengthening

Anteroposterior space can also be created by distal movement of the buccal segments. In the mandibular arch this is mechanically difficult to achieve and is rarely attempted. In the maxillary arch it can be achieved by the use of extraoral traction applied to the first permanent molars, particularly prior to eruption of the second molars or following their extraction. However, even with very good headgear wear, it is difficult to correct a full unit class II molar relationship by distal movement in the absence of favourable maxillary and mandibular growth.

Anteroposterior space can also be created by proclination of the incisors. This would seem an attractive option, particularly in the lower arch where crowding often occurs. In addition, it is mechanically simple to procline the lower incisors with fixed appliances and modern superelastic archwires. However, for the reasons outlined earlier, there is an inherent tendency for these teeth to return to their pre-treatment position in the absence of permanent retention. Moreover, the excessive labial movement of either the upper or lower incisor teeth can have significant negative consequences for facial aesthetics (Fig. 7.18).

Reduction of tooth widths

Space can also be created within a dental arch by reducing the width of individual teeth. This is usually done directly by removing enamel with handheld polishing strips,

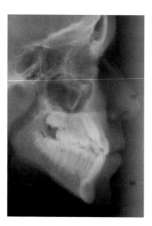 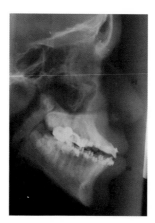 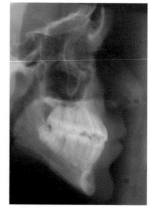

Figure 7.18 A crowded class I case treated with fixed appliances, inappropriate arch expansion and proclination of the labial segments. The mid-treatment radiograph demonstrates the unacceptable position of the incisor teeth. Following the extraction of four first premolars, tooth alignment was maintained, but an acceptable incisor position was achieved following retraction.

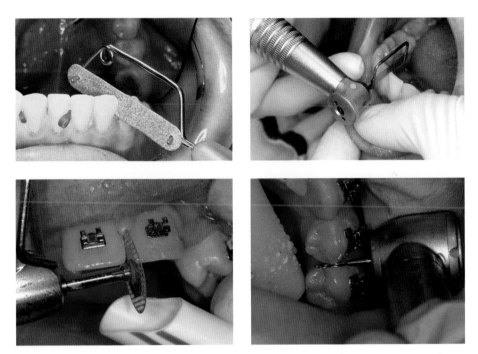

Figure 7.19 Techniques for interproximal reduction of enamel. Handheld or automated strips (top), discs in a contralateral handpiece (bottom left) and air rotor stripping with a tungsten carbide bur (bottom right).

discs with a slow handpiece or fine tungsten carbide and diamond burs with an air turbine (Fig. 7.19). The teeth should be air-cooled during the procedure, as there is a rise in pulp temperature, especially when discs or burs are used. It is also important to leave adequate contact points and no enamel ledges, and therefore should not be undertaken on parallel-sided teeth that have contact points extending subgingivally. Within the buccal segments, up to 1-mm of enamel can be removed at each contact point, but in the labial segments this is less, as the enamel on the teeth is thinner. It appears the newly exposed enamel is no more susceptible to caries, especially if treated with topical fluoride following stripping. The advantage of interdental enamel reduction or stripping, is that a very precise amount of space can be created. However, this is limited and this procedure is only useful in cases with mild crowding.

Planning orthodontic tooth movement

As a general principle, the lower arch dentition is less amenable to change when planning orthodontic treatment, particularly intercanine width and lower incisor inclination. For this reason, the lower arch generally forms the template for any proposed orthodontic tooth movement.

Lower arch

Space is often required in the lower arch for the following:

- Relief of crowding;
- Levelling an increased curve of Spee;
- Correcting a centreline discrepancy; and
- Uprighting distally angulated canines.

Unless all these combined space requirements are mild or the lower incisors are markedly retroclined, extractions will be required to provide the necessary space and the choice will be dictated by the factors outlined above. To relieve lower incisor crowding without proclination, the lower canines will need to be moved distally. The distance the canines need to move will be dictated by the amount of crowding present and this can be measured (Fig. 7.20).

Upper arch

If the dentition is intact and there is no significant discrepancy between the combined size of the maxillary and mandibular tooth crowns, the aim will be to achieve a class I canine and incisor relationship:

- Based upon the position that the lower canines need to be moved to allow alignment of the lower incisors, the necessary movement of the upper canines and anchorage requirements in the upper arch can be planned.
- If the lower arch is being treated non-extraction and the upper canines need to move distally less than half a tooth unit of space, consideration should be given to distal movement of the whole upper buccal segments (certainly in the growing patient). This will usually involve the use of headgear with possible loss of upper second molars.
- If the upper canines need to move distally greater than half a unit of tooth space, first premolar extraction will almost certainly be required in the upper arch, usually with anchorage support. It is possible to generate the space required with distal movement of the upper buccal segments but headgear wear will need to be excellent and growth favourable.

Figure 7.20 To relieve crowding in the lower arch without proclining the lower labial segment, the canines will need to be moved distally. The amount can be gauged by measuring the crowding. The movement required in the maxillary arch to achieve a class I canine relationship can then be estimated.

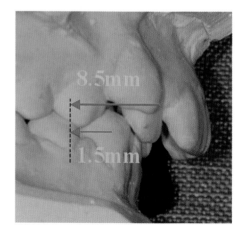

- If the maxillary canines need to move more than a full unit of space, first premolar extraction and distal movement of the buccal segments will be needed.

Buccal occlusion

Correction of the buccal segments will be influenced by the type of malocclusion and may influence the extraction pattern if teeth are to be removed (see Figs 7.9–7.11).

If no extractions are planned in the lower arch and the buccal segment relationship is class I extractions are not indicated in the upper arch. However, if the buccal segment relationship is class II, space will be required to correct this. Depending on how much space is needed, the choice will usually be upper premolar extraction or distal movement of the upper buccal segments. Even in adolescents with good growth, correcting anything greater than a half-unit class II molar relationship by distal movement alone is difficult. Therefore, in the presence of a class II buccal segment relationship, with a well-aligned or only very mildly crowded lower arch where extractions are not planned, extraction of upper premolars is indicated. This will result in a class II molar relationship, which is occlusally and functionally perfectly acceptable.

Incisor relationship

To achieve a class I incisor relationship the following must be achieved:

- Correct overjet;
- Correct overbite; and
- Correct inclination or torque.

The overjet and overbite if increased can be corrected in a growing patient with a functional appliance in the presence of a mild to moderate skeletal class II relationship. Achieving this in the absence of growth or when camouflaging a mild skeletal discrepancy usually requires bodily tooth movement and fixed appliances. As described previously, space will be required in these cases to reduce an increased overjet.

Choice of appliance

Having decided on the tooth movement required to achieve the aims of treatment, the final decision is the appliance system to be used. Orthodontic appliances can be classified as:

- Removable appliances, which can be taken out of the mouth by the patient;
- Functional appliances, which can be either removable or fixed; and
- Fixed appliances, which are attached directly to the teeth.

Generally, removable appliances are used for simple tooth movement, such as individual tipping or limited expansion (see Chapter 8). They can also be used as an adjunct to fixed appliances, particularly during bite opening and molar distalization, or prior to functional appliance therapy to facilitate mandibular postural advancement. Functional appliances are used in the growing patient, often in conjunction with extraoral force, to help correct both sagittal and vertical skeletal discrepancies, usually prior to the use of fixed appliances (see Chapter 8). Fixed appliances are the most popular form of appliance currently in use today because they can effect complex three-dimensional tooth movements in the management of many different types of malocclusion (see Chapter 9).

Limiting factors to orthodontic treatment

At the end of treating planning the orthodontist should have a list of treatment aims and the strategy for their achievement. There are often several options available for any given malocclusion, including no treatment and the factors that may limit what can theoretically be achieved for any given patient should also be considered.

Limiting factors relating to the patient

A number of potential limiting factors will relate directly to the patient:

- Medical health—certain medical conditions will preclude complex appliance therapy.
- Dental health—excellent oral hygiene and an absence of active dental disease are prerequisites prior to orthodontic treatment. Fixed appliances in particular, can exacerbate dental problems. This does not mean precluding patients with a history of periodontal disease from treatment. However, the disease must be controlled and in a period of remission before treatment can be considered (Boyd et al, 1989). If tooth movement is carried out in the presence of active periodontal disease it will hasten bone loss.
- Age of the patient—growth can be utilized in adolescent patients to help correct a skeletal discrepancy; however, in adults the orthodontist must rely upon tooth movement or surgery. A deep bite in a growing individual can be corrected using a bite plane, which allows extrusion of the posterior dentition. In an adult this is unstable because there will be no potential for compensatory growth at the condyle as the lower face height increases.
- Patient compliance—the success of orthodontic treatment is very much dependent on good patient compliance, but this is difficult to measure. It cannot be predicted based on personality or demographics, although patient perception of their own malocclusion and the relationship between patient and orthodontist may give some indication. It is important to tailor treatment to the level of compliance a patient is perceived to be capable of achieving (Fig. 7.21). If appliances that require high-level compliance, such as extraoral traction, are going to be used, these should be fitted initially to assess the patient response prior to the extraction of teeth. It should also be borne in mind that compliance will decline over treatment and is affected by negative experiences in treatment such as pain and discomfort.

Limiting factors relating to the malocclusion

A number of limiting factors will also be influenced by the presenting malocclusion:

- The more severe the skeletal discrepancy, the harder it is to correct with orthodontic tooth movement alone. Tooth movement to camouflage a severe discrepancy may be physically impossible (Handelman, 1996) or may result in unacceptable compromise to the soft tissue profile. This is especially true in class III malocclusion

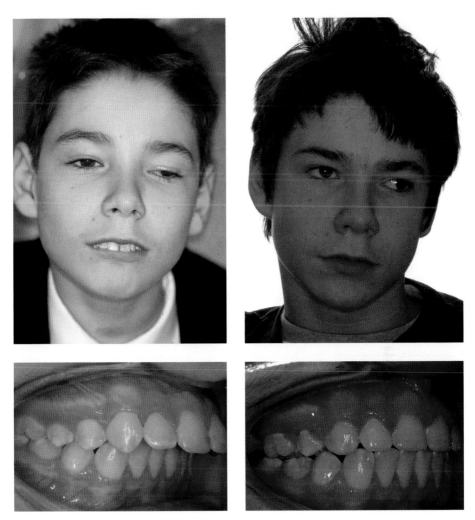

Figure 7.21 Patient with cerebral palsy and an increased overjet associated with a severe class II skeletal base. Orthodontic treatment was limited to the upper arch and there was significant improvement in the occlusion and facial appearance.

and when there is a marked vertical growth pattern such as an anterior open bite, as any further growth will often not be favourable.

- A tooth size discrepancy can compromise obtaining an ideal occlusal fit, especially between the anterior teeth. To obtain a good occlusal fit and an ideal static occlusion, the total mesiodistal dimension of the mandibular dentition should be approximately 92% of that in the maxilla. The ratio of these dimensions was ascertained from ideal occlusions and is called the Bolton ratio after its originator,

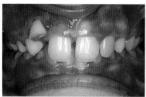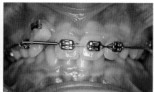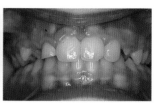

Figure 7.22 Use of an upper fixed appliance to extrude a previously intruded UR2

Wayne Bolton (Bolton, 1958). One of the commonest manifestations of a tooth size discrepancy is a diminutive lateral incisor. This can be clinically masked by a composite buildup of the diminutive teeth or reducing the width of teeth in the opposing arch.

- Hypodontia has implications for space management, especially in the absence of crowding, and space closure can be difficult, especially if numerous teeth are missing.

Orthodontics and dentoalveolar trauma

Trauma to the upper labial segment is very common in childhood and often seen in young children with an increased overjet. Orthodontic attachments can be used in the acute management of trauma, to stabilize teeth following avulsion and to reposition luxated or intruded teeth (Fig. 7.22).

When planning elective orthodontic treatment for a patient with a history of dental trauma, it should be remembered that several long-term complications can occur as a result of orthodontic forces being applied to these teeth:

- Loss of vitality.
- Pulpal calcification, and,
- Root resorption.

Prior to treatment, teeth with a history of trauma need to be carefully assessed both clinically and radiographically, which includes vitality testing and specific periapical radiographs. Traumatized teeth should also be monitored during active treatment, repeating radiographs 6–9 months after commencing tooth movement, and if there is any sign of root resorption, instituting a pause in active treatment of 3 months (Malmgren et al, 1994).

If a tooth is traumatized during or just prior to treatment, a rest period is again recommended, when no active force should be placed on the tooth. This varies in length, depending upon what injury was sustained:

- Uncomplicated crown fracture—3 months.
- Complicated crown fracture—until radiographic evidence of a hard tissue barrier.
- Subluxation—3 months.
- Lateral luxation—3 months.
- Intrusion—12 months.
- Extrusion—12 months.
- Re-implantation—12 months.
- Root fracture—12 to 24 months, if healing of dentine and cementum occurs. If connective tissue healing is present, treat as for teeth with short roots (light forces).

Further Reading

DIBIASE AT (2002). The timing of orthodontic treatment. *Dent Update* 29:434–441.

SARVER DM (2001). The importance of incisor positioning in the esthetic smile: the smile arc. *Am J Orthod Dentofacial Orthop* 120:98–111.

SHAH AA AND SANDLER J (2006). Limiting factors in orthodontic treatment: 1. Factors related to patient, operator and orthodontic appliances. *Dent Update* 33:43–44, 46–48, 51–52.

SHAH AA AND SANDLER J (2006). Limiting factors in orthodontic treatment: 2. The biological limitations of orthodontic treatment. *Dent Update* 33:100–102, 105–106, 108–110.

References

ACKERMAN JL AND PROFFIT WR (1997). Soft tissue limitations in orthodontics: treatment planning guidelines. *Angle Orthod* 67:327–336.

BACCETTI T, REYES BC AND MCNAMARA JA JR (2007). Craniofacial changes in Class III malocclusion as related to skeletal and dental maturation. *Am J Orthod Dentofacial Orthop* 132:171 e1–171 e12.

BOLTON WA (1958). Disharmony in tooth size and its relation to the analysis and treatment of malocclusion. *Am J Orthod* 28:113–130.

BOWMAN SJ AND JOHNSTON LE Jr (2000). The esthetic impact of extraction and nonextraction treatments on Caucasian patients. *Angle Orthod* 70:3–10.

BOYD RL, LEGGOTT PJ, QUINN RS ET AL (1989). Periodontal implications of orthodontic treatment in adults with reduced or normal periodontal tissues versus those of adolescents. *Am J Orthod Dentofacial Orthop* 96:191–198.

HANDELMAN CS (1996). The anterior alveolus: its importance in limiting orthodontic treatment and its influence on the occurrence of iatrogenic sequelae. *Angle Orthod* 66:95–109; discussion 109–110.

HARRISON JE AND ASHBY D (2001). Orthodontic treatment for posterior crossbites. *Cochrane Database Syst Rev* CD000979.

HARRISON JE, O'BRIEN KD AND WORTHINGTON HV (2007). Orthodontic treatment for prominent upper front teeth in children. *Cochrane Database Syst Rev* CD003452.

KIM JH, VIANA MA, GRABER TM ET AL (1999). The effectiveness of protraction face mask therapy: a meta-analysis. *Am J Orthod Dentofacial Orthop* 115:675–685.

KIRSCHEN RH, O'HIGGINS EA AND LEE RT (2000a). The Royal London Space Planning: an integration of space analysis and treatment planning: Part I: Assessing the space required to meet treatment objectives. *Am J Orthod Dentofacial Orthop* 118:448–455.

KIRSCHEN RH, O'HIGGINS EA AND LEE RT (2000b). The Royal London Space Planning: an integration of space analysis and treatment planning: Part II: The effect of other treatment procedures on space. *Am J Orthod Dentofacial Orthop* 118:456–461.

LITTLE RM, RIEDER RA, STEIN A (1990). Mandibular arch length increase during the mixed dentition: Postretention evaluation of stability and relapse. *Am J Orthod Dentofacial Orthop* 97:393–404.

LUTHER F (2007a). TMD and occlusion part I. Damned if we do? Occlusion: the interface of dentistry and orthodontics. *Br Dent J* 202:E2; discussion 38–9.

LUTHER F (2007b). TMD and occlusion part II. Damned if we don't? Functional occlusal problems: TMD epidemiology in a wider context. *Br Dent J* 202:E3; discussion 38–9.

MALMGREN O, MALGREN B, GOLDSTON L (1984). Orthodontic management of the traumatized dentition. In: Andreasen JO, Andreasen FM, eds. Textbook and Colour Atlas of Traumatic Injuries to the Teeth. 3rd edn. Cpenhagen, Mosby. pp. 587–631.

MILLS JRE (1966). Long-term results of the proclination of lower incisors. *Br Dent J* 120:355–363.

MILLS JRE (1968). The stability of the lower labial segment. *Dent Pract* 18:293–306.

O'HIGGINS EA AND LEE RT (2000). How much space is created from expansion or premolar extraction? *J Orthod* 27:11–13.

PAQUETTE DE, BEATTIE JR AND JOHNSTON LE JR (1992). A long-term comparison of nonextraction and premolar extraction edgewise therapy in 'borderline' Class II patients. *Am J Orthod Dentofacial Orthop* 102:1–14.

PARK YC and BURSTONE CJ (1986). Soft-tissue profile–fallacies of hard-tissue standards in treatment planning. *Am J Orthod Dentofacial Orthop* 90:52–62.

RAMOS AL, SAKIMA MT, PINTO ADOS S ET AL (2005). Upper lip changes correlated to maxillary incisor retraction–a metallic implant study. *Angle Orthod* 75:499–505.

RICHARDSON ME AND RICHARDSON A (1993). Lower third molar development subsequent to second molar extraction. *Am J Orthod Dentofacial Orthop* 104:566–574.

RUSHING SE, SILBERMAN SL, MEYDRECH EF ET AL (1995). How dentists perceive the effects of orthodontic extraction on facial appearance. *J Am Dent Assoc* 126:769–772.

THOMAS P AND SANDY JR (1995). Should second molars be extracted? *Dent Update* 22:150–156.

8 Contemporary removable appliances

Removable appliances are not permanently attached to the teeth and can be taken out of the mouth by the patient. During the first half of the twentieth century, orthodontic practice in Europe was based largely on the use of removable appliances. However, over the past few decades there has been a significant decline in their use, primarily as a result of more efficient fixed appliances being available and an increase in numbers of orthodontic specialists able to use them. However, simple removable appliances retain a place in modern orthodontic practice, usually as an adjunct to fixed appliance therapy or for use in the retention phase of treatment. In particular, a group of predominantly removable functional appliances, used primarily in the management of class II malocclusion, have enjoyed a considerable resurgence in popularity in recent years. In addition, new treatment systems using vacuum-formed removable appliances, not only for retention, but also for active tooth movement have been developed.

Tooth movement with removable appliances

A variety of tooth movements can be achieved with removable appliances, either individually or on groups of teeth:
- Tipping;
- Overbite reduction;
- Crossbite correction;
- Extrusion; and
- Intrusion.
  Removable appliances are also useful in maintaining tooth positions during retention.

Tipping
Unlike fixed appliances, which can control the movement of a tooth in three dimensions, the force applied by a removable appliance is mediated by a spring, elastic or piece of acrylic, which can only make point contact with the tooth. As no reactionary force or couple is created, in these situations removable appliances are only capable of simple tooth tipping and apical or bodily movement is not possible. Tipping can be carried out in mesial, distal, buccal or lingual directions, with the rotation occurring about a fulcrum located close to the middle of the tooth root. For the retraction of teeth already mesially inclined, tipping can be an effective tooth movement; but it is inappropriate for teeth that are upright or distally inclined (Fig. 8.1).

Overbite reduction
Incorporating an anterior bite plane on a removable appliance will increase the vertical dimension and allow differential eruption of the posterior teeth, which in a growing patient is an effective way to reduce a deep overbite.

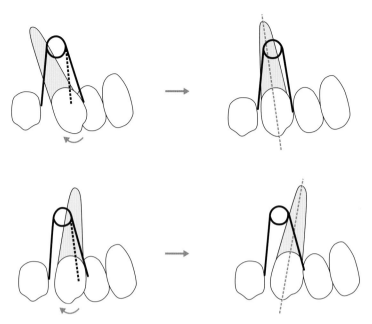

Figure 8.1 Tipping of a tooth with a removable appliance is appropriate if it needs uprighting but inappropriate if the tooth is already angulated in the direction of the intended movement. In this case a mesially angulated canine can be uprighted with an activated spring (upper panels), but this is inappropriate if the tooth is already distally angulated as this would lead to excessive tipping (lower panels).

Anterior crossbite
If space is available, an anterior tooth in crossbite can be pushed over the bite using a removable appliance with an activated palatal spring or screw. Stability will depend upon achieving a positive overbite on the corrected teeth, to prevent them relapsing back into crossbite.

Posterior crossbites
By incorporating a midline expansion screw or spring in an upper removable appliance, the maxillary arch can be widened. This is effective for the correction of posterior crossbites in the mixed dentition, but will produce only tipping of the buccal teeth; the crossbite should therefore be dental not skeletal in origin.

Extrusion
A whip-spring or elastic from a removable appliance can be used to extrude teeth by engaging a fixed attachment on a tooth to generate a vertical component of force. This can be useful for extrusion of an impacted central incisor in the mixed dentition (see Fig. 10.22).

Intrusion
An elastic run underneath a fixed attachment or bracket via a removable appliance can be used to intrude teeth (Fig. 8.2). Good retention is required, as the reaction to any intrusive force will tend to unseat a poorly retained appliance.

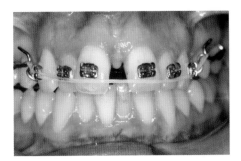

Figure 8.2 Intrusion of the upper labial segment with an elastic attached to an upper removable appliance.

Retention

Removable appliances are routinely used as retainers to maintain the position of teeth following active orthodontic treatment. There are numerous designs available, but the commonest are:

- Hawley;
- Begg;
- Barrer; and
- Vacuum form or Essix.
  Retention is discussed in Chapter 11.

Components of removable appliances

Removable appliances are composed of retentive and active components connected together by a baseplate. When designing a removable appliance, consideration also needs to be given towards anchorage, ensuring that the desired teeth will move under the active force applied by the appliance (Box 8.1).

Retentive components

The retentive components of a removable appliance are concerned primarily with seating it in the correct position, but they can also contribute towards anchorage.

Adams clasp

Adams clasps are constructed in 0.7-mm stainless steel wire and most commonly used on the first molars (Fig. 8.3), although they can be used on premolars and anterior teeth. The arrowheads of the clasp engage undercuts at the mesial and distal corners of the buccal tooth surface and can easily be adjusted at the chairside to increase retention. The bridge of an Adams clasp can also be used by the patient to remove the appliance from the mouth, whilst the orthodontist can use it to attach auxiliary springs or tubes for headgear.

Southend clasp

The Southend clasp is also constructed in 0.7-mm stainless steel wire, but is used for retention on the incisor teeth (Fig. 8.4). This clasp is activated by bending the U-loop towards the baseplate, which carries the clasp back into the labial undercut of the tooth.

Box 8.1   Principles of removable appliance design

The starting point for the design of any removable orthodontic appliance is deciding upon the desired tooth movements and how these will be achieved by the active components. Once these points have been addressed, consideration must be given to retention, anchorage and connecting all the components together using the baseplate. Retention is the mechanism by which the appliance stays in the mouth and is provided by passive components such as clasps and labial bows. Good retention is important to ensure that the active components of the appliance are correctly placed and therefore effective. A retentive appliance is also easier for the patient to wear and therefore optimizes patient compliance.

Anchorage for a removable appliance is provided from either an intra- or extraoral source. Intraoral anchorage comes primarily from the palate and dentition of the same dental arch (intramaxillary); whilst extraoral anchorage is from headgear attached to the appliance. In certain circumstances anchorage is reciprocal when the planned tooth movements for active and reactive components are equal. However, the aim is often for specific teeth to be moved by the appliance, with others remaining stationary. To prevent undesirable tooth movement and anchorage loss, active forces should be kept light and reactionary forces reduced by limiting the number of teeth being moved at any one time. This may mean only activating one spring at a time or providing more than one appliance in order to achieve the treatment aims.

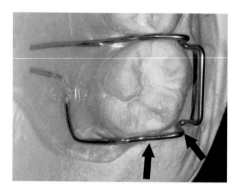

Figure 8.3 Adams clasp. Adjustment at the arrowhead of the clasp (right arrow) will move it horizontally whilst adjustment at the point the wire emerges from the base plate (left arrow) will move the arrowhead vertically.

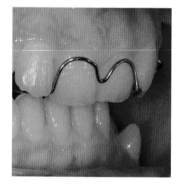

Figure 8.4 Southend clasp.

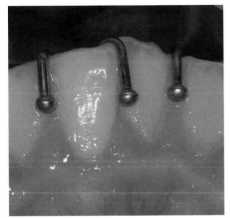

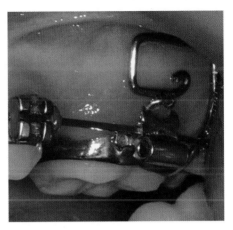

Figure 8.5 Ball-ended clasps.   **Figure 8.6** Plint clasp.

Ball-ended clasp
Ball-ended clasps engage into interproximal undercuts between the teeth (Fig. 8.5) and are activated by bending the ball towards the contact point.

Plint clasp
Plint clasps are useful when using a removable appliance in combination with a fixed appliance (Fig. 8.6). These clasps are constructed in 0.7-mm stainless steel and engage the undercuts on a maxillary molar band.

Labial bow
A labial bow is constructed from 0.7-mm stainless steel wire and can provide retention from the labial surface of the incisor teeth, which can be increased by contouring the wire around these teeth in a fitted labial bow or by placing an acrylic facing on the wire of the bow (Fig. 8.7). The labial bow is afforded flexibility by incorporating U-loops at each end, which allow activation by compression.

Active components
The active components of a removable appliance are responsible for producing the desired tooth movement. They can be categorized as springs, bows, screws and auxiliary elastics.

Springs
Mechanical principles should be considered when applying a force to any tooth with a spring:
- It should be delivered at right angles to the long axis of the tooth and through a surface parallel to it; otherwise, a vertical force is introduced, which will tend to displace the appliance or intrude the tooth.
- It should pass as close to the centre of resistance as possible to reduce rotation.

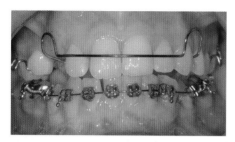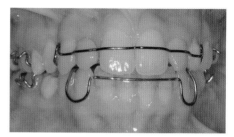

Figure 8.7 Standard (left), fitted (right upper) and acrylic-faced (right lower) labial bows.

The force (F) delivered by a spring is related to the length (L) and thickness or radius of the wire (R), as well as the deflection (D), such that

$$F \propto DR^4/L^3$$

Therefore, lighter forces can be delivered by increasing the length of the wire or reducing its diameter; however, this will make the spring more susceptible to distortion and breakage. This can be prevented to a degree by shielding the arm of the spring with the acrylic baseplate or sheathing it in steel tubing. Springs are usually constructed in stainless steel, either 0.5-mm in diameter, which are activated approximately 3-mm; or 0.7-mm, which are activated by 1-mm to give a similar force.

Palatal finger springs
Palatal finger springs are constructed in 0.5- or 0.6-mm stainless steel wire and used to move teeth mesially or distally along the dental arch (Fig. 8.8). The incorporation of a helix increases the length of the wire and allows the delivery of lighter forces whilst a guard wire will protect the spring from distortion. By convention, the helix is placed such that activation of the spring is achieved as it is tightened and it unwinds as tooth movement occurs; the spring should be positioned at right angles to the planned tooth movement.

Buccal canine retractor
Buccal canine retractors are constructed in 0.7-mm stainless steel, reduced to 0.5-mm if sheathed (Fig. 8.9). These springs can be used to retract buccally placed maxillary canines; however, when activated it is mechanically difficult to apply force directly to the mesial surface of the tooth.

Z-spring
The Z-spring is constructed in 0.5-mm stainless steel wire and generally used to move one or two teeth labially (Fig. 8.10). Activation is achieved by pulling the spring away from the baseplate at an angle of approximately 45°, which will tend to displace the appliance away from the palate; good anterior retention is therefore important.

T-spring
T-springs are constructed in 0.5-mm stainless steel wire and used to move individual teeth either labially or buccally (Fig. 8.11). Activation is again produced by pulling the spring away from the baseplate and therefore retention also needs to be good.

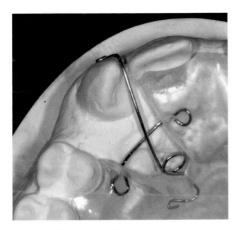

Figure 8.8 Palatal finger spring.

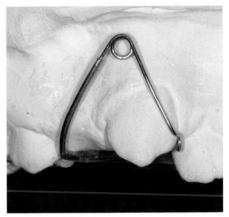

Figure 8.9 Buccal canine retractor.

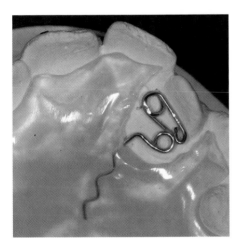

Figure 8.10 Z-spring.

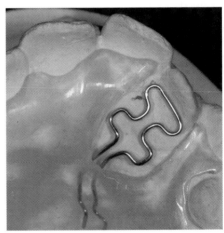

Figure 8.11 T-spring.

Coffin spring

A coffin spring provides a useful alternative to a screw for expansion (Fig. 8.12). This heavy spring is constructed in 1.25-mm wire and activated by pulling the two halves of the appliance apart manually or flattening the spring with pliers. Coffin springs deliver high forces that will tend to displace the appliance and good retention is important.

Active labial bows

An active labial bow can be used to reduce an increased overjet by tipping the teeth palatally if the upper labial segment is proclined and spaced. However, a normal labial bow will only allow a small range of activation and this can be improved either by increasing the amount of wire in the bow, as in a Mills bow, or by constructing it in

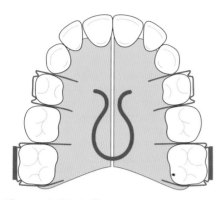

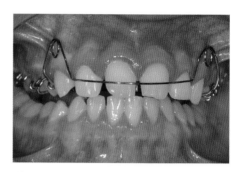

Figure 8.12 Coffin spring in a removable appliance with headgear tubes attached to the first molar cribs.

Figure 8.13 Roberts retractor.

a lighter wire, such as a Roberts retractor (Fig. 8.13). The Roberts retractor is constructed in 0.5-mm stainless steel with buccal arms sheathed in stainless steel tubing. Activation occurs by bending the vertical arms of the bow towards the palate and trimming the acrylic behind the upper incisors to allow palatal movement.

Screws
Screws can be embedded into the baseplate of an appliance and activated by the patient progressively turning a key (Fig. 8.14). Screws can be effective for expansion to correct a posterior dental crossbite, or for distal movement of the buccal segments, often supported by headgear. Each quarter turn of the screw activates it by approximately 0.2-mm and, therefore, should be done by the patient once or twice a week.

Elastics
Elastomeric forces can also be applied from a removable appliance and these can be useful in providing light force, which can be reactivated regularly by the patient. Intra-arch elastics can be used to retract the upper incisors as well as applying an intrusive force in patients with reduced periodontal support (see Fig. 8.2). Inter-arch application of elastics from removable appliances requires good retention to avoid displacement and is generally avoided.

Removable appliance design and use

Comprehensive orthodontic treatment is no longer undertaken with removable appliances alone because the results are invariably inferior to those produced by fixed appliances. However, removable appliances are relatively simple to use (Table 8.1), generally well tolerated by patients and can be used very effectively to correct minor occlusal problems (such as crossbites) in the mixed dentition or provide a valuable adjunct to fixed appliance therapy.

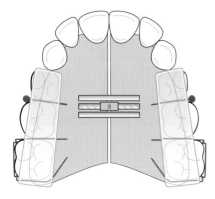

Figure 8.14 Upper removable appliance to correct a posterior crossbite in the mixed dentition. The design includes Adams cribs on the first permanent molars, ball-ended clasps between the deciduous molars, a midline expansion screw and posterior acrylic capping.

Table 8.1 Clinical use of removable appliances

- Impressions taken in alginate;
- Appliance fitted within 2 weeks of the impression to ensure good fit;
- Cribs adjusted for retention, springs activated and acrylic trimmed to allow planned tooth movement;
- Patient given instructions on wear and appliance care;
- Patient reviewed in one month; and
- Signs of good wear include evidence of tooth movement, loosening of the appliance, good speech with the appliance in place and the ability of the patient to insert and remove the appliance unaided.

Expansion

Removable appliances can provide an effective method for expanding the maxillary dental arch, particularly in the mixed dentition (Fig. 8.14):

- The patient activates the appliance by turning a midline screw until the crossbite is overcorrected (the palatal cusps of the maxillary buccal teeth occluding on the incline of the buccal cusps of the mandibular teeth); and
- Following expansion, the posterior capping can be removed and the appliance worn at night for a period of three to six months as a retainer.

Correction of anterior crossbite

Removable appliances are also effective at correcting an anterior crossbite (Fig. 8.15). Palatal Z- or T-springs can be used to correct one or two teeth in anterior crossbite, usually in conjunction with posterior acrylic capping to open the bite and allow movement of the teeth out of crossbite. Occasionally some anterior retention in the form of a Southend clasp may also be required (Fig. 8.16).

Bite plane

In a growing patient, the incorporation of a flat anterior bite plane in a removable appliance allows eruption of the posterior teeth and reduction of a deep overbite (see Fig. 11.15). It can also facilitate earlier placement of a lower fixed appliance without

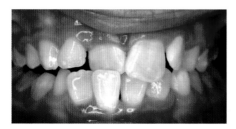 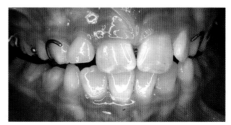

Figure 8.15 Correction of an anterior crossbite with an upper removable appliance.

Figure 8.16 Upper removable appliance to correct an anterior crossbite affecting the UR1 in the mixed dentition. The design includes Adams cribs on the first permanent molars, ball-ended clasps between the deciduous molars, a modified Southend clasp on the UL1, a Z-spring for the UR1 and posterior acrylic capping.

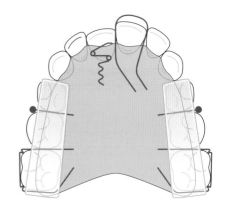

impinging on the occlusion. An inclined bite plane can be useful following functional appliance therapy, either as part of a retainer or as an adjunct during the transition from fixed to functional appliances to help to maintain sagittal correction.

Distal movement of buccal segments

Removable appliances can be used in conjunction with headgear to produce distal movement of the maxillary buccal segments:

- Headgear can be run to a removable appliance via tubes soldered on the molar or premolar cribs (see Fig. 8.12), or via a facebow incorporated directly into the appliance (Fig. 8.17).
- A mechanically more efficient way of applying extraoral traction is directly to fixed bands on the first molars and supplementing this with a removable appliance. The appliance has palatal finger springs placed mesially to the first molars, providing a 24-hour distalizing force and a flat anterior bite plane to aid in overbite reduction (Fig. 8.18). This appliance is often known by the acronym ACCO, standing for *acrylic-cervical-occipital*, depending upon the headgear being used (Cetlin & Ten Hoeve, 1983).

ELSAA

The expansion and *l*abial *s*egment *a*lignment *a*ppliance (ELSAA) is used primarily to align and procline the upper labial segment in class II cases prior to functional appliance therapy. It is particularly useful for creating an overjet when the upper incisors

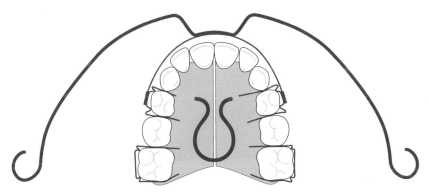

Figure 8.17 The en masse appliance is worn at night and has a headgear facebow directly incorporated. The design includes Adams cribs on the first permanent molars and first premolars, a midline coffin spring and a headgear facebow joined onto tubes on the first premolar cribs.

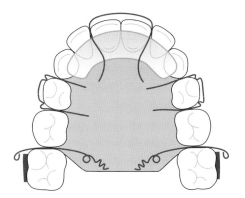

Figure 8.18 THE ACCO appliance to aid molar distalization and reduce a deep overbite. The design includes Adams cribs on the first premolars, a Southend clasp on the upper central incisors, palatal springs mesial to banded first permanent molars and a flat anterior biteplane.

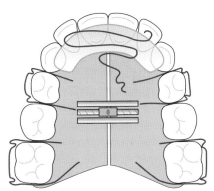

Figure 8.19 The ELSAA appliance to procline the upper incisors, expand the posterior dentition and reduce the overbite. The design includes Adams cribs on the first permanent molars and first premolars, a midline expansion screw, flat anterior bite plane and a re-curved palatal spring behind the upper incisors.

are either upright or retroclined, which usually only takes a few months and then allows good posture of the mandible to be achieved with a functional appliance (Fig. 8.19).

- Incorporation of a midline screw allows for some expansion to prevent a posterior crossbite developing during sagittal correction;
- Palatal springs are activated as the appliance is expanded, which procline and align the incisors; and
- A flat anterior bite plane can also be used to help reduce a deep overbite.

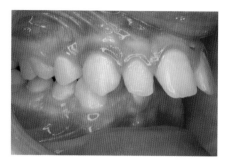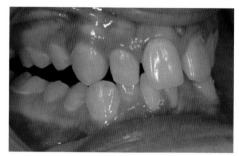

Figure 8.20 Reduction of a large overjet using a functional appliance.

Functional appliances

Functional appliances are a group of largely removable appliances originally developed in Europe during the late nineteenth and early twentieth century. The majority are designed to correct class II malocclusion, primarily by forward posturing of the mandible in a growing child. The term functional jaw orthopoedics was coined for treatment with these types of appliances, which reflected the treatment philosophy underlying their use:

- By changing the functional environment of the dentition, structural adaptation of the orofacial tissues would follow, with an enhancement of growth potential allowing for treatment of sagittal skeletal discrepancies between the jaws.

Whilst this premise is attractive in theory, the mechanism of action associated with functional appliances has remained a matter of some controversy and debate. However, regardless of exactly how they work, it is clear that in certain cases, these appliances can effect a tremendous change in the dental and skeletal relationships of a growing child in a relatively short period of time (Fig. 8.20).

Theories on how functional appliances work
Functional appliances eliminate a sagittal jaw discrepancy by posturing the mandible forward. This postural correction is fundamental to the appliances' mode of action and influences four principle regions:

- Orofacial soft tissues;
- Muscles of mastication;
- Dentition and occlusion; and
- Jaw skeleton.

Orofacial soft tissues
The teeth sit between the tongue on one side and the lips and cheeks on the other. If the balance of these forces is altered, tooth movement can result. Simply correcting the sagittal jaw relationship with a functional appliance can often significantly improve the soft tissue environment surrounding the dentition, particularly in the presence of a lip trap. However, further alteration can also be achieved by incorporating screens or shields constructed in wire or acrylic as part of the appliance, which specifically hold the tongue or cheeks away from the teeth.

Muscles of mastication

Forward posturing of the mandible results in stretch and an alteration in activity of the muscles of mastication, particularly those involved in elevation and retraction of the mandible. These forces will be transmitted to the dentition via the appliance. Electromyographic studies have shown hyperactivity of the lateral pterygoid on protrusion of the mandible (McNamara, 1973). As this muscle is intimately related to the condyle it has been hypothesized that this activity could result in skeletal adaptation. However, some of these earlier studies used cutaneous electromyographic pads and later work using surgically implanted electrodes has shown a reduction in muscular activity on mandibular protrusion (Voudouris et al, 2003), indicating that the lateral pterygoid muscle may not be the primary factor in any skeletal remodelling of the condyle.

Dentition and occlusion

Forward posturing of the mandible also generates an intermaxillary force directed between the maxillary and mandibular dentitions. The class II component of this force can aid significantly with overjet reduction by simply tipping teeth. In addition, the altered mandibular position is also associated with a variable increase in the vertical dimension, which facilitates eruption of the buccal segments. This eruption can be controlled with the use of capping or faceting within the appliance; in particular, allowing eruption of the mandibular buccal teeth in a mesial direction and distal eruption of the maxillary buccal teeth, which aids in the correction of a class II buccal segment relationship and also in overbite reduction (Fig. 8.21).

Jaw skeleton

As a tissue, bone has the capacity to remodel when exposed to functional stimuli, which has been known since the nineteenth century. Sutural growth can be significantly influenced by the application of external force and there is some evidence that the class II force component placed upon the maxilla by a conventional functional appliance can apply some restraint upon forward maxillary growth, particularly when combined with headgear (Vargervik & Harvold, 1985; Wieslander, 1993).

How much effect a functional appliance can have upon growth of the mandible is more controversial. In a primary cartilaginous growth centre, such as the epiphysis of a long bone, growth occurs as a result of proliferation within columns of chrondrocytes and this is under genetic control. A secondary cartilage such as the mandibular condylar cartilage differs, in that stimulating the local functional environment can positively influence cell division and growth. Posturing the mandibular condyle for-

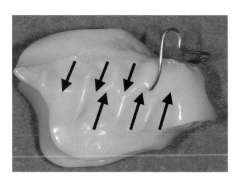

Figure 8.21 Activator appliance. Faceting in the buccal segments encourages differential eruption of the teeth and correction of a class II buccal segment relationship. The lower buccal segments erupt mesially and the upper distally.

wards within the glenoid fossa using a functional appliance should therefore be capable of inducing skeletal change. How much change can be achieved with these appliances has been a subject of great debate within orthodontics for as long as functional appliances have been used. The boundaries of this intellectual spectrum depend upon the relative theories of how facial growth is controlled. If growth is primarily genetically determined, functional appliances will have little effect on the final size of the mandible. However, if one believes that facial growth is controlled by local factors, a functional appliance will change the local environment and exert a significant effect.

Biological effects of functional appliances

The biological effects of functional appliances and mandibular protrusion have been investigated using both animal models and clinical studies.

Animal studies

Various animal models have been used to investigate the effects of functional appliances, including both rodent and primate. Generally, these experiments involve placing fixed splints onto the dentition of these animals, which permanently advance the mandible. There is no doubt that this can produce an increase in proliferation of cells within the condylar cartilage and bony remodelling at the anterior border of the glenoid fossa, and these effects are greater in immature animals that are actively growing (Charlier et al, 1969; McNamara & Bryan, 1987; McNamara et al, 1982; Voudouris et al, 2003; Woodside et al, 1987). However, the applicability of these animal models to humans is somewhat debatable due to differences in morphology, physiology and duration of growth; in particular:

- These experiments often impose an appliance regime on an animal that would not be tolerated by humans;
- Animals grow and mature far more rapidly than humans;
- These experiments often convert a normal occlusion in the animal into a severe malocclusion; and
- Histological, immunohistochemical or gene expression changes induced by an appliance do not necessarily equate to clinically significant growth change.

Clinical evidence

Until relatively recently the majority of clinical evidence associated with the use of functional appliances was obtained from retrospective studies, carried out on small sample groups with poorly matched controls. Cephalometric analysis of these subjects often reported skeletal change and growth as a result of appliance wear, but this was usually based upon cephalometric points difficult to identify and not necessarily representative of true skeletal or soft tissue facial change. This resulted in considerable bias and error; and as such, many of the conclusions of these studies must be viewed with caution (Tulloch et al, 1990).

In the past two decades, several large randomized controlled trials (RCTs) have investigated the effects of early treatment with functional appliances and compared them to untreated controls (Dolce et al, 2007; Ghafari et al, 1998; O'Brien et al, 2003; Tulloch et al, 2004). These trials represent the best current available evidence regarding the clinical use of functional appliances. Three of these studies were carried out in the USA and one in the UK and universally they have shown an initial small but significant increase in mandibular growth in patients undergoing treatment with a functional appliance. However, when these patients were followed through to the end of orthodontic treatment, no significant differences were found between those treated early with a functional appliance and those treated comprehensively later. Any initial growth-related benefits of using a functional appliance were lost in the longer term, a finding that had previously been suggested by retrospective investigations of early functional appliance treatment (Wieslander, 1984, 1993). These RCTs have also demonstrated no significant differences in extraction rates, experience of dentoalveolar trauma or improvements in self-esteem between groups treated with or without a functional appliance. The only significant difference is that the overall treatment time tends to be longer for patients who undergo early treatment with a functional appliance, followed by fixed appliances.

Clinical effects of functional appliances

Numerous types and designs of functional appliance have been described, each with its own treatment philosophy. In essence, all of these appliances have similar effects, with the most significant being dentoalveolar change:

- Retroclination of maxillary incisors;
- Proclination of mandibular incisors;
- Distal tipping of the maxillary dentition;
- Mesial eruption of the mandibular buccal dentition;
- Restraint of forward maxillary development; and
- Forward movement of the mandible due to small additional growth at the condyle and remodelling of the glenoid fossa.

Combined, these effects will result in the correction of a class II dental occlusion, an increase in lower face height and a clockwise rotation of the mandible. Regardless of how a functional appliance corrects a class II discrepancy, their efficiency at doing this can be extremely useful. Converting an occlusion with a class II buccal segment and incisor relationship into one that is class I makes subsequent occlusal detailing with a fixed appliance considerably easier to manage.

Types of functional appliance

There are many different designs of functional appliance, each usually bearing the name of the innovator. They are all designed to posture the mandible forward but they differ in the way this is achieved and how they influence the local soft tissue environment of the jaws and dentition.

Activators

Activators form a group of loosely fitting appliances that come in a single piece or monobloc. They posture the mandible forwards by lingual extension of the acrylic monobloc.

Andresen activator

The activator was originally described by Viggo Andresen and Karl Häupl and consisted of a loose-fitting monobloc appliance that advanced the mandible with lingual flanges (Fig. 8.22). Facets were cut into the acrylic to guide eruption of the mandibular posterior teeth mesially and the maxillary posterior teeth distally and buccally. The original Andresen–Häupl activator was worn at night and had minimal vertical opening. It was

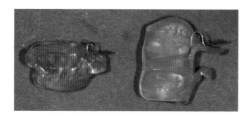

Figure 8.22 Andresen (left) and Harvold (right) activators.

based upon the hypothesis of stimulating increased muscle activity in the mandibular elevator and retractor muscles to act directly on the dentition through the appliance and unload the condyle to allow remodeling and growth.

Woodside or Harvold activator
Later activators such as those described by Donald Woodside (Woodside, 1973) and Egil Harvold (Fig. 8.22) (Harvold & Vargervik, 1971) increased vertical opening beyond the freeway space because these workers believed that the masticatory musculature could not be stimulated during sleep. Therefore to be effective, the appliance had to stretch the orofacial connective tissues, including ligaments and fascial sheets, and direct forces to the teeth and supporting structures. To achieve this a vertical opening of greater than 10-mm was created on protrusion of the mandible, which makes the Woodside and Harvold-type activators more difficult to tolerate and can affect compliance.

Bionator
The Bionator was originally described by Wilhelm Balters and compared to the Andresen activator, the acrylic bulk was considerably reduced to allow increased wear and normal oral function (Fig. 8.23) (Eirew, 1981). A palatal coffin spring was incorporated into the appliance and designed to sit away from the palate, stimulating the tongue to adopt a more anterior position and helping to stabilize the Bionator in the oral cavity. Buccal wire shields were also incorporated to hold the cheeks away from the buccal segments and allow passive expansion of the dental arches.

Activators combined with headgear
Functional appliance wear can encourage a clockwise rotational effect on the dentition and dental bases, which can lead to an increase in the lower face height and greater vertical rather than sagittal change in chin position. To prevent this and optimize skeletal correction in the anteroposterior dimension, headgear can be attached to the appliance. The aim is to restrict anterior and vertical development of the maxilla, whilst encouraging forward mandibular growth.

A number of specific activator-type functional appliance systems which incorporate the use of headgear have been developed. The Teuscher appliance (Teuscher, 1978) (Fig. 8.24) has anterior spurs to torque the upper incisors and prevent their retroclination, allowing the headgear to exert a pull as far forward as possible and prevent the maxilla rotating downwards and backwards. The van Beek appliance (van Beek, 1982) is a modified activator with a headgear directly incorporated into the acrylic, which the patient wears at night and a few hours during the day. The Bass appliance is

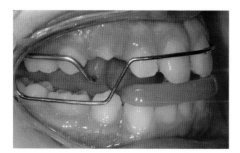

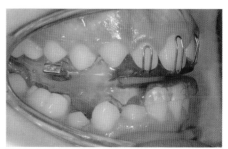

Figure 8.23 Balters bionator.

Figure 8.24 Teuscher appliance.

essentially a maxillary splint to which high-pull headgear is run to restrain maxillary growth, the mandible being guided anteriorly by pads that rest in the lingual sulcus behind the lower incisors (Bass, 1994). Although the logic of using headgear combined with a functional appliance makes some sense, particularly in the presence of skeletal maxillary excess or excessive incisor show in the vertical dimension (a so-called 'gummy' smile) (Orton et al, 1992), the potential benefits are often outweighed by the extra demand placed on compliance.

Medium opening activator (MOA)

The medium opening activator represents a cutback activator with cribs to the maxillary first molars and second premolars to improve retention and make the appliance more tolerable (Fig. 8.25). Mandibular protrusion is achieved via lingual mandibular guidance flanges, with an anterior hole cut into the acrylic to facilitate breathing and speech. The free eruption of mandibular buccal teeth is encouraged, which allows the reduction of a deep overbite at the same time as correcting the overjet.

Fränkel system

A series of removable functional appliances or functional regulators were developed by Rolf Fränkel in what was the German Democratic Republic (Fig. 8.26) (Fränkel, 1980). Fränkel was an advocate of the functional matrix theory of growth, which states that there is no direct genetic influence on the size, shape or position of the skeletal tissues. Rather, bony growth is driven by form and function of the surrounding soft tissues. Fränkel appliances are designed to change the muscular and soft tissue environment of the jaws and therefore modify growth. This is achieved with the use of wires and acrylic shields to displace the cheeks and lips away from the teeth, as well as encouraging forward posture of the mandible. Buccal shields removed pressure from the cheeks to allow for passive arch expansion, whilst theoretically stretching the periosteum to produce additional bony apposition laterally. Lower labial acrylic pads are designed to gently impede activity of the mentalis muscle thought to be an aetiological factor in the increased overjet seen in certain patients. Four types of Fränkel appliances, or functional regulators, have been described for treating class II division 1, class II division 2, class III and anterior open bite malocclusions. The treatment philosophy is based upon full-time wear, but the bulk and fragility of the appliance can make compliance difficult.

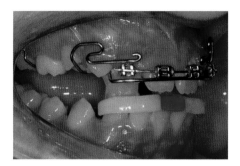

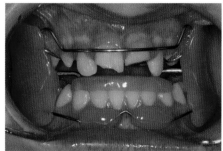

Figure 8.25 Medium opening activator.   **Figure 8.26** Functional regulator 2.

Twin block

William Clark originally described the twin block appliance, which is unusual in consisting of separate upper and lower removable appliances that work in unison (Fig. 8.27) (Clark, 1988). Each appliance incorporates a set of bite blocks that in occlusion posture the mandible forwards. The inclined planes of these blocks are set at approximately 70° with the height greater than 5-mm vertically to ensure that the patient occludes with the lower block in front of the upper and not on it. Overjet reduction can be rapid with a twin block and accompanying changes in the vertical dimension usually do not occur at the same rate, so a lateral open bite is often present at the end of overjet reduction, particularly where the overbite was originally increased (see Fig. 8.20). These open bites can be closed down once the overjet is fully reduced with selective trimming of the upper block to allow eruption of the mandibular first molars, or part-time wear of the appliance. The most significant advantage associated with the twin block is the ease with which it can be worn full-time by a patient and in many respects, this appliance has been responsible for the marked increase in popularity associated with functional appliances in recent years. The twin block also carries a number of other advantages:

- Upper arch expansion can be achieved by incorporating a midline expansion screw;
- Headgear can be easily attached to the upper appliance in cases with maxillary protrusion;
- Fixed appliances can be placed to start alignment of the labial segments without compromising retention of a twin block; and
- This appliance is robust and relatively easy to fabricate.

Herbst appliance

The Herbst appliance is unusual in being a fixed functional appliance cemented or bonded directly to the dentition (Fig. 8.28). Protrusion of the mandible is achieved via a bilateral telescope apparatus attached to maxillary first molar and mandibular first premolar bands. The telescopic arms consist of a tube, plunger and pivot, which allows for opening and some lateral excursion, with these arms advancing the mandible so that the incisors are edge to edge. The fixed nature of this appliance means that effective compliance is not usually an issue and overjet reduction in 6 to 8 months is commonly achieved (Pancherz, 1982). However, potential disadvantages are that the Herbst appliance is expensive to fabricate, is often difficult to tolerate and can be prone to breakage.

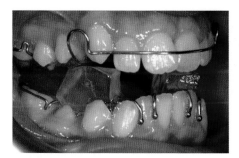

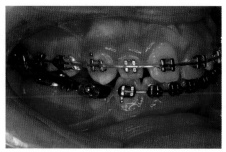

Figure 8.27 Twin block.

Figure 8.28 Herbst appliance. Courtesy of Dirk Bister.

Clinical use of functional appliances

The ideal case for treatment with a functional appliance should have the following clinical features:

- Increased overjet and class II buccal segment relationship;
- Mild to moderate skeletal class II base;
- Average to reduced lower face height;
- Proclined maxillary incisors;
- Retroclined mandibular incisors; and
- Active growth.

Many of the earlier functional appliance systems were developed for treatment without fixed appliances and the patient generally had well-aligned dental arches or only mild crowding. Functional appliances are now often used to correct the skeletal base relationship in the presence of significant crowding, prior to a second phase of treatment with fixed appliances, often in combination with extractions. However, it should be remembered that successful treatment with functional appliances is dependent upon good appliance wear, favourable jaw growth and a well-motivated patient.

Timing of treatment

Functional appliances work most effectively in growing patients; however, the rate of facial and mandibular growth is not constant during childhood and adolescence and can be affected by growth spurts, particularly the pubertal growth spurt. The onset, duration and intensity of the mandibular pubertal growth spurt varies between individuals but generally occurs later in boys than in girls (Box 8.2). Functional appliances appear to have a slightly greater effect on skeletal growth if treatment takes place during this period (Baccetti et al, 2000). However, the precise timing of treatment does not seem to effect the long-term outcome (Tulloch et al, 1997a, b). The advantages of starting treatment in adolescence as opposed to childhood are:

- Skeletal growth will be optimized;
- Treatment will coincide with the late mixed or early permanent dentition;
- It will allow immediate placement of fixed appliances following functional appliance treatment; and
- It will reduce overall treatment and retention time.

Box 8.2 Prediction of adolescent growth

Functional appliances are more effective if their use is timed to coincide with the adolescent growth spurt, or more specifically peak height velocity (PHV) as the peak in adolescent maxillary and mandibular growth occurs at the same time or just after PHV (Baccetti et al, 2000). Generally puberty starts in girls approximately two years before boys and is shorter in duration. The mean PHV occurs at around 12 years of age in girls and 14 in boys (see Fig. 3.3). However, chronological age is a poor predictor as there is a huge range of individual variability. Measurement of height can be used to predict the growth spurt, by taking repeated measurements and plotting them to create a growth curve (Sullivan, 1983). The practical limitation of this method is that it requires several measurements repeated at regular intervals of every four months to construct an individual curve of growth velocity. Measurements must therefore be started at least a year before the earliest possible pubertal spurt, which will be around age 8 in girls and 10 in boys.

To overcome these limitations, various other methods for predicting the timing of PHV have been described, the most popular of which is the use of hand–wrist radiographs. These will give a measure of an individual's skeletal maturity from stages of development of the phalanges and radius, and ossification of the adductor sesamoid of the thumb, which has been reported to precede or coincide with PHV. The predictive value of hand–wrist radiographs appears to improve closer to the PHV, but they need to be obtained at regular intervals to be of use and experience is needed to read them (Houston, 1979). As such, they have fallen out of favour and are rarely used in current orthodontic practice.

Alternate skeletal markers have been described, the most useful of which are the cervical vertebrae. These are usually visible on a lateral skull radiograph and are therefore readily available for examination by the orthodontist. During maturation, the cervical vertebrae increase in height, from wedge-shaped to rectangular and then square, becoming greater in the vertical dimension than horizontal, whilst a concavity also develops on their inferior border (Hassel & Farman, 1995). Their development has been staged and shows good correlation with skeletal maturity as measured from hand–wrist radiographs. Most important are C2, C3 and C4 because PHV and mandibular growth occurs between the times when concavities develop on the inferior borders of C3 and C4 (Franchi et al, 2000). After this point there is a gradual slowing down in adolescent growth.

Earlier treatment starting in the mixed dentition should be considered if there are psychosocial concerns relating to the aesthetic impact of maxillary incisor prominence or there is thought to be a significantly increased risk of trauma due to the increased overjet. Early treatment will necessitate an extended period of retention of any sagittal correction or even re-treatment as there will be a tendency for the original class II

skeletal pattern to reassert itself. The overall treatment time will be therefore significantly increased with no ultimate difference in outcome for the patient compared to
comprehensive treatment started in adolescence. This needs to be explained to the
patient before starting so they can make an informed choice.

Pre-functional stage
To optimize the benefits of using a functional appliance a short period of treatment
prior to fitting the appliance can often be beneficial:
- Maxillary arch expansion to prevent a posterior maxillary lingual crossbite developing following sagittal correction—this can be accomplished using a removable
  appliance with a midline expansion screw. This is not necessary when using a
  functional appliance which allows for maxillary expansion such as a twin block.
- Proclination and alignment of the labial segments if they are retroclined (particularly in a class II division 2 incisor relationship) or if they are crowded—this can be
  done with a removable appliance (see Fig. 8.19) or a sectional fixed appliance run
  either prior to or parallel with the functional appliance (Fig. 8.29).

Impressions and bite
Detailed impressions in alginate should be taken of both dental arches with adequate
extension into the lingual and labial vestibules. This is particularly important if a Fränkel
functional regulator is being prescribed, as the buccal shields and labial pads are made
to actively stretch the mucosa.

All functional appliances posture the mandible forward. To achieve this, they are
constructed on simple articulators with the working models mounted to a postured
bite taken in the mouth. This is usually done in wax, with the mandible as far forwards
as is comfortable (Fig. 8.30).

If the overjet is 10-mm or less this will generally mean the postured bite can be
taken with the incisors in an edge-to-edge relationship. If greater than 10-mm, it is
unlikely that full overjet reduction can be achieved with a single appliance. Rather, the
appliance may need reactivating; either by adjusting it so the mandible is postured
further forwards, or by fabricating a second appliance once the overjet has been
partially reduced (Box 8.3).

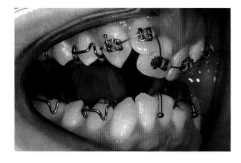

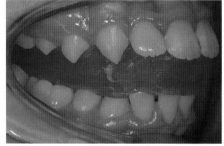

Fig. 8.29 Correction of a class II division 2
incisor relationship with a sectional fixed
appliance and twin block.

Figure 8.30 Wax functional bite.

Box 8.3 One stage versus incremental mandibular advancement

The growth theory subscribed to will affect the clinical use of functional appliances. An example of this is how rapidly the mandible should be advanced with a functional appliance to effect most skeletal change. Advocates of progressive advancement, an increment at a time, argue that this leads to better patient compliance because it is more comfortable and results in greater maintenance of a postured bite during sleep. In addition, a single maximal advancement will generate larger class II forces, which when transmitted to the dentition will result in dentoalveolar rather than skeletal changes (Falck & Fränkel, 1989). Conversely, a single maximum advancement, which stretches the orofacial musculature, should result in a larger physiological response within the muscles and soft tissues, which in turn will generate greater skeletal growth and adaptation. In clinical practice there seems to be little difference in outcomes, either skeletal or dentoalveolar, if the mandible is maximally or incrementally postured forward (Banks et al, 2004). What is probably more important is retention of overjet reduction following active treatment, to allow consolidation of any remodelling within the glenoid fossa and condyle.

Vertically there should be approximately 2-mm of separation between the incisors. The exceptions to this are for Harvold-type activators, which are constructed to open the bite beyond the freeway space and for twin blocks, which require at least 5-mm of vertical separation in the buccal segments to allow for the inclined occlusal planes.

Appliance fitting and review
Appliances should be fitted within two weeks of the impressions being taken to ensure a good fit, as a poorly fitting appliance will negatively impact on compliance.
- The patient should be shown the appliance before fitting.
- Once fitted full instructions, including the minimal hourly wear required per day, should be given.
- The patient should be allowed to practice inserting and removing the appliance. Some clinicians advocate a gradual buildup of hours over several weeks to let the patient get used to wearing the appliance.
- The use of a calendar to record the hours worn may improve compliance and wear.
- The patient should be reviewed one month following appliance fitting and if no problems are reported and the appliance is being worn as instructed, bimonthly thereafter.
- At each visit, the overjet and buccal segment relationship should be recorded. In addition, the overjet should also be recorded in maximum protrusion. The difference between this and the overjet should remain roughly the same, indicating that any overjet reduction is physical as opposed to postural.

- If no change of the overjet or buccal segments is seen within six months of the appliance being fitted, the treatment plan should be reviewed. It is usually due to the appliance not being worn as instructed and unless compliance improves dramatically, continuing with functional appliance treatment will not be successful. Other signs of poor wear are continued problems with speech, a pristine appliance with no signs of wear and numerous breakages due to repeated removal by the patient.

End of treatment with functional appliance and retention

Once the overjet is corrected, wear of the appliance should be continued on a part-time basis to retain the sagittal correction and allow occlusal settling. This is especially relevant when using an appliance such as the twin block, which does not allow free eruption of the buccal segments and often results in a transient lateral open bite at the end of treatment.

- Further records should be collected to help plan any subsequent treatment. This will include a cephalometric lateral skull radiograph, which will help determine how the correction of overjet was achieved. In most cases, further treatment with fixed appliances will be planned to align the dentition and detail the occlusion.
- Unless early treatment was carried out in the mixed dentition, at the end of the functional phase of treatment, the patient will be in the permanent dentition, allowing direct transfer into fixed appliances.
- Further treatment must be planned to consolidate the class II correction achieved with the functional appliance, whilst addressing any undesirable effects such as marked proclination of the lower labial segment. Strategies to achieve this include:
  - Extractions;
  - Reinforcing maxillary anchorage with headgear;
  - Maintaining bite correction with supplementary wear of a removable appliance with an inclined anterior bite plane; and
  - Use of class II elastics.
- Due to the tendency of the original growth pattern to re-establish itself following treatment, retention should be continued until the end of adolescent skeletal growth and incorporate a postural component to maintain the class II correction. This can include part-time wear of a cut-down functional appliance or a removable appliance with an inclined anterior bite plane.

Clear orthodontic aligners—the renaissance of removable appliances

The past decade has seen the introduction of several removable appliance systems, which use a combination of thermoplastic formable materials and three-dimensional computer modelling to treat tooth malalignment. Clear plastic aligners have been available for many years as retainers and small tooth movements are possible by repositioning teeth on the dental study cast or by altering the shape of the aligner with a specially heated instrument.

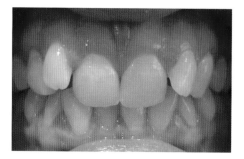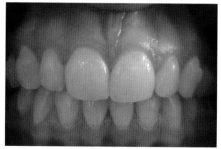

Figure 8.31 Alignment of mild crowding using Invisalign® removable appliances. Courtesy of Mohit Khurana.

More recently, computer technology has allowed high-accuracy dental impressions to be scanned and the creation of a virtual model of the malocclusion, which can then be manipulated (Invisalign®). From these manipulations, a series of removable aligners are fabricated, which the patient wears for approximate two-week intervals. These aligners can be effective for expansion, intrusion and the alignment of mild crowding (Fig. 8.31). Significantly, they are virtually invisible and can be removed by the patient, proving popular with adults. However, whilst they can be combined with fixed attachments for more complex tooth movement they cannot close space and are therefore inappropriate for cases where the degree of crowding warrants tooth extraction.

Further reading

AELBERS CMF AND DERMAUT LR (1996). Orthopedics in orthodontics: part 1, fiction or reality – a review of the literature. *Am J Orthod Dentofacial Orthopedics* 110:513–519.

BISHARA SE (1989). Functional appliances; a review. *Am J Orthod Dentofacial Orthop* 95:250–258.

COZZA P, BACCETTI T, FRANCHI L, ET AL (2005). Mandibular changes produced by functional appliances in Class II malocclusion: a systematic review. *Am J Orthod Dentofacial Orthop* 129:599.e1–599.e12.

MEIKLE MC (2005). Guest editorial: what do prospective randomized clinical trials tell us about the treatment of class II malocclusions? A personal viewpoint. *Eur J Orthod* 27:105–114.

ORTON HS (1990). *Functional Appliances in Orthodontic Treatment* (London: Quintessence).

VIG PS AND VIG KWL (1986). Hybrid appliances: a component approach to dentofacial orthopedics. *Am J Orthod Dentofacial Orthop* 90:273–285.

References

BACCETTI T, FRANCHI L, TOTH LR, ET AL (2000). Treatment timing for Twin-block therapy. *Am J Orthod Dentofacial Orthop* 118:159–170.

BANKS P, WRIGHT J AND O'BRIEN K (2004). Incremental versus maximum bite advancement during twin-block therapy: a randomized controlled clinical trial. *Am J Orthod Dentofacial Orthop* 126:583–588.

BASS NM (1994). Update on the Bass appliance system. *J Clin Orthod* 28:421–428.

CETLIN NM AND TEN HOEVE A (1983). Nonextraction treatment. *J Clin Orthod* 17:396–413.

CHARLIER JP, PETROVIC A and HERRMANN-STUTZMANN J (1969). Effects of mandibular hyperpropulsion on the prechondroblastic zone of young rat condyle. *Am J Orthod* 55:71–74.

CLARK WJ (1988). The twin block technique. A functional orthopedic appliance system. *Am J Orthod Dentofacial Orthop* 93:1–18.

DOLCE C, MCGORRAY SP, BRAZEAU L, ET AL (2007). Timing of Class II treatment: skeletal changes comparing 1-phase and 2-phase treatment. *Am J Orthod Dentofacial Orthop* 132:481–489.

EIREW HL (1981). The bionator. *Br J Orthod* 8:33–36.

FALCK F AND FRANKEL R (1989). Clinical relevance of step-by-step mandibular advancement in the treatment of mandibular retrusion using the Frankel appliance. *Am J Orthod Dentofacial Orthop* 96:333–341.

FRANCHI L, BACCETTI T AND MCNAMARA JA JR (2000). Mandibular growth as related to cervical vertebral maturation and body height. *Am J Orthod Dentofacial Orthop* 118:335–340.

FRÄNKEL R (1980). A functional approach to orofacial orthopaedics. *Br J Orthod* 7:41–51.

GHAFARI J, SHOFER FS, JACOBSSON-HUNT U, ET AL (1998). Headgear versus function regulator in the early treatment of Class II, division 1 malocclusion: a randomized clinical trial. *Am J Orthod Dentofacial Orthop* 113:51–61.

HARVOLD EP AND VARGERVIK K (1971). Morphogenetic response to activator treatment. *Am J Orthod* 60:478–490.

HASSEL B AND FARMAN AG (1995). Skeletal maturation evaluation using cervical vertebrae. *Am J Orthod Dentofacial Orthop* 107:58–66.

HOUSTON WJ (1979). The current status of facial growth prediction: a review. *Br J Orthod* 6:11–17.

MCNAMARA JA JR (1973). Neuromuscular and skeletal adaptations to altered function in the orofacial region. *Am J Orthod* 64:578–606.

MCNAMARA JA JR AND BRYAN FA (1987). Long-term mandibular adaptations to protrusive function: an experimental study in *Macaca mulatta. Am J Orthod Dentofacial Orthop* 92:98–108.

MCNAMARA JA JR, HINTON RJ AND HOFFMAN DL (1982). Histologic analysis of temporomandibular joint adaptation to protrusive function in young adult rhesus monkeys (*Macaca mulatta*). *Am J Orthod* 82:288–298.

O'BRIEN K, WRIGHT J, CONBOY F, ET AL (2003). Effectiveness of early orthodontic treatment with the Twin-block appliance: a multicenter, randomized, controlled trial. Part 2: Psychosocial effects. *Am J Orthod Dentofacial Orthop* 124:488–494; discussion 494–495.

ORTON HS, SLATTERY DA AND ORTON S (1992). The treatment of severe 'gummy' Class II division 1 malocclusion using the maxillary intrusion splint. *Eur J Orthod* 14:216–223.

PANCHERZ H (1982). The mechanism of Class II correction in Herbst appliance treatment. A cephalometric investigation. *Am J Orthod* 82:104–113.

SULLIVAN PG (1983). Prediction of the pubertal growth spurt by measurement of standing height. *Eur J Orthod* 5:189–197.

TEUSCHER U (1978). A growth-related concept for skeletal class II treatment. *Am J Orthod* 74:258–275.

TULLOCH JF, MEDLAND W AND TUNCAY OC (1990). Methods used to evaluate growth modification in Class II malocclusion. *Am J Orthod Dentofacial Orthop* 98:340–347.

TULLOCH JF, PHILLIPS C, KOCH G, PHILLIPS C (1997a). The effect of early intervention on skeletal pattern in Class II malocclusion: a randomized clinical trial. *Am J Orthod Dentofacial Orthop* 111:391–400.

TULLOCH JF, PROFFIT WR, PHILLIPS C (1997b). Influences on the outcome of early treatment for Class II malocclusion. *Am J Orthod Dentofacial Orthop* 111:533–542.

TULLOCH JF, PROFFIT WR AND PHILLIPS C (2004). Outcomes in a 2-phase randomized clinical trial of early Class II treatment. *Am J Orthod Dentofacial Orthop* 125:657–667.

VAN BEEK H (1982). Overjet correction by a combined headgear and activator. *Eur J Orthod* 4:279–290.

VARGERVIK K, HARVOLD EP (1985). Response to activator treatment in class II malocclusions. *Am J Orthod* 88:242–251.

VOUDOURIS JC, WOODSIDE DG, ALTUNA G, ET AL (2003). Condyle-fossa modifications and muscle interactions during Herbst treatment, Part 2. Results and conclusions. *Am J Orthod Dentofacial Orthop* 124:13–29.

WIESLANDER L (1984). Intensive treatment of severe Class II malocclusions with a headgear-Herbst appliance in the early mixed dentition. *Am J Orthod* 86:1–13.

WIESLANDER L (1993). Long-term effect of treatment with the headgear-Herbst appliance in the early mixed dentition. Stability or relapse? *Am J Orthod Dentofacial Orthop* 104:319–329.

WOODSIDE DG (1973). Some effects of activator treatment on the mandible and the midface. *Trans Eur Orthod Soc* 443–447.

WOODSIDE DG, METAXAS A AND ALTUNA G (1987). The influence of functional appliance therapy on glenoid fossa remodeling. *Am J Orthod Dentofacial Orthop* 92:181–198.

9

Contemporary fixed appliances

Most orthodontic treatment is carried out using fixed appliances, directly attached to the teeth. Development of these appliance systems began in the USA at the turn of the twentieth century and they have become progressively more sophisticated. Fixed orthodontic appliances are required for accurate tooth positioning. The brackets, archwires and auxiliary components that make up a fixed appliance are responsible for mediating tooth movement and this takes place at the tooth–bracket interface.

The evolution of fixed appliances

The predominant fixed appliance system in use today is based around a bracket with a rectangular edgewise slot and an in-built prescription for each individual tooth position. A number of modifications on this basic design now exist, largely concerned with the method of attaching the archwire within the bracket slot and either positioning the bracket on the labial or lingual surface of the tooth. However, another group of fixed appliance light wire systems have also been developed, which allow much greater amounts of tooth tipping during the early stages of treatment.

The standard edgewise appliance

The standard edgewise appliance originated from the work of Edward Angle, who experimented with a series of systems before developing the edgewise slot, on which most fixed appliances are now based (Angle, 1928). Initially placing the slot vertically, Angle found that by laying it horizontally within the bracket, greater control of the teeth could be obtained (Fig. 9.1): the interaction of a rectangular wire in a rectangular slot providing precise three-dimensional control of tooth position. The standard edgewise appliance became the fixed appliance of choice up until the late 1970s (Fig. 9.2), but it did suffer from several disadvantages. In particular, the passive bracket slot meant that final detailing of tooth position in rectangular wires was dependent upon many bends being placed within the archwire for each individual tooth (Fig. 9.3). This was time-consuming and required considerable skill on the part of the orthodontist. The presence of these bends also meant that space closure had to be carried out with closing loops, which were also complicated to bend (see Fig. 9.2). In addition, teeth are moved bodily along the archwire through alveolar bone using an edgewise appliance, which is demanding upon anchorage.

Light wire appliances

In an effort to overcome the high anchorage demand associated with the standard edgewise appliance, an Australian orthodontist, P. Raymond Begg developed a fixed

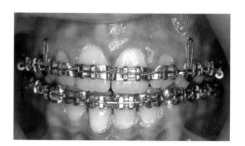

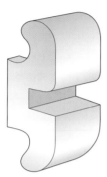

Figure 9.1 Edgewise slot.

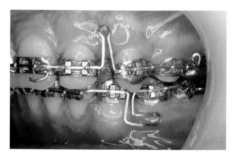

Figure 9.2 Fully banded standard edgewise appliances with space-closing loops in the upper and lower archwires.

Figure 9.3 Typical finishing archwire incorporating individual tooth bends for an edgewise appliance.

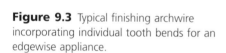

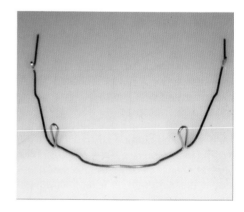

appliance system where tooth movement was based around the concept of differential force (Fig. 9.4) (Begg, 1956):

- The tooth crowns are initially tipped into their desired position using intermaxillary elastics; and
- The roots are then uprighted as a separate procedure using auxiliary springs.

It is much easier to tip a tooth than move it bodily and this requires less force, so the Begg technique was much lighter on anchorage and became very popular during the 1960s and 1970s (Fig. 9.5). Begg treatment mechanics are compartmentalized

Pre-treatment   Stage II end   End of treatment

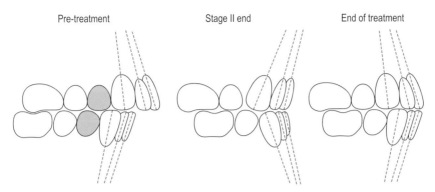

Figure 9.4 Begg treatment involves the concept of differential force. The tooth crowns are first tipped into the desired position and then the roots are uprighted. This differential tooth movement requires less anchorage than bodily moving teeth.

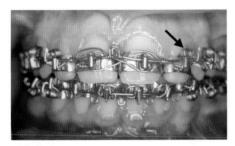 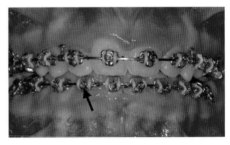

Fig. 9.5 A fully banded Begg appliance (left) and bonded Tip-Edge® appliance (right). Both these appliances use auxiliary springs (arrowed) to upright the teeth during the final stage of treatment.

into three stages, each with specific objectives that have to be achieved before progressing (Cadman, 1975a, b) (Box 9.1). However, because it only uses round archwires, precise finishing is difficult and the use of auxiliaries in the final stages of treatment to upright teeth that often have been tipped through quite significant distances proved to be quite complex, difficult to control and also time-consuming. In an effort to address this, the Tip-Edge appliance was developed by Peter Kesling in the late 1980s (Kesling, 1988; Kesling et al, 1991). This appliance also tips the teeth during the initial phase of treatment, but allows later uprighting with more rigid three-dimensional control by closing the slot down around full-size rectangular archwires (Fig. 9.5).

The preadjusted edgewise appliance

After studying a large sample of untreated ideal occlusions, Lawrence Andrews published his six keys of occlusion (see Box 1.2) (Andrews, 1972) and introduced an edgewise bracket system that has revolutionized fixed appliance orthodontics (Andrews, 1979). The preadjusted edgewise or 'straight-wire' appliance that Andrews described is the most popular fixed appliance system in use today (Fig. 9.6). Unlike standard edgewise brackets, which are identical for each tooth and require bends within the archwire to generate individuality of tooth position, each tooth in the preadjusted

Box 9.1   Stages of Begg treatment

The Begg technique is divided into three separate and distinct stages of treatment, each with specific goals that should all be achieved before moving into the next stage. For all of these stages there is an emphasis upon overcorrection of tooth position.

- Stage 1
  - Crowding and irregularity of the teeth are corrected;
  - Spaces between anterior teeth are closed;
  - Rotations of all teeth are overcorrected;
  - Overbite or open bite and overjet are corrected to place the incisor teeth in an edge to edge relationship;
  - Molar relationship is corrected; and
  - Coordination of the dental arches is completed.
- Stage 2
  - All extraction spaces are closed; and
  - The objectives achieved in stage 1 are maintained.
- Stage 3
  - The labiolingual, buccolingual and mesiodistal axial inclinations of the teeth are corrected; and
  - Space closure and the corrected molar relationship are maintained.

Figure 9.6 Preadjusted edgewise appliance.

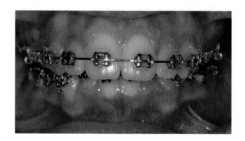

edgewise system has a customized bracket. This built-in prescription was based around Andrews' measurements from the untreated sample of ideal occlusions he studied and included a number of features (Fig. 9.7):

- Pre-angulated slots for correct mesiodistal tooth angulation or tip;
- Bracket bases inclined for correct inclination or torque; and
- Variable distance from base of slot to base of bracket for correct in/out position.

In this preadjusted system, the work in accurately positioning the teeth is done by the bracket prescription, significantly reducing the amount of wire bending required. A further advantage is that it also allows groups of teeth to be moved and spaces closed by sliding them in unison along a rigid archwire; because once tooth alignment has been achieved, the archwire sits passively in each bracket slot.

The original Andrews bracket prescription is still available, although there have been adaptations made as the appliance system has been developed clinically (Box 9.2). In

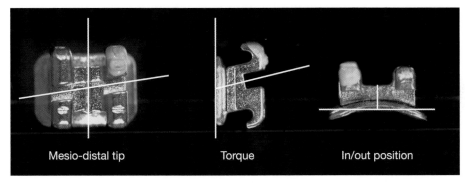

| Mesio-distal tip | Torque | In/out position |

Figure 9.7 Pre-adjusted Siamese edgewise brackets showing twin design and contoured base. The bracket prescription will position the tooth in three dimensions, generating mesiodistal tip, torque and in/out positioning.

Box 9.2 Bracket prescriptions

Lawrence Andrews described the original bracket prescriptions for his preadjusted appliance based upon data he obtained measuring tooth positions from untreated ideal occlusions (Andrews, 1972). As experience was obtained with this appliance during clinical use, Andrews went on to describe several different bracket series for extraction and non-extraction cases, in addition to series for use with different amounts of crowding. The extraction series brackets included adjustments for tip and rotation to counter the effects of space closure (Andrews, 1976), but overall these different series significantly complicated stock management for the orthodontist.

In contrast, Ronald Roth recommended a single series based on the Andrews extraction prescription. This prescription had extra torque in the upper labial segment because the edgewise slot does not express the full torque value of the bracket, particularly as the upper labial segment is retracted during space closure. Roth also placed a greater emphasis on functional occlusion and gave the canines greater tip to facilitate cuspal guidance. There was also greater torque in the maxillary molar region to prevent dropping of the palatal cusps and eliminate non-working side interferences (Roth, 1976).

More recently, Richard McLaughlin, John Bennett and Hugo Trevisi have developed the MBT prescription, which has increased torque in the upper labial segment and lingual crown torque in the lower labial segment. This was designed to minimize proclination of the lower incisors during treatment. The MBT prescription also has reduced tip, most notably in the upper arch, to reduce anchorage requirements. In addition, reduced torque in the lower molar region helps to prevent lingual rolling of lower molars as they are moved along the archwire (McLaughlin & Bennett, 1990).

particular, it was found that some of the torque prescriptions in the original Andrews appliance were not being fully expressed, most notably in the upper incisors due to the 'slop' or free space that inevitably exists between the wire and bracket slot. Therefore, many later prescriptions have increased torque values in the upper labial segment to compensate for this. Biological and anatomical variation, as well as mechanical deficiencies associated with the appliance, mean that one overall prescription does not fit all cases. A variety of modifications in bracket prescription and occasionally some wire bending are often required during the normal clinical use of a preadjusted appliance. These may be needed to overcome errors in bracket positioning, significant variations in tooth structure or position, and the presence of marked skeletal discrepancies (Creekmore & Kunik, 1993; Thickett et al, 2007).

Lingual appliances

One of the biggest problems associated with labial fixed appliance systems are the poor aesthetics. To overcome this, lingual appliance systems were introduced in the USA in the 1970s (Alexander et al, 1982). However, these proved to be clinically very difficult to use and with the introduction of aesthetic labial brackets, lingual orthodontics virtually disappeared from clinical practice in the USA. However, in Europe and Asia, several systems have been developed more recently and the technique is growing in popularity (Fig. 9.8) (Wiechmann, 2002). The principle advantages of lingual appliances are the improved aesthetics, lack of labial decalcification in cases with poor diet or plaque control and better bite opening due to a bite plane effect of the brackets. Disadvantages for the patient include problems with speech, soreness of the tongue and increased cost; whilst for the orthodontist, there is the inherent difficulty and time required for chairside adjustment.

Components of fixed appliances

Fixed orthodontic appliances consist of three main components:

- Brackets and molar tubes, which are bonded directly to the tooth crowns, or in the case of molar tubes, often welded to stainless steel bands that fit around the tooth;
- Archwires, which are attached to the brackets and pass through the molar tubes; and
- Auxiliaries, which will vary between appliance types, but include bracket ligatures, pins, elastics, uprighting and torquing springs, ligature wires and fixed devices for anchorage reinforcement or arch expansion.

Brackets

Orthodontic brackets are fixed to the tooth crown and mediate forces applied by the archwire and auxiliaries on the tooth. Brackets are either routinely cast or injection-molded from stainless steel; although to reduce the chance of allergic reaction, nickel-free brackets made from titanium or cobalt chromium are now available. Bonding techniques rely on a physical interaction being established between the bracket base and an etched enamel tooth surface. Bracket bases are therefore roughened or sand-blasted to improve this bond (Fig. 9.9) and often curved in both the horizontal and

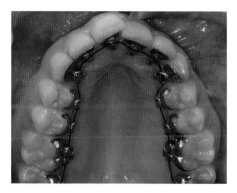

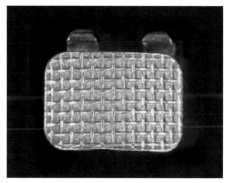

Figure 9.8 Incognito® lingual fixed appliance.

Figure 9.9 Mesh design bracket base to improve bond strength.

vertical planes, which aids in bracket location and seating on the tooth crown (see Fig. 9.7).

Edgewise brackets
Edgewise brackets have rectangular slots, which are deeper in the horizontal as opposed to vertical plane. Slot and archwire dimensions have traditionally been described empirically, with the original dimensions being 0.022 inches vertically and 0.028 inches horizontally to accommodate gold archwires, which were quite soft. Once stiffer stainless steel archwires were introduced, slot size was reduced to 0.018 inches vertically and 0.025 inches horizontally. However, with greater uptake of pre-adjusted edgewise systems, there has been a move back to the original slot dimension. This allows increased dimensions of the working archwire and provides better overbite and torque control during space closure with sliding mechanics. Edgewise brackets are fabricated with a single archwire channel and two tie-wings (see Fig. 9.1); or more commonly as Siamese or twin brackets, which have four tie-wings (see Fig. 9.7). Siamese designs have an increased bracket width, which produces better control of tooth rotations and root position; whilst the presence of two separate tie-wings allows partial ligation of crowded teeth during initial alignment. However, the increased width of Siamese brackets results in a reduced interbracket span and some compromise in flexibility of the archwire during early alignment.

Aesthetic edgewise brackets
A significant disadvantage of metallic orthodontic brackets is their poor aesthetics; edgewise bracket systems that are transparent, or more closely resemble natural tooth colour, have therefore been developed (Fig. 9.10). The early aesthetic brackets were made of acrylic and polycarbonate, which discolored quite rapidly and were prone to both permanent deformation and failure. To overcome these problems, plastic brackets were made in polyurethane or polycarbonate reinforced with ceramic or fiberglass fillers.

Figure 9.10 Ceramic preadjusted edgewise bracket. Note the excessive composite 'flash' around a number of these brackets. This should be removed to prevent plaque accumulation in these areas.

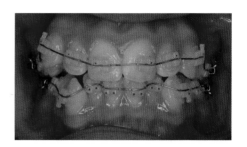

Ceramic brackets were introduced in the 1980s and provide higher strength, more resistance to wear and deformation, better colour stability and superior aesthetics. They are manufactured from aluminium oxide and are described as either mono- or polycrystalline, depending upon whether they are made from one or many crystals. Although the aesthetics are significantly improved, they are not without disadvantages compared to metal brackets (Russell, 2005). Ceramic brackets have low fracture toughness, which can lead to higher bracket breakage. There is also greater friction between the archwire and bracket slot, which can be reduced by the incorporation of a metal slot. Excessively high bond strengths, particularly in the earlier brackets, also increased the risk of enamel damage on bracket removal. One final problem is the fact that ceramics are harder than enamel. This can result in significant enamel wear if brackets are placed in a position of occlusal contact with the natural dentition, commonly the lower incisors in cases with an increased overbite. Despite these problems, adult patients often request ceramic brackets because of the improved aesthetics.

Light wire appliance brackets

The original light wire appliance was the Begg appliance, which utilized a simple bracket that was identical for each tooth. Begg brackets incorporate a narrow open-ended slot, into which a stiff round archwire is placed from the gingival aspect and held in position by the insertion of a small metallic auxiliary lock pin (Fig. 9.11). The loosely fitting round wire allows considerable scope for the teeth to tip under the influence of light intermaxillary elastic traction, which in combination with anchor bends placed in rigid archwires, allows rapid reduction of both overbite and overjet during initial treatment. Following this, a variety of auxiliary springs are required to upright and torque the teeth into the correct position. Unfortunately, this stage of treatment is quite complicated and the nature of the bracket slot means that precise control of tooth position is difficult. For these reasons, the Begg appliance has diminished in popularity during recent years.

The Tip-Edge bracket has been modified from an edgewise design to facilitate the advantages of free tooth-tipping on round wires during early treatment, followed by accurate tooth positioning on rectangular wires during the later stages. This has been achieved by designing a narrow preadjusted edgewise bracket with wedges removed from each side of the archwire slot, which allow the bracket to tip up to 25° either mesially or distally. Lateral extensions or wings on the bracket provide good rotational control of tooth position and as the bracket tips, the dimensions of the slot increase. This allows the subsequent placement of rectangular wires; as the teeth are then uprighted with auxiliary side-winder springs, the slot dimension closes down and the prescribed tip and torque within the bracket is expressed (Fig. 9.12) (Parkhouse, 1998).

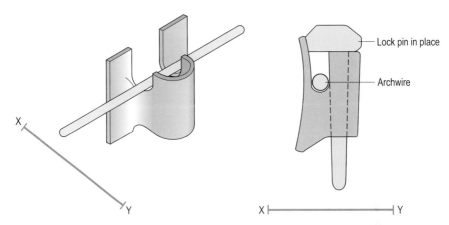

Lock pin in place

Archwire

Figure 9.11 Begg light wire bracket.

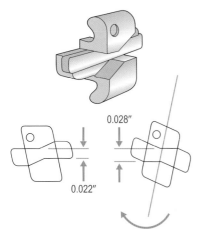

0.028″

0.022″

Figure 9.12 Tip-Edge® bracket. As the tooth tips, the bracket slot dimension increases from 0.022 inches to 0.028. Uprighting on rectangular wires under the force of an auxiliary spring during the final stages of treatment closes down the slot and allows the bracket prescription to be expressed in three dimensions.

More recently, the Tip-Edge PLUS bracket has been introduced, which eliminates the need for auxiliary springs by incorporating a tunnel deep to the main bracket slot (Fig. 9.13). A superelastic auxiliary archwire placed into this tunnel during the final stages of treatment provides the uprighting forces necessary for the bracket prescription to be expressed (Parkhouse, 2007).

Self-ligating brackets
Friction between the bracket and the archwire can theoretically result in a loss of anchorage and slower tooth movement. In addition, individual bracket ligation with conventional edgewise appliances is time-consuming for both patient and orthodontist. In an attempt to reduce friction and appointment times, a range of brackets whose slot is closed by the use of a metal gate or clip are now available (Fig. 9.14). This technique is referred to as self-ligation, as the ligation system is built into the bracket.

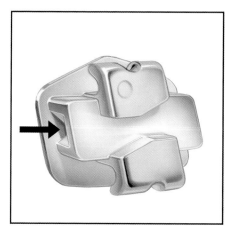

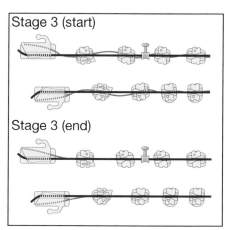

Stage 3 (start)

Stage 3 (end)

Figure 9.13 Tip-Edge PLUS® bracket with auxiliary tunnel (arrowed) deep to the main bracket slot. A flexible nickel titanium archwire passes through the auxiliary tunnels and collectively does the work of individual side-winders. This allows simultaneous torque and tip delivery to be maintained as the teeth upright. During the final stage (three) of treatment, a passive rectangular archwire maintains arch shape and ensures correct torque delivery as a flexible superelastic archwire running through the auxiliary tunnels acts to provide the necessary uprighting tip. This tip brings the finishing surfaces of the main archwire slots into full contact with the rectangular main archwire and therefore, both tip and torque are corrected. Reproduced with permission from Parkhouse (2008) *Tip-Edge Orthodontics* (St Louis: Mosby Elsevier); and with thanks to Richard Parkhouse. ®TP orthodontics, Inc. – La Porte, Ind. USA.

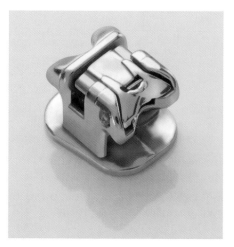

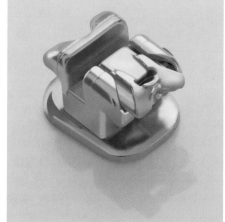

Figure 9.14 Damon MX® self-ligating bracket with the gate closed (left) and open (right). Courtesy of David Birnie and Andy Price. ®Ormco corporation.

The concept is not new, having been originally pioneered in the 1930s. However, these bracket systems have undergone a renaissance over the past two decades, largely because of enhanced ingenuity and reliability. Self-ligating brackets provide a number of theoretical advantages over conventional appliances (Harradine, 2003):

- Reduced friction;
- More robust ligation;
- More efficient tooth movement and sliding mechanics;
- Enhanced rotational control; and
- Reduced chairside adjustment time.

Archwires

The original archwires used in orthodontics were made of gold but metallurgical advances have meant that a wide range of metal alloys are now available. These different alloys all offer a variety of physical properties, which can be defined (Box 9.3). The ideal properties required of an orthodontic archwire will depend upon the stage of treatment and the type of tooth movements being carried out and no archwire material will offer all of these together (Kapila & Sachdeva, 1989). For this reason, a number of different archwires are required during a course of orthodontic treatment and these will vary in both the type of metal used and the dimensions. The particular sequence that an orthodontist chooses is often down to personal preference.

Tooth alignment during the initial stages of treatment requires the following properties:

- Large springback;
- Low stiffness;
- High stored energy;
- Biocompatibility; and
- Low surface friction.

For this reason, round nickel titanium, stainless steel multistrand or coaxial wires are generally used and these will progress in diameter from 0.012 to 0.018 inches, depending upon the degree of irregularity associated with the dentition. These are often followed by a short period with a rectangular nickel titanium archwire to begin torque expression.

Once initial alignment has been achieved, wires of increasing stiffness are used to complete the process of levelling the dentition, begin overbite reduction and allow sliding of teeth along the archwire. These are usually round stainless steel wires, which provide the necessary stiffness over a range of diameters from 0.016 to 0.020 inches.

During the later stages of treatment, the process of overbite reduction is completed and if necessary, space closure is carried out by moving blocks or individual teeth, either along the archwire with sliding mechanics under force provided by auxiliaries or with the archwire under force provided by closing loops. In both circumstances, the archwire will require the following properties:

- High stiffness;
- Low stored energy;
- Biocompatibility;
- Low surface friction; and
- Good joinability.

Box 9.3   Physical properties of an archwire

The physical properties of an archwire material can be described in relation to a plot of stress (force per unit area) versus strain (deflection per unit length) as it is loaded under tension (see Figure).

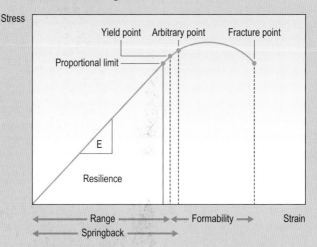

Plot of stress versus strain.

- Stiffness is the force delivered by a wire and is represented by the gradient of the straight line on a stress–strain curve or Young's modulus (E) where the wire is demonstrating elastic deformation. The steeper the line, the stiffer the wire.
- Range is the amount of deflection that a wire can achieve within the proportional limit, the point at which the wire will return to its original dimension on removal of the load. In practice, range is often measured to the yield point, where the wire no longer behaves elastically and 0.1% permanent deformation takes place on removal of the load.
- Springback is the range of activation of a wire, or how far it can be bent and still return to its original shape. The flatter the line on a stress–strain graph, the greater the springback in the wire. In practice, clinically useful springback can still be achieved with some permanent deformation of the archwire. Therefore springback is usually measured in relation to some arbitrarily selected point of loading.
- Formability is the ability of a wire to be bent into a desired configuration or the amount of permanent deformation that can take place before the wire fractures. On the stress–strain graph it is the distance between the yield point and fracture point.
- Resilience is the energy stored in the wire to move teeth when it is deformed. It is represented by the area under the line describing elastic deformation of the wire up to the proportional limit.

A number of other features of an archwire should be considered, although they cannot be identified on a stress–strain graph.

- Biocompatibility is the biological tolerance to materials within the wire, which includes resistance to corrosion.
- Environmental stability is the maintenance of properties following the manufacture of a wire.
- Joinability is the ability to solder or weld auxiliaries to a wire.
- Friction is the resistance to tooth movement associated with a wire.
- Annealing is the heating and cooling of wire to reduce stiffness and increase ductility.
- Ductility is the ability of a wire to undergo a large permanent deformation under tensile stress without failure.
- Cold-working is the repeated deformation or bending of a wire whilst cold. It increases the hardness but also brittleness, making the alloy more prone to fracture.
- Flexibility is the ability of a wire to undergo a large deformation when subjected to low levels of stress.

For sliding mechanics, the frictional properties of the archwire will also have a significant influence on the efficiency of tooth movement, whilst for space closure with looped archwires, good formability will be important. Archwires used during the later stages of overbite reduction and for space closure tend to be made of rectangular stainless steel.

Archwire materials
The metal alloys currently used for the fabrication of orthodontic archwires include stainless steel, nickel titanium, cobalt chromium and beta titanium.

Stainless steel
Stainless steel is an alloy consisting of iron, chromium and nickel, which has a large modulus of elasticity. As such, stainless steel archwires are generally stiff and resist deformation, which makes them ideal as working archwires, providing support as teeth are moved along the wire. However, this stiffness makes them poor for initial alignment; it is difficult to tie a stainless steel archwire into a crowded dentition and if this is achieved, it is often accompanied by permanent deformation. Stainless steel wires used in orthodontics consist of iron (70%), chromium (17 to 20%), nickel (8 to 12%) and a maximum of 0.08% carbon. These are known as '18-8' stainless steels, reflecting the amount of chromium and nickel in the alloy. Chromium makes the wire resistant to corrosion in the oral environment, whilst nickel increases ductility. Stainless steel can be softened by annealing, hardened by cold-working during manufacture and springback can be improved by increasing the length of wire between brackets, achieved by incorporating loops (Fig. 9.15). Alternatively, the flexibility of stainless steel archwires can be increased by winding several smaller wires together to form large multistrand or twistflex wires; or wrapping smaller wires around a larger central wire to produce a coaxial wire. This is because the

force delivered by a wire is related to the radius of the individual wires that make up an archwire.

Cobalt chromium

Commercially marketed as Elgiloy, cobalt chromium has a greater formability than stainless steel and similar stiffness, but with greater friction. It can be hardened by heat-treating in the laboratory and is used for the construction of auxiliaries, such as an intrusion arch or quadhelix.

Beta titanium

Introduced in the 1980s, beta titanium wires have good formability, with a stiffness of around one-third that of stainless steel; but they are also associated with higher friction. These archwires are used in the final stages of treatment, when finishing bends may be required to detail individual tooth position and achieve settling of the occlusion.

Nickel titanium

Nickel titanium or 'NiTi' archwires are characterized by high flexibility and the delivery of low force over long range. They also exhibit the phenomenon of shape memory; when deformed they will tend to return to their original shape; and superelasticity, the wire delivering the same force over a large range of deformation (Fig. 9.16). This

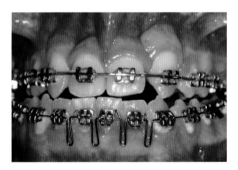

Fig. 9.15 Looped steel archwire to align the lower incisors. This is time-consuming and technically demanding, can result in difficulty with oral hygiene and can produce soft tissue trauma. This technique has been superseded by the advent of superelastic archwires.

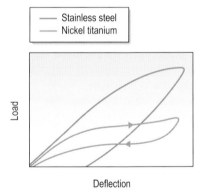

Figure 9.16 Plot of stress versus strain for a nickel titanium wire compared to stainless steel. The plateau on the nickel titanium graph represents a phase shift in the crystalline structure of the metal on loading and unloading. The result is that the wire will deliver the same force over a large range of deformation, a property known as superelasticity. In addition, the deactivation plateau is lower than that for activation; less force is delivered on unloading than is required to activate the wire, a property known as hysteresis.

behaviour occurs because nickel titanium undergoes a phase transition of crystalline structure on loading and unloading. These two phases are represented by the low stiffness martensitic crystal structure and the higher stiffness austenitic, with the superelasticity of NiTi archwires correlated to the coexistence of these two phases. It is also important to note that the deactivation plateau is lower than the activation, a phenomenon called hysteresis, which means that the force delivered by the wire to the tooth is lower than that needed to activate it.

Nickel titanium was originally developed by the Naval Ordinance Laboratory in the USA in the early 1960s as nitinol and was introduced into orthodontics a decade later. The early wires had their crystalline structure stabilized or fixed in the martensitic form by cold working and exhibited greater flexibility but no shape memory. Later nickel titanium wires exhibited a phase shift in crystalline structure, induced by either mechanical stress such as ligation into a displaced tooth (pseudoelastic) or temperature change on placement into the oral cavity (thermoelastic). In combination, these properties give the wire its shape memory. The transitional temperature can be altered by changing the composition of the alloy, in particular by partially replacing the nickel with copper. In modern wires it is set at around body temperature. The wire outside the mouth is in the martensitic form and very flexible, allowing easy engagement into displaced teeth. As the wire reaches body temperature on placement in the mouth, the reverse occurs and it transforms into the austenitic form, returning to its original shape and imparting a gentle aligning force on the teeth. This force remains light because the pseudoelastic property of the wire ensures that when it is engaged in the bracket slot of a displaced tooth, the deflection of the wire (if it is sufficient enough) will generate a local martensitic transformation. As it unloads in these areas, the force will be lowered as the wire becomes superelastic, as exhibited by the plateau of the force–deflection graph (Fig. 9.16). Once the tooth is aligned, the reduction in wire deflection will restore the stiffer austenitic phase.

These wires are ideal for aligning teeth during the initial stages of treatment. However, the properties of low stiffness and poor formability make nickel titanium an unsuitable material for later stages of treatment where a stiffer archwire is required for space closure and overbite control.

Auxiliaries

A variety of auxiliary components are also required for the successful use of fixed appliances. These include both elastomeric and metallic products (Fig. 9.17).

- Elastomeric products are commercially available and are generally made from latex or polyurethane. These include small elastomeric ligatures to hold the archwire within the bracket slot; lengths of elastomeric chain, which can be stretched and used for moving single or multiple groups of teeth; elastomeric thread for the application of traction to individual teeth; elastomeric tube for covering exposed sections of an archwire; elastic bands for the application of inter- and intramaxillary force; and more robust extraoral elastics for headgear.
- Metallic products include lengths of coiled spring made from stainless steel, cobalt chromium or nickel titanium, which in an open configuration is described as push-coil. This is threaded around the archwire and used to create space by pushing teeth apart (see Fig. 9.28). In a closed configuration nickel titanium coil springs can be stretched to provide a light continuous force for space closure and tooth

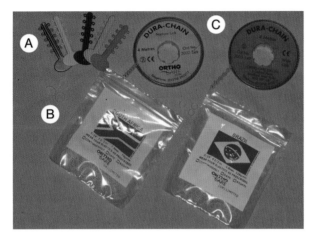
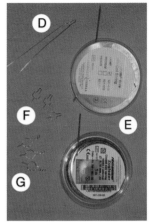

Figure 9.17 Elastomeric and metallic auxiliaries used with fixed appliances. Elastomerics include (A) ormolasts or modules; (B) elastics; (C) powerchain. Metallic auxiliaries include (D) long ligatures; (E) open and closed coil; (F) short ligatures; (G) Kobyashi ligatures.

movement. Soft-grade stainless steel ligatures can be used in short form around individual brackets to provide more secure ligation to the archwire than elastomeric ties or in long form to ligature groups of teeth together or lace them back. Stainless steel auxiliary springs are used primarily in conjunction with light wire appliances such as Begg and Tip-Edge, being threaded through a vertical slot in the bracket and used to apply uprighting or rotational force onto individual teeth (see Fig. 9.5).

Palatal and lingual arches

Palatal and lingual arches consist of a rigid stainless steel wire soldered onto molar bands. The orthodontist fits the relevant molar bands in the mouth but does not cement them in place. An impression is taken with the bands in situ and they are transferred with the impression, to be cast up on the working model by the technician who then constructs the relevant arch. The appliance is then cemented into place within the mouth.

- A transpalatal arch is constructed from a 0.9-mm stainless steel wire that traverses the hard palate and is attached to bands cemented onto the first or occasionally second molar teeth (Fig. 9.18). The arch fixes the maxillary intermolar distance, theoretically preventing these teeth from moving mesially into a smaller archform, and reinforcing their anchorage value. In reality, these arches are not particularly effective for anteroposterior anchorage, but can provide useful vertical anchorage; when mechanically erupting an impacted tooth or using an intrusion arch. A palatal arch will also prevent maxillary molars from flaring buccally when using high-pull headgear and can also be activated to de-rotate molars.
- Nance palatal arches extend towards the palatal vault and incorporate an acrylic button that lies on the palatal mucosa (Fig. 9.18). This also acts to fix the upper arch length and can be used for anchorage support. However, these auxiliaries can

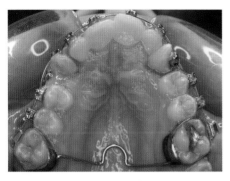

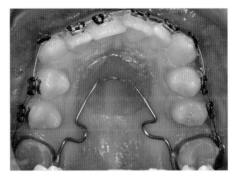

Figure 9.18 Palatal arch (left) and palatal arch incorporating a Nance button (right).

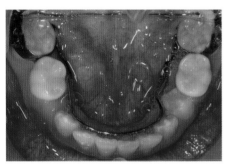

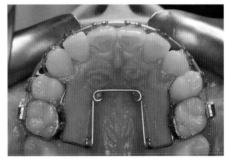

Figure 9.19 Lingual arch.

Figure 9.20 Quadhelix.

cause soft tissue irritation if the acrylic button embeds into the palatal mucosa, especially if left in situ during overjet reduction.

- Lingual arches are used in the mandibular arch and are also constructed from 0.9-mm stainless steel wire (Fig. 9.19). The wire extends behind the cingulae of the lower incisors and extends to bands cemented onto the lower first molars. Lingual arches are generally used as space maintainers; either to prevent forward movement of the permanent molars following early loss of deciduous molars or to maintain the leeway space during the transition from mixed to permanent dentition.

Fixed expansion arches

Fixed expansion arches are also fabricated in the laboratory and require a cast model of the maxillary arch incorporating orthodontic bands for their construction in a manner similar to that of palatal and lingual arches.

- A quadhelix is made from either 0.9 to 1.0-mm stainless steel or 0.95-mm cobalt chromium wire and extends across the palate from bands cemented onto the first molars, but also incorporates helices to increase the range of action (Fig. 9.20). The quadhelix is activated by approximately one molar tooth width and produces

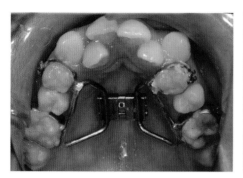
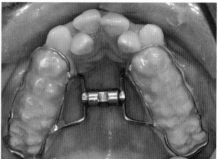

Figure 9.21 Banded RME with HYRAX screw (left) and bonded RME with SUPERscrew (right).

300–400 g of force, which gives mostly dental expansion (up to 4 mm), although in a preadolescent child it can produce some skeletal change.

- A HYRAX (*hy*genic *ra*pid expansion) or SUPERscrew telescopic expander, either attached to the first molar and first premolar teeth via cemented bands or cemented directly to the buccal dentition by acrylic capping (Fig. 9.21), can provide significant expansion of the maxillary dental arch. Each turn of the screw is approximately equal to 0.25-mm and for rapid maxillary expansion (RME) it is turned between 2 and 4 times per day until the maxillary arch is overexpanded. This generally equates to the maxillary palatal cusps occluding on the lingual inclines of the mandibular molar buccal cusps. Expansion is mostly skeletal before the age of 16 when there is patency of the midpalatal suture. Following expansion, the appliance is left in place for approximately three months as a retainer. Up to 10 kg of force can be achieved with these appliances and initially, up to 80% of the expansion achieved will be skeletal, more so anteriorly. However, over the longer term, a lot of this will relapse, with ultimately only around 50% being skeletal. RME can be effective in producing up to 10-mm of maxillary expansion.

Placement and manipulation of fixed appliances

Prior to the development of direct bonding in the 1980s, the only way to place a fixed appliance was by spot-welding the brackets to stainless steel bands and individually banding all the teeth, including the incisors (see Figs 9.2 and 9.5). In current practice, it is possible to bond all the teeth, but molars are still commonly banded.

Molar banding

Molars are generally banded because their restricted access can make moisture control and accurate positioning for bonding more difficult. In addition, the increased forces of mastication associated with the molar dentition can lead to increased bond failures in these regions. A number of specific indications exist for banding instead of bonding molar teeth:

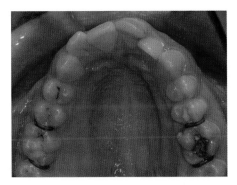

Figure 9.22 Separating elastics placed to create space to allow the placement of bands.

- Auxiliaries, such as palatal and lingual arches, are attached to the lingual surface of a band;
- Headgear should only be used in conjunction with banded molars because extraoral force will increase the chances of bond failure and a risk of injury to the patient; and
- Large coronal restorations and a lack of enamel can make bonding difficult.

To create space for the placement of bands, the contact points need to be opened by placing separators between the teeth for a few days (Fig. 9.22). The most common separators are small elastomeric rings; however, if a contact point is particularly tight, or a restoration is in the way, metal separators can also be used. The separators are removed immediately prior to band placement and the opened contact point facilitates easy band placement around the tooth. Orthodontic bands are seamless and come preformed in various sizes. The appropriate size is selected and the band fitted by finger pressure and then occlusal force as the patient is asked to bite down on a bite-stick, which seats the band in the correct position. Once the correct band has been selected and tried in, it is removed and then cemented in place. Glass ionomer cement is recommended, as it chemically bonds to enamel and releases fluoride, which helps prevent demineralization.

Bracket placement

Both standard edgewise and Begg brackets are simply placed at a specific distance from the occlusal edge of the tooth crown. However, this does not provide a consistent reference point, as the bracket position is determined primarily by the size of the crown. With contemporary preadjusted appliances, the aim is to place the bracket at the centre of the anatomical crown and parallel to the long axis of the tooth. This means that the bracket prescription will be expressed correctly in relation to mesiodistal tip, torque and in/out position, irrespective of the size and form of the tooth. Bracket positioning can be achieved in two ways:

- Direct bonding places the brackets on the teeth individually at the chairside; and
- Indirect bonding places the brackets on study models in the laboratory and these are transferred to the teeth using a positioning tray. The advantage is greater accuracy of bracket positioning; however, the extra cost and time involved make this process less popular for routine orthodontics with labial appliances, although it is used when placing lingual fixed appliances.

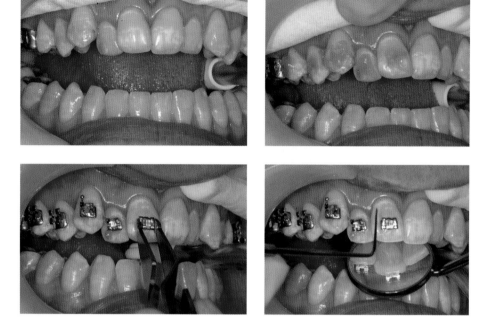

Figure 9.23 Direct bonding. Moisture control is obtained, acid etch placed, the tooth surface washed and dried, and brackets positioned. Excess composite flash is removed and the composite either cures chemically or via the application of an external light source.

Orthodontic brackets are generally bonded to enamel using mechanical locking created by acid-etching the enamel surface of the teeth. The steps involved in bonding are as follows (Fig. 9.23):

- Cleaning the tooth surface, to remove any pellicle using a slow hand piece and prophy brush or cup;
- Acid-etching the enamel surface using 37% phosphoric acid for 20–30 seconds;
- Washing and drying the tooth surface;
- Placing unfilled primer on the etched area of the tooth;
- Placing composite resin on the bracket base;
- Positioning the bracket on the tooth crown;
- Cleaning up excess composite from around the bracket base; and
- Curing the composite, either chemically or with a blue light source.

It is very important to clean up excess composite or 'flash' (see Fig. 9.10) as this can create problems in maintaining high levels of oral hygiene and result in demineralization around the bracket, a major risk of fixed appliance therapy.

Wire placement

In conventional fixed appliances the orthodontic archwires are held in place with ligatures that pass over the archwire and under the bracket tie-wings. These ligatures can be elastomeric or steel, the latter providing securer ligation and reduced friction, but taking longer to place. Self-ligating bracket systems use a variety of methods to mechanically lock the archwire into the bracket slot.

Removal of appliances

Bands are removed using special pliers, which exert an occlusally directed force from the gingival margin (Fig. 9.24). Because of the anatomy of molar teeth, the force is applied from the palatal aspect in the maxillary arch and buccally in the mandible.

In contrast to bands, the bond strength for bondable attachments must be higher to prevent repeated failures. The aim upon removal of a bonded fixed appliance is for the failure to occur between the bracket base and composite junction, and not at the junction between enamel and composite, to avoid the risk of enamel fracture. To achieve this, a shear force is applied across the bracket base with debonding pliers (Fig. 9.25). This distorts the bracket base and causes failure at the junction between bracket base and composite. Residual composite is removed from the tooth, ideally using a tungsten carbide fissure burr in a slow handpiece.

Ceramic brackets initially had very high bond strengths, which resulted in a significant risk of enamel fracture on debonding. To overcome this, most contemporary systems have a failure point built into the bracket base, which means that when a

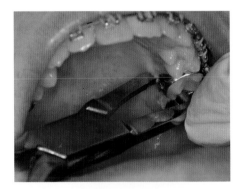

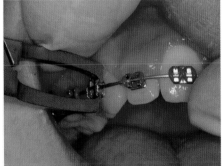

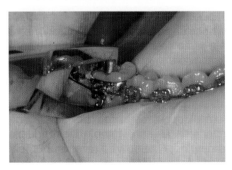

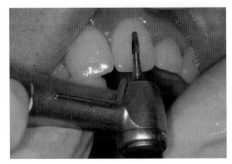

Figure 9.24 Band removal.

Figure 9.25 Bracket debonding and removal of composite with a tungsten carbide fissure burr.

shear force is applied, the bracket fractures down the midline, collapsing the tie-wings of the bracket that can then be easily removed.

Stages of fixed appliance treatment

Treatment with fixed orthodontic appliances can be separated into a number of phases, each with a list of specific objectives.

Levelling and aligning

The first phase in all fixed appliance treatment is to align and level the dentition. Levelling means the correction of marginal ridge discrepancies as opposed to definitive overbite control. To achieve this, small-diameter flexible nickel titanium or multistranded steel arch wires are used (Figs 9.26 and 9.27).

The aligning archwires are initially ligated into all the brackets, either fully or partially, unless a tooth is severely crowded and short of space. In this case, space will need to be created before the tooth can be aligned. This can be achieved by aligning the other teeth first and then placing a more rigid wire, such as stainless steel. A length of compressed coil spring placed on this archwire is then used to create space for the crowded tooth (Fig. 9.28). Once space has been created, the tooth can be aligned by placing a lighter, more flexible archwire as described earlier.

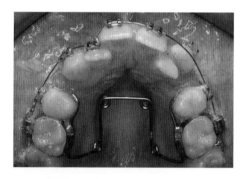
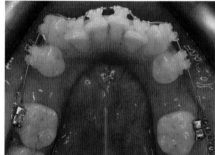
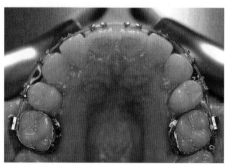
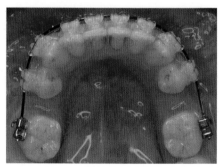
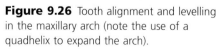

Figure 9.26 Tooth alignment and levelling in the maxillary arch (note the use of a quadhelix to expand the arch).

Figure 9.27 Tooth alignment and levelling in the mandibular arch.

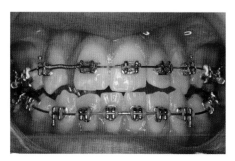
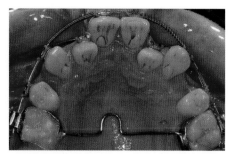

Figure 9.28 Space creation with push coil on round stainless steel archwire.

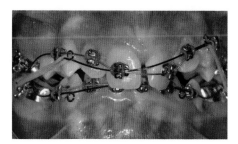
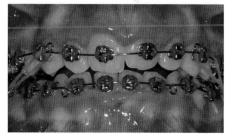

Figure 9.29 Overbite and overjet reduction with a Tip-Edge® appliance.

The alignment stage of treatment is completed when the working archwire is fully engaged in all the brackets. The working archwire when using a 0.022 × 0.028 inch bracket slot is usually a 0.019 × 0.025 inch stainless steel archwire. This provides sufficient rigidity for overbite reduction and control, and for space closure using sliding mechanics.

Overbite control

A number of techniques for facilitating overbite reduction are available and these vary between appliance systems. The Begg and Tip-Edge techniques are characterized by an initial stage of treatment concerned with tooth alignment that takes place simultaneously with both overbite and overjet reduction. This is achieved by using a combination of rigid steel archwires that bypass the premolar teeth and light intermaxillary elastic traction to tip the labial teeth. The steel wires have tip-back anchorage bends to create an intrusive force on the labial dentition, whilst the intermaxillary elastics have an extrusive effect on the molars. In combination, these mechanics are very effective in helping to reduce a deep overbite (Fig. 9.29).

Edgewise and preadjusted edgewise appliances begin the process of overbite reduction following initial tooth alignment and use continuous rigid archwires, often with a reverse curve of Spee in the lower archwire (Fig. 9.30 and see Fig. 11.15). The working archwire is usually rectangular and composed of stainless steel. Care needs to be taken to prevent lower incisor proclination with these archwires and lingual crown torque is usually placed in the labial segment of the wire to prevent this. Much like the Begg and Tip-Edge appliances, the use of class II intermaxillary elastics can

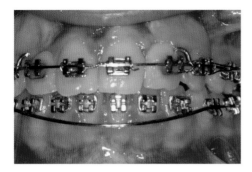

Figure 9.30 Reverse curve of Spee in the lower archwire to reduce the overbite.

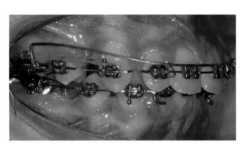 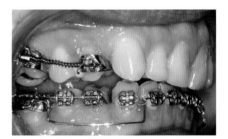

Figure 9.31 Burstone-type intrusion arch (left) and Ricketts utility arch (right) to reduce overbite.

also aid in bite opening, as the vertical component of force will produce molar extrusion.

Edgewise appliances can also use utility arches and segmental mechanics to aid overbite reduction. Utility arches are auxiliary archwires that bypass the buccal segments and provide an intrusive force direct to the labial dentition. These arches are stabilized for anchorage posteriorly and act directly to intrude the incisors, being tied directly into the incisor bracket slots (Ricketts utility arch) or above an archwire that has been sectioned distally to the lateral incisors (Burstone intrusion arch). Utility arches are mechanically efficient, but do create a step in the archwire; they are also complex to fabricate and require triple tubes attached to the molar bands. However, they can be a useful adjunct in cases with deep bites (Fig. 9.31).

Space closure and overjet correction

One of the great advantages of contemporary preadjusted edgewise systems is the use of sliding mechanics for space closure, which is impossible when using standard edgewise brackets because of the numerous bends that must be placed in the archwire to achieve tooth positioning. Therefore, for standard edgewise appliances, loops are bent into the wire (see Fig. 9.2), which pull the opposing segments together and close space. Whilst loop mechanics benefit significantly from reduced friction, the disadvantages include:

- Wire bending;
- High forces;
- Limited range of activation; and
- Poor control of labial torque.

In preadjusted edgewise appliances, the first-, second- and third-order bends are incorporated within the bracket prescription; therefore following tooth alignment the archwire is both flat and straight. This facilitates space closure by simply sliding the teeth along the archwire (Fig. 9.32). The advantages of sliding mechanics are:

- Simple mechanics;
- Low forces required; and
- Good labial torque control.

Force can be applied using simple elastics, elastomeric chain or coiled nickel titanium springs. However, a significant disadvantage of sliding mechanics is friction between the bracket and archwire as the tooth slides. Any applied force must overcome this before tooth movement can take place.

Anchorage support is often required during overjet correction. This can be provided by the use of class II or class III intermaxillary elastics (Fig. 9.33). These will have an extrusive effect on the molar dentition, which can result in a clockwise rotation of the occlusal plane and therefore should be avoided in cases with an increased maxillary–mandibular planes angle.

Finishing

With earlier edgewise systems, considerable time had to be spent at the end of treatment placing artistic bends into the archwires to compensate for the standard bracket placed on each tooth. This was time-consuming and imprecise. With the introduction of preadjusted systems, the bracket prescription does a lot of the work in achieving

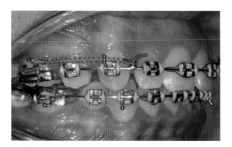 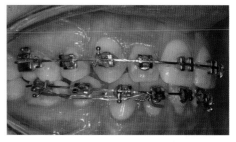

Figure 9.32 Space closure using sliding mechanics.

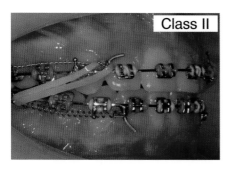 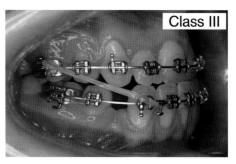

Figure 9.33 Class II and III intermaxillary traction provided by elastics.

Figure 9.34 Settling elastics.

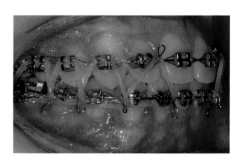

the correct in/out position, angulation and torque for each tooth relative to its neighbours within the dental arch. Finishing has become less reliant upon wire bending and more of a reflection of correct bracket positioning. However, even with precise bracket positioning, a period of finishing to achieve an optimal aesthetic and occlusal result is often required. This usually involves removing the heavy rectangular steel working archwires, and replacing them with lighter wires that allow some occlusal settling. A good wire for this is beta titanium, which is not as stiff as stainless steel and has excellent formability. This is often supplemented with the use of intermaxillary settling elastics, which help to create maximum interdigitation by gently extruding the teeth (Fig. 9.34).

Further reading

BEGG PR AND KESLING PC (1977). *Orthodontic Theory and Technique*, 3rd edn (Philadelphia: WB Saunders).

BENNETT JC AND MCLAUGHLIN RP (1997). *Orthodontic Management of the Dentition with the Preadjusted Appliance* (Oxford: Isis Medical Media).

IRELAND AJ AND MCDONALD F (2001). *The Orthodontic Patient: Treatment and Biomechanics* (Oxford: Oxford University Press).

MCLAUGHLIN RP, BENNETT JC AND TREVISI HJ (2001). *Systemized Orthodontic Treatment Mechanics* (St Louis: Mosby).

PARKHOUSE R (2008). *Tip-Edge Orthodontics* (St Louis: Mosby Elsevier).

WILLIAMS JK, COOK PA, ISAACSON KG ET AL (1995). *Fixed Orthodontic Appliances* (Oxford: Wright).

References

ALEXANDER CM, ALEXANDER RG, GORMAN JC, ET AL (1982). Lingual orthodontics. A status report. *J Clin Orthod* 16:255–262.

ANDREWS LF (1972). The six keys to normal occlusion. *Am J Orthod* 62:296–309.

ANDREWS LF (1976). The straight-wire appliance. Extraction brackets and 'classification of treatment'. *J Clin Orthod* 10:360–379.

ANDREWS LF (1979). The straight-wire appliance. *Br J Orthod* 6:125–143.

ANGLE EH (1928). The latest and best in orthodontic mechanisms. *Dent Cosmos* 70:1143–1158.

BEGG PR (1956). Differential force in orthodontic treatment. *Am J Orthod* 42:481–510.

CADMAN GR (1975a). A vade mecum for the Begg technique: technical principles. *Am J Orthod* 67:477–512.

CADMAN GR (1975b). A vade mecum for the Begg technique: treatment procedures. *Am J Orthod* 67:601–624.

CREEKMORE TD AND KUNIK RL (1993). Straight wire: the next generation. *Am J Orthod Dentofacial Orthop* 104:8–20.

HARRADINE NW (2003). Self-ligating brackets: where are we now? *J Orthod* 30:262–273.

KAPILA S AND SACHDEVA R (1989). Mechanical properties and clinical applications of orthodontic wires. *Am J Orthod Dentofacial Orthop* 96:100–109.

KESLING PC (1988). Expanding the horizons of the edgewise arch wire slot. *Am J Orthod Dentofacial Orthop* 94:26–37.

KESLING PC, ROCKE RT AND KESLING CK (1991). Treatment with Tip-Edge brackets and differential tooth movement. *Am J Orthod Dentofacial Orthop* 99:387–401.

MCLAUGHLIN RP AND BENNETT JC (1990). [Development of standard Edgewise apparatus for a pre-torqued and pre-angulated bracket system]. *Inf Orthod Kieferorthop* 22:149–163.

PARKHOUSE RC (1998). Rectangular wire and third-order torque: a new perspective. *Am J Orthod Dentofacial Orthop* 113:421–430.

PARKHOUSE RC (2007). Current products and practice: Tip-Edge Plus. *J Orthod* 34:59–68.

ROTH RH (1976). Five year clinical evaluation of the Andrews straight-wire appliance. *J Clin Orthod* 10:836–850.

RUSSELL JS (2005). Aesthetic orthodontic brackets. *J Orthod* 32:146–163.

THICKETT E, TAYLOR NG AND HODGE T (2007). Choosing a pre-adjusted orthodontic appliance prescription for anterior teeth. *J Orthod* 34:95–100.

WIECHMANN D (2002). A new bracket system for lingual orthodontic treatment. Part 1: Theoretical background and development. *J Orofac Orthop* 63:234–245.

10

Management of the developing dentition

A number of developmental anomalies can affect both the deciduous and permanent dentitions. These include variations in the number of teeth or their individual morphology, the position they attain within the dental arches and the composition of their constituent hard tissues. The aetiological basis of these abnormalities can be genetic, environmental or multifactorial, but they can all impact upon the developing occlusion, either directly or indirectly. In this chapter the aetiology and management of malocclusion in the developing dentition is discussed.

Early loss of deciduous teeth

The early loss of deciduous teeth is usually the result of extraction due to caries or trauma and can have implications for the developing occlusion: in particular, future space distribution and symmetry within the affected dental arch. The degree of space loss and potential occlusal disruption will be influenced primarily by:

- Age—the earlier the deciduous tooth is lost, the more potential for crowding will exist;
- Crowding—the more inherent crowding already present within the dental arch, the more potential space loss will occur as a result of premature deciduous tooth loss;
- Tooth type—the position of the affected tooth within the dental arch will also influence subsequent space distribution:
  - Deciduous incisors rarely affect space in the permanent dentition unless they are lost very early as a result of trauma or early resorption secondary to crowding.
  - Deciduous canines are not often lost prematurely; but when they are, this can lead to a centreline shift towards the affected side in unilateral cases, particularly in a crowded dentition (Fig. 10.1).
  - Deciduous first molars can also produce a centreline shift when lost prematurely and unilaterally. In the presence of crowding, early loss of these teeth can also result in space loss through forward movement of the buccal segments and accentuate premolar crowding.
  - Deciduous second molars less commonly affect the centreline when lost prematurely, but they do influence the position of the first permanent molar. Early loss can result in forward bodily movement of this tooth if it is unerupted, or tipping and rotation if it is erupted. This can result in space loss and premolar crowding (Fig. 10.2), the severity reflecting the amount of forward movement that has occurred.

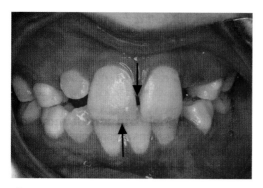

Figure 10.1 The lower centreline has shifted to the right following early loss of the LRC.

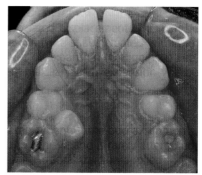

Figure 10.2 Crowding of maxillary second premolars as a result of early loss of the second deciduous molars. The UL5 remains impacted in the palate whilst the UR5 has erupted palatally.

The timing of deciduous tooth extraction can also influence the eruption rate of permanent successors. Very early loss of deciduous teeth can delay successional tooth eruption, whilst later extraction can have the opposite effect.

Balancing and compensating extractions

Balancing and compensating extractions aim to preserve arch symmetry and occlusal relationships by extracting teeth opposing those requiring enforced extraction.

- A balancing extraction is the removal of a tooth from the opposite side of the same dental arch to preserve the centreline by maintaining arch symmetry; and
- A compensating extraction is the removal of a tooth from the opposing quadrant to maintain the buccal occlusion by allowing molar teeth to drift forwards in unison.

The decision to carry out a balancing or compensating extraction will depend upon a number of factors (Box 10.1). However, before the elective extraction of any deciduous tooth is instituted, a radiographic screen should be carried out to check for the presence, position and normal formation of the developing permanent dentition. Any other deciduous teeth of questionable prognosis should also be considered as candidates for balancing or compensating extraction, particularly if general anaesthesia is required. It can be more difficult to justify these extractions if local anaesthesia is used for the elective extraction of a single symptomatic tooth and cooperation for further extractions may be poor.

Space maintenance

A space maintainer is a removable or fixed orthodontic appliance that preserves space within the dental arches (Fig. 10.3). These appliances are most commonly used in the mixed dentition to prevent forward drift of the first permanent molars following early loss of deciduous second molar teeth, or to maintain space and serve as a prosthesis in the labial segment after traumatic loss of permanent incisors.

> **Box 10.1 Which deciduous teeth require balancing and compensating extractions?**
>
> - It is not necessary to balance or compensate the loss of a deciduous incisor from either dental arch.
> - The premature and unilateral loss of a deciduous canine is often associated with a centreline shift and a balancing extraction can help to preserve the centreline; however, compensating extractions are not required in this situation.
> - First deciduous molars can also induce a centreline shift if lost unilaterally and a balancing extraction may be required to preserve the centreline, particularly in a crowded arch.
> - If mandibular first deciduous molars are to be lost, some consideration can be given to compensating extractions in the maxillary arch to preserve the buccal segment relationship, particularly if these teeth have any question regarding their long-term prognosis.
> - Second deciduous molars do not require balancing extractions; however, if the loss of these teeth is required bilaterally in either dental arch, and this may contribute to a significant alteration in the molar relationship, then compensating extractions may be indicated.

A space maintainer in the posterior dentition can be useful in the following situations:
- In an occlusion with only mild crowding where any further space loss would result in the need for more complex orthodontic treatment; and
- In an occlusion with severe crowding where any further space loss would result in more than a single tooth unit of space being required.

It should always be remembered that a tooth is the ideal space maintainer and every effort should be made to preserve deciduous teeth until the time of their natural exfoliation (Fig. 10.3). If a space maintainer is to be used it should be in a mouth with good oral hygiene and ideally, a low risk of further caries. Unfortunately, cases requiring elective tooth extraction due to dental caries are often the least suitable for long-term space maintenance.

Prolonged retention of deciduous teeth

Considerable variation can exist in the timing of deciduous tooth exfoliation and the subsequent eruption of permanent successors. The presence of marked asymmetry in the retention of deciduous teeth should be investigated radiographically.

Occasionally a permanent successor will erupt having failed to resorb the roots of the overlying deciduous tooth (Fig. 10.4). The patient should be encouraged to exfoliate these retained deciduous teeth themselves and if this is not possible, they should be extracted under local anaesthetic.

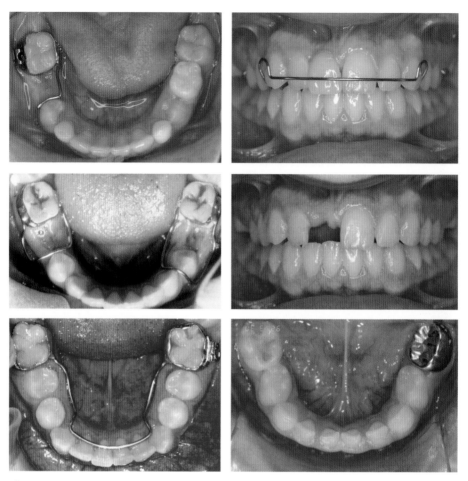

Figure 10.3 Lower fixed space maintainers to preserve the arch length (left panels), preservation of labial segment position with a removable retainer (upper right and middle panels) and restoration of a LLE with a stainless steel crown to prevent space loss (lower right panel) (lower right panel courtesy of Evelyn Sheehy).

Crowding, or an ectopic position affecting the permanent successor, can also lead to prolonged retention of the overlying deciduous tooth.

- Management is dictated principally by the amount of space available within the dental arch and the position of the unerupted permanent tooth. If space is at a premium, maintenance may be required following removal of the deciduous tooth, or alternatively space will need to be created.
- If space is available, extraction of the deciduous tooth alone can often lead to successful eruption if the permanent tooth is in a favourable position.
- If the position is less favourable, exposure of the permanent tooth (with or without the application of orthodontic traction) may also be required.

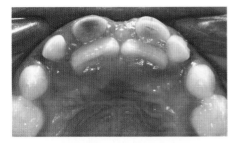

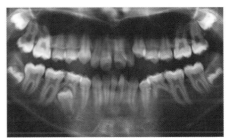

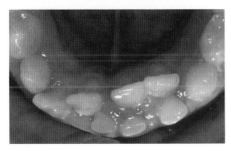

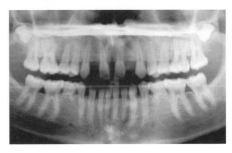

Figure 10.4 Retained deciduous incisors. The permanent incisors have failed to resorb their deciduous predecessors and erupted palatally (upper panel) and lingually (lower panel).

Figure 10.5 Retained deciduous molars in association with congenital absence of the second premolar. In the upper radiograph, the LLE has a good long-term prognosis. In the lower radiograph, extensive root resorption means a poor prognosis for both the retained lower Es.

- Extraction of the permanent tooth may be considered if the position is poor, either in isolation or in combination with other teeth as part of an orthodontic treatment plan. The decision to extract will also be influenced by the type of tooth under consideration.

Another cause of deciduous tooth retention is congenital absence of the permanent successor. For most of these deciduous teeth, the long-term prognosis is poor and they will either be lost naturally or ultimately require extraction. However, they can often act as useful maintainers of arch space or alveolar bone in the shorter term.

Retained second deciduous molars

The second deciduous molar can often be retained due to congenital absence of the second premolar. If this is the case, several treatment options should be considered:

- Extraction to facilitate space closure;
- Extraction and prosthetic replacement; and
- Retention of the second deciduous molar.

Treatment planning will depend primarily upon future space requirements for the correction of any underlying malocclusion and the long-term prognosis of the second deciduous molar. Clinical and radiographic examination of the crown, root and associated alveolar bone will give a useful indication of this (Fig. 10.5). Any of the following features, either alone or in combination, will demonstrate a potentially poor prognosis:

- Caries;
- Root resorption;
- Bone resorption;
- Periapical or interradicular pathology;
- Ankylosis;
- Infraocclusion; and
- Gingival recession.

Second deciduous molars can have an excellent long-term prognosis if they are in good condition and will match the lifespan of many prostheses. Indeed, if they survive to twenty years of age, continued long-term function can be anticipated (Bjerklin & Bennett, 2000; Sletten et al, 2003).

Ankylosis and infraocclusion

A tooth becomes ankylosed when the periodontal ligament is lost and direct fusion occurs between root dentine and the surrounding alveolar bone. Ankylosis most commonly affects deciduous molars, occurring in up to 9% of children (Kurol, 1981). A number of factors are thought to contribute:

- Genetic predisposition;
- Failure of normal resorption by the permanent successor;
- Congenital absence of the permanent successor;
- Trauma; and
- Infection.

A consequence of ankylosis can be the apparent 'submergence' or infraocclusion of the affected tooth relative to the occlusal plane (Fig. 10.6). This occurs in the growing child because alveolar bone and occlusal height increase with development, whilst the position of the ankylosed tooth remains fixed.

- In the presence of a permanent successor and minimal infraocclusion, the ankylosed tooth can usually be left under observation to exfoliate naturally.
- If the infraocclusion becomes greater this can lead to displacement, tipping and overeruption of adjacent teeth. In these circumstances, consideration should be given to either restoring the vertical dimension or extracting the affected tooth.

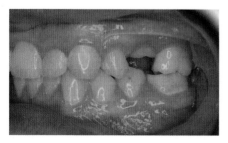 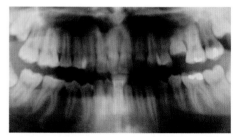

Figure 10.6 Infraocclusion of the ULE in association with congenital absence of the UL5.

- In the absence of a permanent successor, a decision will need to be made regarding long-term management of the hypodontia. However, the presence of ankylosis or infraocclusion in a growing patient will often make extraction more likely.

Hypodontia

The congenital absence of one or more teeth is a relatively common anomaly in human populations.

- Nonsyndromic or familial hypodontia occurs as an isolated trait; and
- Syndromic hypodontia occurs with accompanying genetic disease.

The term hypodontia is generally used to describe congenital tooth absence, but the definitions are actually quite specific (Fig. 10.7):

- Hypodontia refers to a lack of one to six teeth, excluding third molars;
- Oligodontia refers to a lack of more than six teeth, excluding third molars; and
- Anodontia refers to a complete absence of teeth in one or both dentitions.

Nonsyndromic hypodontia

Nonsyndromic hypodontia can either appear sporadically within a member of a family or be inherited. This form can follow autosomal dominant, autosomal recessive or autosomal sex-linked patterns of inheritance, with considerable variation in both penetrance and expressivity. This is by far the most common type of congenital tooth absence and can be further categorized based upon clinical presentation:

- Localized incisor–premolar hypodontia (OMIM 106600), which affects only one or a few of these teeth. This is the most common form and is seen in around 8% of Caucasians (Nieminen et al, 1995).
- Oligodontia (OMIM 604625) occurs in around 0.25% of Caucasians and can involve all classes of teeth (Sarnas & Rune, 1983).

Within these clinical entities, certain teeth fail to develop more often than others:

- Third molars are the most commonly absent tooth;
- These are followed by mandibular second premolars and maxillary lateral incisors (around 2%) and mandibular central incisors (0.2%) in Caucasians (Neal & Bowden, 1988); and
- Congential absence of canines, first and second molars, is rare (Simons et al, 1993).

Nonsyndromic hypodontia can be associated with other developmental anomalies affecting the dentition, which provides evidence of a genetic influence (Table 10.1). However, a multifactorial model has also been suggested (Brook, 1984), with the phenotypic effect being related to certain thresholds, themselves influenced by both genetic and environmental factors. Clearly, within this model, the mutation of a major gene may be a significant enough event to result in inherited tooth loss (Box 10.2).

Syndromic hypodontia

Congenital tooth absence is also seen in association with other recognizable structural defects or abnormalities (Table 10.2).

- One of the commonest causes of syndromic hypodontia is Down syndrome (OMIM 190685), which results from the presence of an extra copy of all or part of chromosome 21.

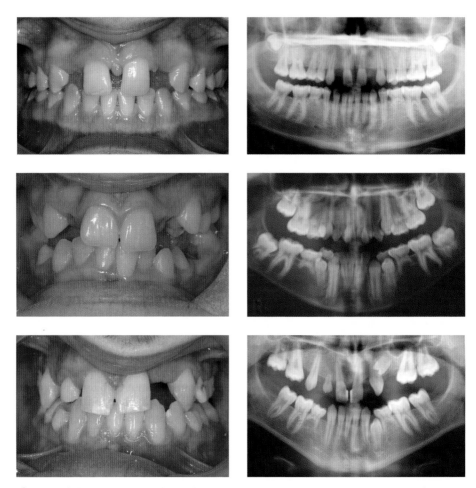

Figure 10.7 Hypodontia and oligodontia. In the upper case there is hypodontia with UR2, UL2, LL8, LL5, LR5 and LR8 absent. In the middle case there is more severe hypodontia, with UR8, UR5, UR4, UL4, UL5, UL8, LR8, LR5, LL5 and LL8 absent. In the lower case there is oligodontia, with UR8, UR5, UR4, UR2, UL2, UL5, UL8, LL8, LL4, LL1, LR4, LR5, and LR8 absent.

Table 10.1   Dental anomalies associated with hypodontia

- Reduced crown and root size
- Conical crown shape
- Enamel hypoplasia
- Molar taurodontism
- Delayed eruption
- Prolonged retention of primary teeth
- Infraocclusion of primary teeth
- Tooth impaction (particularly maxillary canines)
- Ectopic eruption
- Transposition
- Lack of alveolar bone
- Reduced vertical dimensions
- Increased overbite

Box 10.2   Candidate genes for nonsyndromic human hypodontia

Targeted deletion of many genes in mutant mice can disrupt tooth formation and these have provided a reference point in the search for candidate genes in human populations. However, given the large number of potential genes available, it is somewhat surprising that only three have been positively identified in human familial hypodontia (Cobourne, 2007):

- Mutations in the human *MSX1* gene have been predominantly associated with familial oligodontia (Vastardis et al, 1996). Associations between *MSX1* and the more common form of incisor–premolar hypodontia are rarer.
- Mutations in the human *PAX9* gene have been identified in association with variable forms of oligodontia that particularly affect the molar dentition.
- The identification of a Finnish family affected by autosomal dominant oligodontia has provided an unexpected further insight into the genetics of inherited tooth loss. Within this pedigree, those individuals affected by oligodontia were also found to carry a significant risk of developing colorectal neoplasia. *AXIN2* was identified as the candidate gene for this condition because it was located in the correct chromosomal region, had a known association with colorectal carcinoma and encoded a protein that regulates the Wnt signalling pathway. Wnt proteins have a wide-ranging role during embryonic development and demonstrate expression in the tooth. Suppression of Wnt signalling in mutant mice can inhibit tooth development and crucially, all the affected family members had a mutation which produced a loss of function of the AXIN2 protein (Lammi et al, 2004).

Table 10.2 Syndromic conditions associated with hypodontia

Syndrome	Gene
Anhidrotic ectodermal dysplasia (OMIM 305100)	EDA
Adult (OMIM 103285)	TP73L
Ehlers Danlos (OMIM 225410)	ADAMTS2
Incontinentia pigmenti (OMIM 308300)	NEMO
Limb mammary (OMIM 603543)	TP63
Reiger (OMIM 180500)	PITX2
Witkop (OMIM 189500)	MSX1
Ellis–van Creveld (OMIM 225500)	EVC or EVC2

- Mutations in the homeobox gene *MSX1* have been associated with a syndromic condition demonstrating various combinations of CLP, CP and hypodontia (van den Boogaard et al, 2000) and with Witkop syndrome (OMIM 189500), a form of ectodermal dysplasia (Jumlongras et al, 2001). Thus, *MSX1* represents a candidate gene for both syndromic and nonsydromic hypodontia (see Box 10.2).

Management

The management of congenital tooth absence will involve either:

- Space closure; or
- Maintenance or opening of space, followed by prosthetic replacement of missing tooth units.

Milder forms of hypodontia can usually be managed within an orthodontic treatment plan in consultation with either the general dental practitioner or restorative specialist and is usually carried out in the permanent dentition (see Chapter 11). More severe hypodontia or oligodontia requires complex multidisciplinary treatment and is usually carried out within a specialist centre.

Supernumerary teeth

Supernumerary teeth are teeth present in addition to the normal complement and can occur within either dentition.

- In Caucasians, supernumerary teeth are seen more commonly in the permanent dentition, affecting around 4% of the population;
- In the deciduous dentition, the range is less than 1%; and
- In the permanent dentition, supernumerary teeth are twice as common in males and five times more common in the maxilla than in the mandible.

In common with hypodontia, supernumerary teeth also occur either as an isolated trait or as a manifestation of a clinical syndrome (Table 10.3), but they are usually classified according to morphology and location:

Table 10.3 Syndromic conditions associated with supernumerary teeth

Syndrome	Gene
Cleft lip and palate	
Cleidocranial dysostosis (OMIM 119600)	*RUNX2*
Gardner (OMIM 175100)	*APC*
Ellis–van Creveld (OMIM 225500)	*EVC; EVC2*
Incontinentia pigmenti (OMIM 308300)	*NEMO*

Box 10.3 Managing the mesiodens

The mesiodens is one of the commonest forms of supernumerary tooth and is often detected in the anterior maxilla as a chance radiographic finding. Whilst removal is indicated if they interfere with the eruption, position or proposed orthodontic movement of adjacent teeth, quite often they are asymptomatic and in these circumstances, they should be left alone (Kurol, 2006). The potential risks associated with leaving these teeth in situ, such as follicular enlargement, cystic formation and resorption of maxillary incisor roots, would appear to be small (Tyrologou et al, 2005). In addition, if the mesiodens subsequently erupts, it can be removed with a relatively simple extraction under local anaesthesia.

- Conical supernumeraries are small peg-shaped teeth with normal root formation. When located in the midline of the anterior maxilla these teeth are known as mesiodens (Box 10.3); whilst in the maxillary molar region they are known as paramolars (buccal, lingual or interproximal to the second and third molars) or distomolars (distal to the third molar) (Fig. 10.8).
- Tuberculate supernumeraries are characterized by a multicusped coronal morphology and a lack of root development (Fig. 10.9). These teeth are usually found palatal to the maxillary permanent incisors, often occur in pairs and frequently prevent eruption of the permanent incisors (Fig. 10.10).
- Supplemental supernumeraries represent the duplication of a tooth within a series and can be difficult to differentiate from the normal tooth (Fig. 10.11). These teeth are usually found at the end of a series and can be seen in the incisor, premolar and molar fields. They represent the most common type of supernumerary found in the primary dentition (Fig. 10.12).
- Odontomes are developmental malformations that contain both enamel and dentine (Fig. 10.13), and can be compound (containing many small separate tooth-like structures usually situated in the anterior jaw) or complex (a large mass of disorganized enamel and dentine usually situated in the posterior jaw).

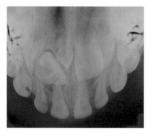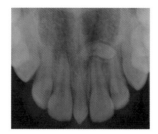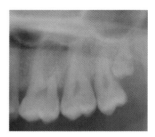

Figure 10.8 Conical supernumeraries. Mesiodens positioned in the anterior maxilla, either vertically (left and middle) or horizontally (middle). Distomolar erupting behind the UL8 (right).

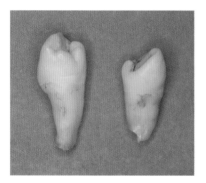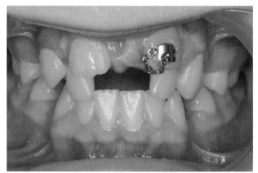

Figure 10.9 Extracted tuberculate supernumeraries and the effect of these teeth on the developing dentition.

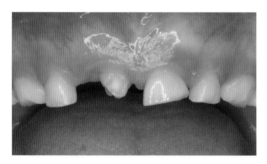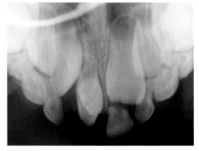

Figure 10.10 Erupted tuberculate supernumerary. The URA has been exfoliated and the UR1 is unlikely to erupt whilst the supernumerary is in situ.

Supernumerary teeth occur individually or in groups and can be unilateral or bilateral. These teeth are found most frequently in the anterior maxilla, but are also seen in the premolar and molar regions. In the permanent dentition, the majority fail to erupt and are asymptomatic, only being discovered during routine radiographic screening. However, they can also cause dental problems, which include:

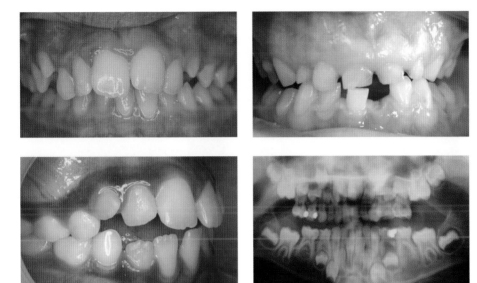

Figure 10.11 Supplemental UR2's.

Figure 10.12 Supplemental URB. Courtesy of Thantrira Porntaveetus.

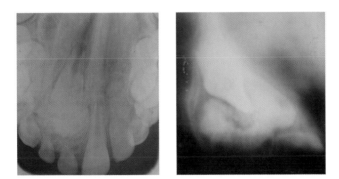

Figure 10.13 Complex odontome in the anterior maxilla. The Scanora view on the right reveals the full extent of the odontome overlying the UR1.

- Failure of tooth eruption—the presence of a supernumerary can prevent the eruption of a permanent tooth (Fig. 10.14). In these circumstances, the supernumerary should be removed and provided space is available and the tooth is in a good position, there is a high chance the impacted tooth may well erupt unaided. However, exposure of the tooth is often undertaken at the same time, particularly in older children so orthodontic traction can be applied to the tooth to mechanically erupt it into the dental arch if it does not erupt spontaneously (see Fig. 10.22).
- Crowding—supernumerary teeth can contribute to dental crowding, either directly as a result of eruption (particularly for supplemental teeth) or indirectly by causing

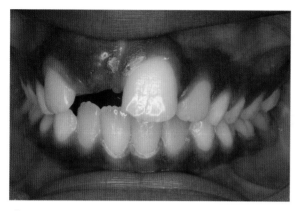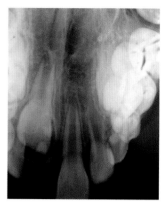

Figure 10.14 Supernumerary preventing eruption of the UR1.

displacements or rotations of adjacent erupted teeth (Fig. 10.15). These supernumerary teeth will usually require extraction as part of a definitive orthodontic treatment plan. When extracting these teeth, care must be taken to ensure the most poorly formed is removed.

- Spacing—supernumeraries can also produce spacing between erupted teeth, particularly a mesiodens producing a maxillary diastema between the central incisors. If orthodontic space closure is planned, these supernumeraries will require extraction.
- Cystic formation—as with any unerupted tooth, cystic formation can occur. Any evidence of follicular enlargement or cystic formation and these teeth should be removed.

Asymptomatic supernumerary teeth not affecting the occlusal relationships of the erupted dentition can be left in situ. These teeth should be kept under periodic radiographic review to ensure they are not damaging any adjacent structures or undergoing cystic change.

Abnormalities of tooth size

Teeth either larger or smaller than the normal population range for dimensions are usually referred to as megadont or microdont, respectively. These variations in tooth size can affect either the crown or root in isolation, or the whole tooth. Little is known about the aetiology of tooth size variation but it is almost certainly genetic.

- Megadontia most frequently affects the maxillary permanent incisors (Fig. 10.16) or mandibular second premolars and is often symmetrical. These teeth can be differentiated from double teeth by the absence of coronal notching and presence of normal pulpal morphology. Extraction of megadont teeth is often indicated, particularly with maxillary central incisors, because the aesthetics can be poor. Depending upon the space requirements, either the lateral incisors can be approximated and adjusted restoratively to look like central incisors or space maintained for prosthetic replacement.

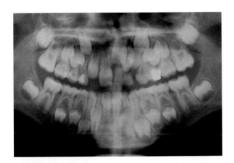 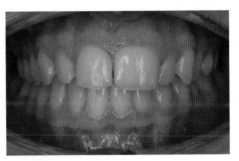

Figure 10.15 Supplemental UL2 causing crowding of the UL1 and UL2.

Figure 10.16 Megadont UL1.

- Microdontia is commonly associated with hypodontia and can affect the whole dentition or individual teeth. The maxillary permanent lateral incisor is one of the commonest teeth to be affected, often having a characteristic peg-shaped crown morphology (Fig. 10.17) and this has a causal association with palatal impaction of the maxillary canines. Whether a microdont maxillary lateral incisor is retained or extracted depends not only on the underlying malocclusion and the need for extractions, but also on the shape and form of the lateral incisor and whether it can ultimately be an aesthetic and functionally viable tooth. If this tooth is to be retained, the crown will require restorative buildup to improve the aesthetics and symmetry if it is unilateral. Space will often need to be created to allow this, which usually necessitates fixed appliances. If the lateral incisor is extracted, space will also need to be created if prosthetic replacement is planned, as these teeth are usually smaller than the space required for suitable pontics.

Abnormalities of tooth form

A number of anomalies associated with tooth form have been described. These conditions are generally rare, occurring with prevalence well below 5% of Caucasians, and with the exception of double teeth, they generally affect the permanent dentition more commonly than the deciduous.

- Double teeth can range from a slightly enlarged tooth with minor coronal notching to almost complete separation of two normally formed teeth. They are most commonly seen in the labial region of the mandibular deciduous dentition (Fig. 10.18), but can also affect permanent teeth. In the deciduous dentition, it is important to establish whether a double tooth is associated with hypodontia because this can indicate possible tooth absence affecting the permanent teeth. Conversely, if the double tooth is part of a normal complement, supernumerary teeth may be seen in the permanent dentition. Localized crowding or spacing can be seen in association with double teeth in both dentitions but in the deciduous, extraction is rarely indicated. Permanent double teeth can be managed restoratively if the coronal

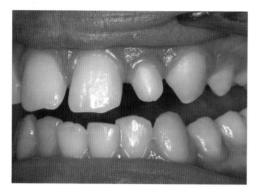
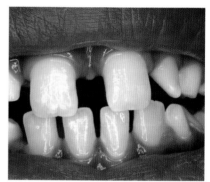

Figure 10.17 Microdont UL2's.

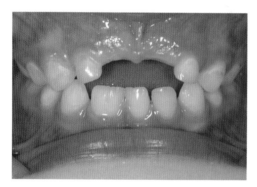
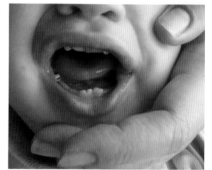

Figure 10.18 Double incisor teeth in the deciduous dentition with minor (left) and marked (right) coronal notching. Right panel courtesy of Rudi Keane.

portion is not too large; however, those with more deviant anatomy may require extraction followed by space closure or prosthetic replacement.

- Accessory cusps are quite a common finding in both the deciduous and permanent dentition. Talon cusp, which can affect the maxillary permanent incisors, occasionally causes occlusal problems and tooth displacement. Treatment usually involves cusp removal, either with selective grinding or in combination with pulpotomy (Fig. 10.19).

- Invaginated teeth are characterized by the presence of an enamel-lined cavity, normally situated within the coronal portion of the tooth. These cavities can range from a simple pit in an otherwise normal tooth, to a deep fissure associated with marked distortion of tooth form. Treatment depends upon severity of the invagination; pulpal infection will require endodontics, whilst more severely distorted teeth will often require extraction.

- Evaginated teeth have an external enamel-covered projection on the surface of the tooth. The size of these evaginations and the degree of pulpal involvement can vary greatly. Treatment choices are comparable with those for accessory cusps.

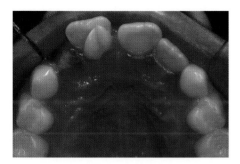

Figure 10.19 Talon cusp. Courtesy of Evelyn Sheehy.

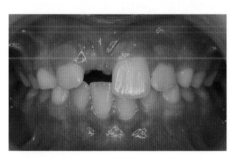

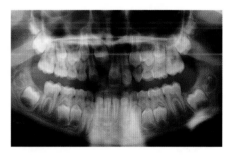

Figure 10.20 The UR1 is dilacerated as a result of previous trauma to the URA and has failed to erupt.

- Dilaceration is an abnormal angulation between the crown and root of a tooth, usually affects maxillary incisors, and can occur as a consequence of intrusive trauma to their deciduous predecessors, although in the majority of cases there is no history of trauma (Stewart, 1978) (Fig. 10.20 and see Fig. 10.23). The most common scenario is a failure of the affected incisor to erupt and unless the dilaceration is mild, these teeth usually require extraction.
- Taurodont (OMIM 272700) or bull-like teeth have a pulp chamber enlarged at the expense of the roots (Fig. 10.21). This condition is seen in around 2.5–5% of adult Caucasians and can occur in isolation, or in association with amelogenesis imperfecta.

Abnormalities of eruption

A number of systemic conditions are associated with delayed eruption and these can affect both dentitions (Table 10.4). In the permanent dentition, great individual variation can exist in the timing of tooth eruption, with symmetrical deviation of anything up to two years from the mean not necessarily being a cause for concern. In the majority of children, local factors will be the main cause of any eruption disturbances that do occur (Table 10.5).

Primary management relies upon ensuring adequate space exists in the dental arch to accommodate the unerupted tooth and removing any potential obstruction. In these

Figure 10.21 Taurodont first permanent molars (LR6 is also carious).

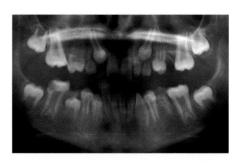

Table 10.4 Systemic conditions associated with delayed tooth eruption
• Down syndrome • Cleidocranial dysostosis • Turner syndrome • Hereditary gingival hyperplasia • Cleft lip and palate

Table 10.5 Local factors causing disturbances of tooth eruption
• Crowding • Trauma • Ectopic position of the tooth germ • Supernumerary teeth • Retained deciduous teeth • Early extraction of deciduous teeth • Transposition • Local pathology

circumstances, the majority of teeth will erupt. If this fails to happen, or the unerupted tooth is ectopic from its normal path of eruption, surgical exposure, with or without orthodontic traction, may be required to accommodate the affected tooth into the dental arch (Box 10.4).

Unerupted permanent maxillary incisor

A discrepancy in eruption between contralateral maxillary incisors of greater than six months, or eruption of lateral incisors before the centrals warrants radiographic investigation. Delayed eruption of maxillary incisors is most commonly associated with the presence of supernumerary teeth (particularly tuberculate), retained deciduous incisors or dilaceration. Obstruction secondary to a supernumerary tooth is by far the commonest cause.

- In the absence of a central incisor the lateral incisors can very rapidly drift towards the midline, particularly in the presence of crowding. If space needs to be created this can be achieved with a simple removable or sectional fixed appliance, often with extraction of the deciduous canines to provide some space in the labial segment.

Box 10.4   Surgical exposure of impacted teeth

In the labial regions of the maxilla, and both labially and lingually in the mandible, the alveolar crest is covered by a keratinized, firmly attached gingiva, which is replaced by a more mobile, non-keratinized alveolar mucosa at the mucogingival junction. In contrast, on the palatal side of the maxilla there is no alveolar mucosa, the attached gingiva and palatal mucosa are both keratinized and firmly attached to the underlying bone, with no recognizable boundary between them. It is important for an impacted tooth to erupt through attached gingiva because this tissue provides a firm attachment at the dentogingival junction, is robust enough to maintain integrity of the periodontium during masticatory function and provides the best potential for long-term periodontal health. This will influence the method of exposure for teeth impacted in different areas of the jaws.

Impacted teeth are surgically exposed using one of two basic techniques:

- Open eruption—the crown is surgically uncovered and the tooth left exposed within the oral cavity; it is then allowed to erupt naturally, or the orthodontist places an attachment directly to guide eruption. Open eruption either involves removal of the overlying mucosa accompanied by any necessary bone (window technique), or an apically repositioned flap (a modification for labially impacted teeth that relocates the flap apically, covers the cervical margin of the exposed tooth with attached gingiva and ensures that this tissue accompanies the tooth into its final eruptive position). The main advantage of an open technique is that the orthodontist can directly visualize the tooth following exposure. However, for less accessible teeth, particularly maxillary canines situated high in the palate, the wound can rapidly re-epithelialize if the post-surgical dressing is lost prematurely, which may necessitate a second surgical procedure. The presence of an open wound can also result in more postoperative discomfort for the patient.
- Closed eruption—the crown is surgically exposed, an orthodontic attachment is placed and the overlying mucosa is replaced. A chain or wire extends from the attachment through the mucosa, which allows the orthodontist to place traction in a manner that is generally more comfortable for the patient. This method attempts to simulate normal tooth eruption and foster good long-term periodontal health. However, it can be a lengthy overall procedure, moisture control is often difficult at surgery and the attachment can become detached during traction, which may necessitate further surgery to replace.

The open window or closed techniques are suitable for teeth impacted beneath attached gingiva. Those situated below non-keratinized alveolar mucosa require either an apically repositioned flap or closed eruption.

- For those associated with a supernumerary tooth, if sufficient space is present and the incisor is superficially placed, it will usually erupt within twelve months of removing the supernumerary. For incisors impacted in a higher position the supernumerary should also be removed. For children under the age of ten, the permanent incisor follicle should be left undisturbed and eruption monitored. If the tooth fails to erupt, it can be exposed and bonded when it is more mature. In those over ten, exposure with placement of a bracket and gold chain should be carried out at the time of supernumerary extraction. The incisor should erupt spontaneously and the bracket and chain can then be removed (see Fig. 10.9). If it fails to erupt, orthodontic traction can be applied without the need for further surgery.
- In the absence of any supernumerary, a mature impacted incisor delayed more than six months should have a bracket and gold chain placed and be observed for six months. Surgery on immature incisors should be delayed until apexification is complete and observed for twelve months before applying traction.
- Dilacerated incisors can only be accommodated if the degree of dilaceration is mild; more severe cases may result in the root perforating the maxillary labial plate if the crown is aligned (Fig. 10.23).

Unerupted permanent maxillary canine

The permanent maxillary canine fails to erupt in approximately 2% of Caucasian children and these teeth will often require orthodontic management (Bishara, 1992; Ferguson, 1990). Deviation from the normal path of eruption is usually associated with subsequent impaction and in the vast majority of cases this occurs in a palatal direction, although the canine can also impact on the buccal side or within the line of the dental arch. A number of reasons have been suggested to explain the particular vulnerability of the maxillary canine to deviation from its normal eruptive path:

- A developmental position that begins high in the maxilla and results in a long path of eruption;

Figure 10.22 The impacted UL1 has been exposed, bonded with a gold chain and traction applied using a removable appliance. Fixed appliances were subsequently used to detail the permanent dentition.

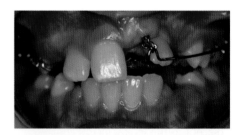
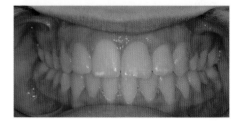

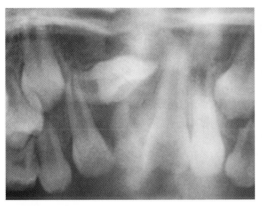 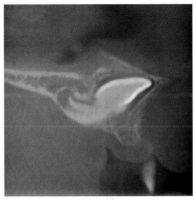

Figure 10.23 A conventional panoramic view (left) and cone beam CT sagittal section (right) through a severely dilacerated UR1.

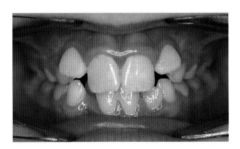

Figure 10.24 Maxillary permanent canines palpable in the buccal sulcus. The canine position is given away by the inclination of the permanent lateral incisor crowns.

- Reliance upon the maxillary lateral incisor root for guidance of eruption, which can be lacking if these teeth are diminutive or congenitally absent (Brin et al, 1986);
- Retention of the deciduous canine obstructing normal eruption;
- Chronology of eruption, in the maxillary arch the canine often erupts after the first premolars; therefore space can be at a premium; and
- A genetic susceptibility (based upon observations that demonstrate a familial tendency, occurrence of other dental anomalies in association with ectopic maxillary canines and a female predilection) (Peck et al, 1994).

Clinical examination

At the age of 10 years, the maxillary canine should be palpable in the buccal sulcus adjacent to the lateral incisor root (Fig. 10.24). If it is not, or if there is any asymmetry in palpation, then an abnormal path of eruption should be suspected and radiographic investigation instigated (Ericson & Kurol, 1986). Other clinical features, which may alert the clinician to possible impaction include:

- A palatal bulge;
- Delayed eruption, marked distal angulation or retroclination, microdontia or absence of the permanent lateral incisor; and
- A firm deciduous canine (particularly beyond the age of 14 years) indicating a lack of resorption.

Radiographic examination

Radiographic examination is required to demonstrate the presence of the canine, its position within the maxillary arch, the condition of adjacent teeth (particularly the degree of resorption associated with the deciduous canine or presence of any resorption associated with the permanent incisors) and any other pathology. The position of the canine should be evaluated in all three planes of space:

- Buccopalatal relationship to the dental arch;
- Height relative to the occlusal plane;
- Angulation relative to the mid-sagittal plane; and
- Distance from the mid-sagittal plane.

Two films are required to definitively establish canine position and the parallax (or tube-shift) technique is commonly used to achieve this (Jacobs, 1999). Parallax is the apparent displacement of an object when observed from two different positions and, in radiological terms, relies upon taking two views with the X-ray tube in a different position for each view. Horizontal parallax uses a horizontal shift in the X-ray tube (usually with successive periapical views taken with the tube moved horizontally), whilst vertical parallax uses a vertical shift in the tube (usually achieved with a panoramic and anterior occlusal view). The advantage of the parallax technique is that it always involves an intraoral view, which gives good detail of the canine and incisors (Fig. 10.25). More recently, the use of cone beam CT has been described to precisely locate the position of ectopic canines (Walker et al, 2006) (see Box 6.5).

Interceptive treatment

An impacted canine can be associated with a significant risk of damage to adjacent teeth, particularly the lateral and occasionally the central incisors (Fig. 10.26) and often requires surgical intervention combined with prolonged orthodontic treatment in order to accommodate it in the maxillary arch. Some evidence exists from prospective studies to suggest that early extraction of the deciduous canine can help prevent a palatally ectopic permanent canine becoming impacted (Fig. 10.27) (Ericson & Kurol, 1988; Power & Short, 1993), particularly if there is a lack of crowding or headgear is used to create space (Leonardi et al, 2004). Whilst this evidence is weak (Parkin et al, 2009), with radiographic evidence of an ectopic position and a lack of normal resorption associated with the deciduous canine, consideration should be given to elective extraction of this tooth. The best results seem to be obtained under the following conditions:

- Patient aged between 10 and 13 years and in the mixed dentition;
- Canine positioned distal to the midline of the lateral incisor root and less than 55° to the mid-sagittal plane; and
- An absence of crowding in the maxillary arch.

If radiographic evidence of an improvement in canine position is not evident within 12 months of extraction, further treatment should be considered.

Management

The maxillary canine is a large tooth, possessing the longest root in the dentition and forming an important aesthetic and functional component of the occlusion. Every effort should be made to try and accommodate this tooth in the dental arch. However, a number of general factors should be taken into consideration when treatment planning for an impacted canine:

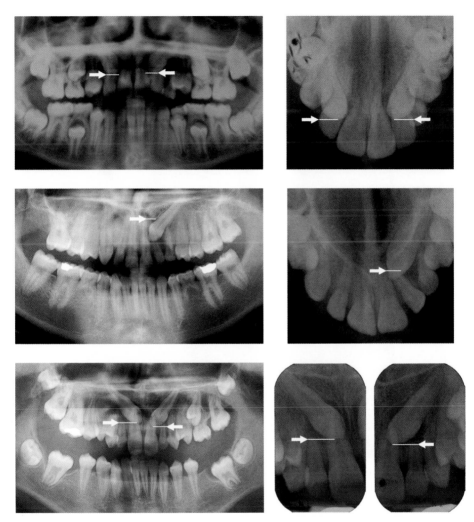

Figure 10.25 Vertical parallax to localize maxillary canine position. In the upper radiographs, the coronal tip of both maxillary canines lie midway along the roots of the lateral incisors on the panoramic radiograph; whilst on the anterior occlusal radiograph they are clearly midway along the crowns of the lateral incisors. These canines have moved down as the X-ray tube has moved up and are therefore buccally positioned. In the middle radiographs, the UL3 is situated below the root apex of the UL2 on the panoramic radiograph; whilst on the anterior occlusal radiograph it is now situated above the tip. The canine has moved up as the X-ray tube has moved up and is therefore positioned palatally. In the lower radiographs the coronal tips of both maxillary canines are situated just below the apices of the lateral incisors on the panoramic radiograph; whilst on the periapical radiographs they are in a similar position. These canines have not moved significantly as the X-ray tube has moved and are therefore situated in the line of the dental arch.

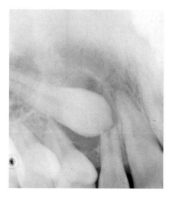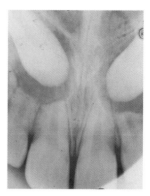

Figure 10.26 Resorption of the UR2 (left) and the UR2, UR1 and UL2 (right) root apices in association with impacted maxillary canines. Left panel courtesy of Jackie Silvester.

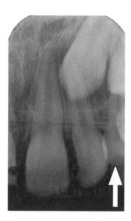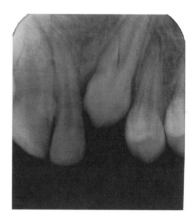

Figure 10.27 Improvement in the position of an impacted maxillary canine after extraction of its deciduous predecessor (arrowed).

- Patient attitude to treatment;
- Position of the canine;
- Presence of any associated pathology; and
- Underlying malocclusion.

The treatment of choice is generally surgical exposure followed by orthodontic alignment. However, the patient may not wish to undergo the extended orthodontic treatment that might be required to accommodate a canine following surgical exposure, or the canine may be in such a poor position that orthodontic alignment is not practical. In this case, autotransplantation of the tooth directly into the correct position is a further option. Alternatively, a decision can be made to extract the impacted canine or more rarely, leave it in situ.

Surgical exposure and orthodontic alignment

Surgical exposure aims to remove any hard or soft tissue obstruction that may be impeding eruption and can be enough to induce the canine to erupt, particularly those in more

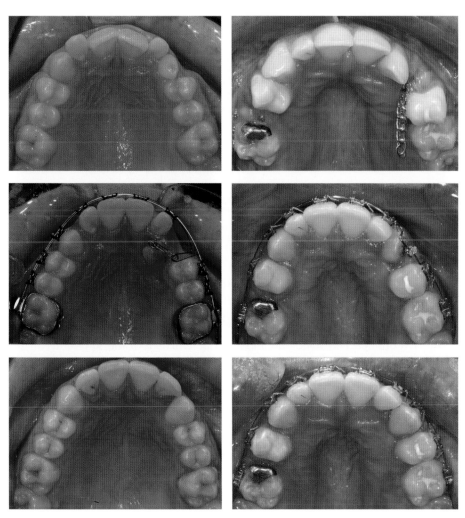

Figure 10.28 Surgical open (left panels) and closed (right panels) exposure and of a palatally impacted UL3 followed by orthodontic alignment.

favourable positions. For those that fail to respond or are more displaced, orthodontic alignment will also be required (Fig. 10.28). When embarking upon the prescription of surgical exposure and orthodontic alignment, the following should be remembered:

- This treatment usually involves fixed appliances and can be time-consuming; therefore patient motivation and compliance must be high.
- The canine must be in a position that makes orthodontic alignment an achievable goal. In particular, those situated as high as the apical third of the incisor roots, beyond the lateral incisor towards the midline or at an angle of greater than 55° to the mid-sagittal plane can be more difficult to align (Fig. 10.29).
- Space needs to be available in the maxillary arch for the canine. If this is lacking it will need to be generated, by either distal movement of the buccal segment or

Figure 10.29 The prognosis for successful orthodontic alignment of a palatally impacted maxillary canine is influenced by the position of this tooth. As the height increases, distance towards the dental midline reduces or angle to the mid-sagittal plane increases beyond 55°, the prognosis worsens.

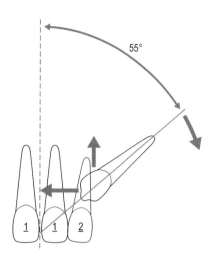

extraction. If the lateral incisor is diminutive, some consideration can be given to extracting this tooth; however, first premolars are the usual choice. It is desirable to ascertain that an impacted canine will erupt before extracting a premolar, but this is not always practical.

The site of impaction will be an important determinant of the surgical technique used for exposing a maxillary canine (see Box 10.4):

- For those on the labial side, the aim is for the tooth to be erupted through attached gingiva. Therefore, if the crown is located below the mucogingival junction, an open procedure is appropriate and the crown simply uncovered. For canines above the mucogingival junction, a closed exposure and bonding with gold chain is the treatment of choice unless the canine is labial to the lateral incisor; in these cases an apically repositioned flap will provide the best chance of the tooth erupting through an attached gingiva (Kokich, 2004).
- For palatally impacted canines an open or closed technique can be used, depending on the position of the tooth. In terms of outcome there is little evidence that one technique is significantly better than the other (Parkin et al, 2008).

A variety of techniques that allow orthodontic traction to be placed on an impacted canine have been described, but all will usually involve direct bonding of an orthodontic bracket (see Box. 10.4). Either removable or fixed appliances can be used to apply traction, but for either technique space is required in the dental arch. For canines in less favourable positions, fixed appliances are essential and as this process can be quite anchorage demanding, reinforcement should be considered. Using fixed appliances, traction can be applied with flexible piggyback archwires, elastomeric chain or string, rigid buccal arms or even magnets. The choice of technique will depend largely upon canine position and preference of the orthodontic operator.

Autotransplantation

Autotransplantation involves the surgical removal of an impacted canine and subsequent implantation into its normal position within the maxillary alveolus. Space will need to be available to accept the transplant and a short period of orthodontic treat-

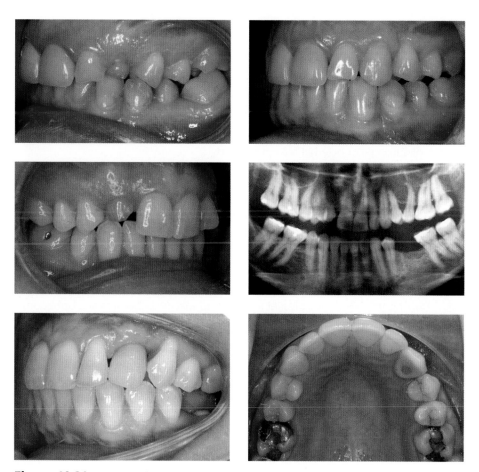

Figure 10.30 Autotransplantation of an impacted UL3 in an adult patient. Fixed appliances were used to create some space for this tooth prior to transplantation (upper panels). A retained URC with a poor long-term prognosis and aesthetics in a 43-year old woman who previously had the impacted UR3 extracted as a teenager (even though the UR2 was congenitally absent) (middle panels). Implant restoration to replace a previously extracted UL3 after orthodontic treatment to create space (Lower panels). Transplant and implant placement carried out by Jerry Kwok.

ment may be needed to generate this, particularly if a deciduous canine has been retained; but this process will generally be less time-consuming than aligning a canine with orthodontic traction (Fig. 10.30). If the position of the ectopic canine prevents any initial orthodontic treatment, the canine can initially be removed and 'parked' under the buccal mucosa whilst the necessary orthodontics is undertaken. Once space has been created for the tooth, a secondary surgical procedure can be undertaken to autotransplant the tooth.

A disadvantage of autotransplantation is that these teeth can be susceptible to subsequent ankylosis or external root resorption and generally have a reduced long-term prognosis in comparison to canines aligned orthodontically. In addition, the success of this technique is highly dependent upon the skill of the surgical operator.

- Surgical removal of the canine should be as atraumatic as possible (which can be difficult because these are often the very canines that are in the worst position) to avoid subsequent ankylosis;
- The canine should be kept out of occlusion and semi-rigidly splinted for a maximum of three weeks following the transplant;
- Once the splint is removed, the canine should be root canal treated to reduce the risk of subsequent external resorption; and
- Orthodontic movement of transplanted canines is possible but often limited in scope.

Extracting the canine or leaving it in situ

If a decision is made not to accommodate the impacted canine, then it can be extracted or left in situ. In either case, if the deciduous canine remains, the patient should be aware of the long-term prognosis and the likely need for eventual replacement of this tooth (see Fig. 10.30, middle panels). Alternatively, if the deciduous canine is not retained, a good contact between the lateral incisor and first premolar should be established (see Fig. 7.14). This may already be present if there is no spacing in the arch and orthodontic treatment may be avoided. However, if there is any residual spacing, either space closure or prosthetic replacement will be necessary and in both cases, some orthodontic treatment may be required (particularly if there is also an underlying malocclusion). A number of factors should be remembered when extracting a permanent canine:

- If it is in a poor position, this will almost certainly involve a general anaesthetic.
- If the extraction is prescribed because the patient has declined orthodontic treatment, any options to accommodate the canine in the future will be lost.
- If the extraction is part of an orthodontic treatment plan, either unilaterally or in combination with other teeth, space distribution will need to be considered within the context of the whole malocclusion. Ideally, space should be closed and a contact between the lateral incisor and first premolar established (Box 10.5). However, this may not be possible in the absence of crowding or an increased overjet.
- If space is not to be closed, prosthetic replacement of the canine with a single unit bridge or implant will be required.
- In the presence of severe resorption and a poor long-term prognosis associated with any incisor teeth (see Fig. 10.26), canine extraction should be avoided and ideally, this tooth accommodated in the dental arch (Fig. 10.31).

The option to leave a maxillary canine in situ is usually made on the basis that the patient is happy with their dental appearance and does not wish to have any form of treatment.

- Ideally, the canine should not be closely associated with the erupted dentition;
- There should be no evidence of any pathological change or root resorption affecting the adjacent teeth;
- Regular radiographic review is recommended in the growing patient because incisor roots can be vulnerable to resorption; and
- Longer term pathological change, such as follicular enlargement and cyst formation, should also be monitored radiographically.

Box 10.5 Putting a first premolar in the canine position

The morphology of the maxillary first premolar differs from that of the canine in several respects:
- The root is smaller and often bifid, lacking the characteristic wide and prominent labial surface seen in the canine.
- The crown is also smaller from the buccal aspect and there is an additional palatal cusp.

However, from the buccal aspect the premolar crown does resemble that of the canine and this tooth can make an excellent substitute, which can be enhanced by a few modifications:
- The premolar root should be placed more buccally in the maxilla to create a canine eminence.
- The crown can also be rotated mesiopalatally which increases the mesiodistal width, helps to hide the palatal cusp and improves the occlusal relation with the mandibular canine.
- The palatal cusp can also be ground to reduce its prominence.
- Group function in lateral excursion is preferable to guidance, which avoids heavy loading of the less robust premolar root.

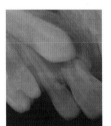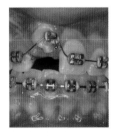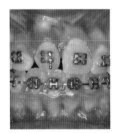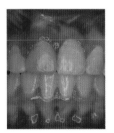

Figure 10.31 Marked resorption of the UR1 in association with an impacted canine. The UR1 was extracted, the canine brought down into the arch and then modified with composite to resemble the central incisor.

Unerupted permanent mandibular canine

The permanent mandibular canine fails to erupt less commonly than the maxillary and when this does occur, it is usually a consequence of crowding. These teeth are often vertically orientated, labially placed and will erupt spontaneously once space is available in the arch. If surgical exposure is required, care should be taken to ensure these teeth erupt through attached gingiva. Occasionally an impacted mandibular canine can fail to erupt and migrate within the mandible, particularly if it is orientated horizontally (Fig. 10.32) (Peck, 1998). These teeth are not generally amenable to orthodontic traction and the options are then extraction or autotransplantation.

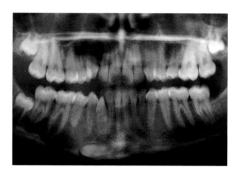

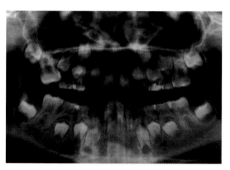

Figure 10.32 Retained LLC and horizontally displaced LL3. Courtesy of Jackie Silvester.

Figure 10.33 Impaction of the UR6 against the URE.

Impacted maxillary first permanent molar

Impaction of a maxillary first permanent molar against the second deciduous molar (Fig. 10.33) occurs in around 4% of the population and is usually indicative of crowding in the posterior maxilla (Kurol & Bjerklin, 1982).

- Clinical examination often reveals only the distal part of the offending first permanent molar erupted in the oral cavity; and
- Radiographic examination shows a mesially angulated first permanent molar impacted against the resorbing distal surface of the second deciduous molar.

Occasionally these teeth will spontaneously erupt but if this does not occur within 6–12 months, some intervention is indicated:

- A separating elastic, spring or brass wire placed below the contact point between the permanent and deciduous molars, or distal grinding of the second deciduous molar can help to disimpact the first molar.
- Extraction (or early loss due to resorption) of the second deciduous molar will relieve the impaction, but usually results in space loss affecting the second premolar region as the permanent molar drifts forwards into the space vacated by the deciduous molar. Orthodontic intervention may then be required to upright a mesially angulated first permanent molar and regenerate the lost premolar space.

Primary failure of eruption

Primary failure of eruption (PFE) is an isolated condition associated with a localized failure of tooth eruption:

- The molar dentition is more commonly affected than the incisor;
- Affected teeth may erupt into initial occlusion and then cease to erupt, or may fail to erupt entirely;
- Both deciduous and permanent teeth may be affected;
- Involvement may be unilateral or bilateral;
- Involved permanent teeth tend to become ankylosed; and
- Application of orthodontic force leads to ankylosis rather than normal tooth movement.

Diagnosis of PFE is usually made when there is an absence of any clear genetic, pathological or environmental factor responsible for preventing the eruption of an affected tooth (Fig. 10.34).

Management

Management of PFE is difficult because active orthodontic extrusion will normally result in ankylosis and a failure to bring an affected tooth into occlusion. Extraction, followed by either orthodontic space closure or prosthetic replacement, is usually indicated. Alternatively, localized bony osteotomy and orthodontic extrusion of the whole segment can be attempted. If some eruption of the tooth has occurred, a localized coronal buildup may be the treatment of choice to improve the vertical position. Cases where multiple teeth are involved are more difficult to manage, the only available method of bringing them into occlusion being a segmental osteotomy.

Transposition

Dental transposition is the complete positional interchange of two adjacent teeth, or the development, or eruption of a tooth in a position normally occupied by a non-adjacent tooth.

- Transposition can affect the maxillary or mandibular dentition, either unilaterally or bilaterally but is rare, occurring in below 1% of most populations; and
- The canine tooth is almost always affected, with the majority of cases involving the canine and first premolar in the maxilla (Fig. 10.35), or canine and lateral incisor in the mandible (Table 10.6).

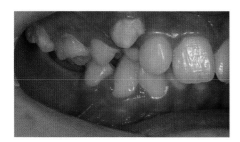 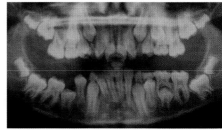

Figure 10.34 Primary failure of eruption affecting the LR6.

Table 10.6 Classification of dental transposition[a]
Maxilla
<ul><li>Maxillary canine first premolar (Mx.C.P1)</li><li>Maxillary canine lateral incisor (Mx.C.I2)</li><li>Maxillary canine first molar (Mx.M1)</li><li>Maxillary lateral incisor central incisor (Mx.I2.I1)</li><li>Maxillary canine central incisor (Mx.C.I1)</li></ul>
Mandible
<ul><li>Mandibular lateral incisor canine (Md.L2.C)</li><li>Mandibular canine transmigration (Md.C.trans)</li></ul>
[a]Peck et al, 1993, 1998.

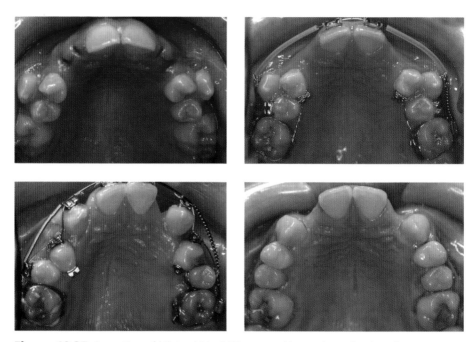

Figure 10.35 Correction of bilateral Mx.C.P1 transpositions using a fixed appliance.

Several mechanisms to account for the phenomenon of dental transposition have been proposed:

- The positional interchange of developing tooth buds;
- Alteration of tooth eruption paths;
- Retention of deciduous teeth; and
- Trauma.

However, many types of transposition are often associated with factors that have a genetic basis:

- Female predilection;
- Unilateral and left-sided dominance;
- Hypodontia;
- Peg-shaped maxillary lateral incisor teeth;
- Retained primary teeth; and
- Down syndrome.

On this basis it has been suggested that the primary aetiological basis of transposition is genetic, within a model of multifactorial inheritance (Peck et al, 1993, 1998).

Management

Interceptive extraction of an overlying deciduous tooth may be considered if a transposition is identified early enough and this may facilitate correction, particularly if the transposition is not fully established. Definitive treatment of an established transposition will involve either:

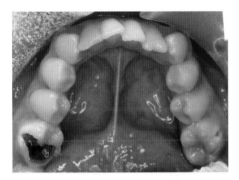

Figure 10.36 Carious mandibular first permanent molars.

- Correcting the order of affected teeth;
- Accepting the transposed order; and
- Extracting one of the affected teeth.
   These options need to be evaluated as part of the overall treatment plan for each individual malocclusion and will often require fixed appliances (Ngan et al, 2004).

Early loss of first permanent molars
The decennial National Children's Dental Health Survey has clearly shown a progressive reduction in dentinal caries experience in the permanent dentition of children aged between 8 and 15 years over the past thirty years (Pitts et al, 2006). However, in those children who do experience dental caries, first permanent molars can be susceptible to progressive and rapid decay (Fig. 10.36). In addition, combined first molar–incisor hypomineralization (MIH) is a recognized condition of unknown aetiology seen in around 15% of Caucasian children, which can significantly affect the long-term prognosis of first permanent molars in more severe cases (Koch et al, 1987). The increased use of fixed orthodontic appliances has meant that a good occlusal result can be obtained following the enforced loss of these teeth in a wider range of cases (Sandler et al, 2000). However, those children who require first molar extraction are often the least suitable for subsequent fixed appliance treatment because of high caries susceptibility and low potential compliance.
   Ideally, premature loss of first molars should be followed by successful eruption of the second molars to replace them, ultimately followed by third molars to complete the molar dentition (Fig. 10.37). If any space is required within the arches to correct an underlying malocclusion, the first molar extraction sites should provide this. However, extraction of these teeth often results in a large amount of space being created at some distance from those sites where it is required to relieve incisor crowding or reduce an overjet. In these circumstances, fixed appliances will be required to control this.
   First permanent molars are never the ideal choice of teeth to extract because significant occlusal complications can result, particularly if they are removed before the age of 8 years:
- There is often no radiographic evidence of third molar development at this stage and if these teeth fail to form, the molar dentition will be compromised;
- The unerupted mandibular second premolar can drift distally and tip from its position below the apices of the deciduous second molar;

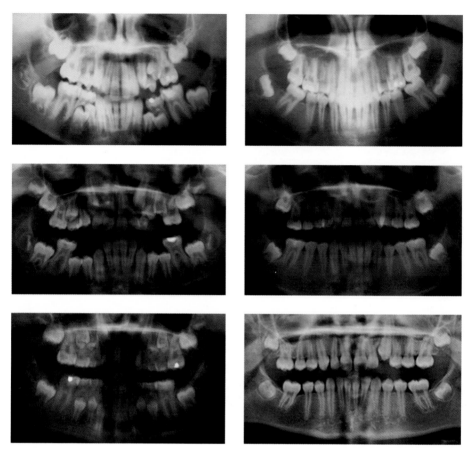

Figure 10.37 Good occlusal results following extraction of the lower first permanent molars (upper panels) and all four first permanent molars (middle and lower panels). The second molars are at a good angulation with minimal spacing and there is evidence of third molar development.

- The lower labial segment can retrocline, resulting in an increased overbite; and
- The maxillary second molar will often erupt into a good position, but space loss can be rapid, which can have consequences if there are potential space requirements elsewhere in the maxillary arch

Delayed extraction, during the later stages of second molar eruption, can also result in occlusal problems (Fig. 10.38):

- The mandibular second molar can tip mesially and rotate mesiolingually, producing spacing, poor mesial contact with the second premolar and occlusal interferences;
- The erupted mandibular second premolar can also tip distally towards the second molar, worsening the contact point relationships; and

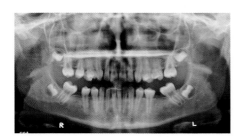

Figure 10.38 A poor occlusal result following extraction of the lower first permanent molars. The second permanent molars are spaced and mesially angulated after late extraction of the first molars.

- Significant loss of alveolar bone can occur in these regions of spacing, which can make subsequent orthodontic space closure difficult.

However, in many cases the poor prognosis associated with carious, hypoplastic or heavily restored first molars will dictate that extraction is required. Indeed, radiographic evidence of caries into dentine affecting first permanent molars should elicit consideration of their elective extraction. The best spontaneous occlusal results are obtained in the following circumstances:

- The child should be aged around 9 years;
- All permanent teeth (including third molars) are present;
- There is a class I occlusion;
- Minimal incisor or moderate buccal segment crowding is present; and
- The mandibular second molar roots should be approximately half-formed, with evidence of early dentine calcification within the bifurcation.

In most circumstances, not all of the first permanent molars will have a poor prognosis and the need for balancing or compensating extractions will have to be evaluated. Generally, extraction of a mandibular first molar may require compensatory extraction of the opposing maxillary molar to prevent overeruption of this tooth. This decision is more difficult if space is required in the maxillary arch to correct a malocclusion (Box 10.6):

- If the patient is not ready for definitive treatment, attempts can be made to delay the compensating extraction and either monitor or actively prevent any potential overeruption of the maxillary first molar.
- Alternatively, the first molar can be extracted and the space maintained if the second molar is present, for use during later treatment. However, patients with a history of extensive dental caries do not represent the most appropriate cases for long-term wear of space maintainers.
- If definitive treatment can begin immediately there is less need for compensating extraction unless the maxillary first molar has a reduced prognosis. With a sound first molar, extraction of a premolar may be considered, particularly if space is required to reduce an overjet.

Balancing first molar extractions are rarely required to preserve a centreline. However, these extraction decisions will need to be made as part of the overall treatment plan for the whole occlusion.

Early loss of the maxillary central incisor

Traumatic loss of a maxillary central incisor is seen in around of 3% of children and usually occurs unilaterally, in the mixed dentition and in a child with an increased

Box 10.6   Treatment planning for the loss of first permanent molars

Class I Malocclusion
- Minimal incisor or moderate premolar crowding—aim for extraction at the optimal time for good spontaneous eruption of second molars, relief of crowding and space closure.
- More severe crowding (particularly in the incisor regions)—either delay extraction until the second molars have erupted and use the extraction space for tooth alignment with fixed appliances; or extract at the optimal time for spontaneous space closure and treat the crowding once the permanent dentition is established. However, if premolar extractions are likely to be required, third molars should be present and of good morphology.

Class II Division 1 Malocclusion
- Space will be required to relieve any crowding and reduce the overjet. Timing of maxillary first molar extraction is important because of the need for overjet reduction.
- Extract maxillary first molars at the optimal time and correct the sagittal discrepancy early with a functional appliance, or a removable appliance and headgear. Fixed appliances can then be used to detail the occlusion.
- Extract maxillary first molars at the optimal time but wait for second molar eruption. Then treat with either a functional appliance, second molar distalization or premolar extraction in combination with fixed appliances. However, for premolar extraction the third molars should ideally be present and of good morphology.
- Extract maxillary first molars after second molar eruption and use the space for overjet reduction with fixed appliances.

Class II Division 2 Malocclusion
- Requirements are similar to those for a class 2 division 1, space being required to relieve crowding and correct the incisor relationship. However, overbite reduction can be difficult if large extraction spaces need to be closed in the mandibular arch and these should therefore be avoided. If mandibular first molars need to be extracted this should be done at the optimal time to avoid spacing associated with erupted second molars, even if this may result in some worsening of the overbite.

Class III Malocclusion
- For those class III malocclusions that will be treated with orthodontics alone, space will often be required to relieve crowding in the maxillary arch and for incisor retraction in the mandible and this should ideally be provided by extracting the first molars after the second molars have erupted.

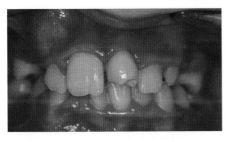 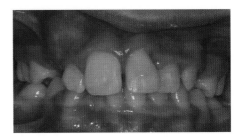

Figure 10.39 Premolar transplanted into the central incisor position and built up with composite Courtesy of Joanna Johnson.

overjet (Jarvinen, 1978). Reimplantation should always be attempted if possible, because regardless of the long-term prognosis, these teeth will serve as a useful maintainer of both arch space and alveolar bone. If they are subsequently lost, longer term space maintenance can be achieved with a simple upper partial denture. If these teeth are not reimplanted, a decision will need to be made regarding space management. Long-term space maintenance can be achieved with a partial denture; however, this can be associated with a loss of alveolar bone height, which can make subsequent prosthetic replacement more difficult. Alternatively, the space can be allowed to close and reopened in the permanent dentition prior to prosthetic replacement. This allows preservation of alveolar bone, but will require fixed appliance treatment and often space creation in the upper arch.

Management
Unilateral loss of a maxillary central incisor will usually require prosthetic replacement, with either a resin-retained bridge or implant, because a lateral incisor rarely makes a good unilateral substitute for the central incisor. If space is required elsewhere in the maxillary arch, this is usually dealt with on its own merit. Occasionally, if premolar extractions are planned to correct any underlying malocclusion, autotransplantation and subsequent coronal modification of one of these teeth can provide a further option for replacing the maxillary incisor (Fig. 10.39).

In cases of bilateral loss, if space is required to reduce an overjet or relieve crowding and the lateral incisors are of a reasonable size and form, consideration can be given to moving them into the position vacated by the centrals (Fig. 10.40), although it can be difficult to obtain good aesthetics without modifying their coronal morphology restoratively.

Maxillary midline diastema
A maxillary midline diastema can be a normal feature of dental development and will often improve following eruption of the permanent canine teeth. However, a number of other causes also exist (Fig. 10.41):
- Spacing of the dentition;
- Proclination of the upper incisors (often in association with a digit sucking habit);
- Congenital absence (or microdontia) of maxillary lateral incisors;
- Midline supernumerary;
- Pathological change in the anterior maxilla (rarely); and
- A prominent labial frenum.

Figure 10.40 Lateral incisor teeth as the centrals following traumatic loss.

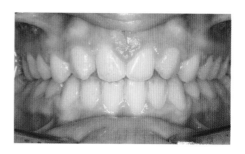

Figure 10.41 Maxillary diastema.

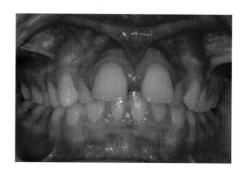

Management

Management of a midline diastema will depend primarily upon the underlying cause. In the absence of any obstruction, pathology or marked reduction in the amount of tooth tissue within the anterior maxilla, active orthodontic treatment to close a diastema is usually carried out in the permanent dentition and unless small, normally requires bodily movement of the incisors with a fixed appliance. The propensity of a closed maxillary diastema to reopen following brace removal means that long-term retention is usually mandatory. For this reason, particularly for a minor diastema, persuading the patient that it is a feature of individuality that does not require closing can be advantageous.

A prominent labial frenum can be suspected in the following circumstances:

- It can often be seen between the maxillary central incisors on direct visualization;
- Blanching in the region of the frenum can occur when tension is applied by lifting the upper lip; and
- A spade-shaped or notched intermaxillary segment can be visible on radiographic examination.

The relative contribution of a prominent labial frenum in the aetiology of a diastema is controversial. However, if it is present, removal (or frenectomy) can be prescribed as part of the orthodontic treatment plan to close a diastema. Opinions vary as to the optimal time to carry out a frenectomy:

- Improved surgical access and the theory that scar tissue contraction can help approximate the maxillary incisors argues in favour of frenectomy before orthodontic closure; and
- A tendency for superior remodelling of the labial frenum on closure of a diastema means frenectomy should be delayed until after the diastema is closed.

On balance it would seem sensible to delay any frenectomy until orthodontic closure of the diastema has been completed, which should be carried out in the permanent dentition, following eruption of the maxillary canines.

Digit sucking

A prolonged digit sucking habit can give rise to a number of characteristic features as part of a malocclusion and these often manifest in the late deciduous or early mixed dentitions (see Fig. 1.10):

- Proclination of the upper incisors;
- Anterior open bite (often with a degree of asymmetry);
- Narrow maxillary arch;
- Posterior crossbite; and
- Increased lower face height.

These features are associated directly with the habitual placement of the digit and indirectly with the reduced tongue position and negative intraoral pressure generated with the habit. The underlying pattern of facial growth will also influence the malocclusion, any tendency toward vertical excess and a posterior mandibular growth rotation will potentially worsen the effects of any habit, or even make a more significant contribution than the habit itself.

Digit sucking occurs quite commonly in children below the age of 10 years and will often cease spontaneously. In most of these cases, the anterior open bite will resolve, although correction of the crossbite may require some maxillary arch expansion. However, in a minority of cases the habit can persist into the teenage years and can be the main contributing factor in the aetiology of a significant malocclusion. These children should be encouraged to stop the habit, ideally without intervention, although a variety of commercial aids are also available. If these fail occasionally a simple removable or fixed orthodontic appliance may be required to finally break the habit.

Crowding

As the permanent incisors are larger than their deciduous predecessors, space must be made available in the dental arches if they are to erupt without crowding. Spacing between the deciduous incisors can provide some of this (see Box 4.5 and Fig. 4.15); but the permanent incisors commonly erupt into crowded positions, particularly in the lower arch. A small improvement in this crowding can sometimes occur prior to eruption of the permanent canines, due largely to incisor proclination during eruption and some transverse expansion into the canine regions (Lundy & Richardson, 1995). However, once the permanent canines have erupted, there will almost certainly be no further improvement in incisor alignment and often an increase in crowding.

A variety of interceptive measures for alleviating incisor crowding during the mixed dentition, including arch expansion, extraction of the deciduous canines and serial extraction, have been described. Expansion across the intercanine width is largely unstable, particularly in the lower arch and is not recommended. Extraction of the deciduous canines will result in some short-term improvement in lower incisor alignment; however, whilst this can be effective for labiolingual displacements, it is less so for rotations. In addition, the incisors may tip lingually, which can reduce arch length and result in greater crowding in the long-term. Despite these limitations the extraction of deciduous canines can be a useful strategy in the following circumstances:

- Preventing the maxillary lateral incisors erupting into crossbite;
- Helping to align a labially standing lower incisor and preventing any gingival recession;
- Aiding in the correction of a class III incisor relationship;
- Providing space for alignment and crossbite correction associated with a crowded maxillary incisor; and
- As an interceptive procedure to prevent impaction of the maxillary canine.

Serial extraction

The use of serial extraction as an interceptive orthodontic procedure was originally popularized by Bjerger Kjellgren at the Eastman Dental Institute in Stockholm (Kjellgren, 1947). Serial extraction aims to produce a well-aligned dentition in cases with a full complement of teeth and no significant sagittal discrepancy, without the need for orthodontic appliances. Essentially, serial extraction involves:

- Extraction of all the deciduous canines as the permanent lateral incisors are erupting, which provides space for these teeth to align;
- Extraction of first deciduous molars around twelve months later to encourage eruption of first premolars in advance of the permanent canines; and
- Ultimately, extraction of the first premolars as the permanent canines are beginning their eruption, as this allows for their spontaneous alignment.

Serial extraction borrows space in the mixed dentition for early alignment of the labial segments and ultimately repays this by extraction of four first premolars. As a complete sequence it is no longer recommended for a number of reasons:

- The child undergoes progressive extraction of twelve teeth;
- In the maxilla, premolars usually erupt before the permanent canines anyway;
- Extraction of first deciduous molars can result in significant buccal segment space loss if the permanent canine does erupt before the first premolar;
- An aberrant position of the maxillary canine can mean a failure to erupt even after premolar extraction; and
- A fixed orthodontic appliance may be needed anyway to produce good final alignment and close any residual space. It is easier, simpler and more predictable to wait until the early permanent dentition before undertaking premolar extraction and orthodontic alignment.

Crossbites

Teeth can erupt into a position of crossbite during the mixed dentition, either individually or within a group. Early correction is indicated, particularly if the crossbite is associated with a mandibular displacement or periodontal damage, and this can be achieved relatively easily during the mixed dentition.

Posterior crossbite

A posterior crossbite in the mixed dentition can be an early manifestation of a skeletal discrepancy, or be related to a persistent digit-sucking habit and can occur unilaterally or bilaterally. There is a weak association between posterior crossbite with displacement and the later development of temporomandibular dysfunction (Mohlin & Thilander, 1984); whilst asymmetric muscular activity associated with an established mandibular displacement can be perpetuated from the primary and mixed into the

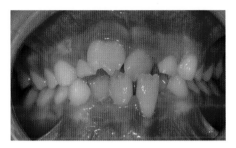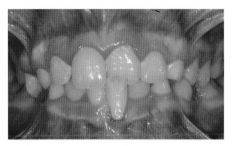

Figure 10.42 Gingival recession affecting the LL1 in two cases of anterior crossbite.

permanent dentition. For these reasons, it is considered appropriate to correct a posterior crossbite and eliminate the displacement as early as possible (Harrison & Ashby, 2001) and a number of relatively simple methods are available to do this.

Removable appliances
Correction can occasionally be achieved by occlusal grinding in the primary dentition; however, more commonly a removable appliance with a midline expansion screw can be used in the early mixed dentition (see Fig. 8.14).

Fixed appliances
Fixed palatal expanders such as a quad- or trihelix can be used for expansion in the mixed dentition, especially if some skeletal change is also desired.

Anterior crossbites
An anterior crossbite can cause gingival recession associated with the lower incisors if there is a displacement on closing, particularly if these teeth are displaced labially (Fig. 10.42). This is an indication for treatment in the mixed dentition and correction can be achieved with removable or fixed appliances. In the presence of a positive overbite, a corrected anterior crossbite will usually be self-retaining.

Removable appliances
If space is available in the dental arch, a removable appliance can be used to push the upper incisor teeth over the bite using simple palatal springs (see Fig. 8.16). This tipping movement will also usually result in some reduction of the overbite, which is often beneficial. Occlusal interferences usually need to be eliminated before overbite correction can take place, especially with an increased overbite, and posterior occlusal capping can be incorporated into the appliance to achieve this.

Fixed appliances
If space or bodily tooth movement are required to correct an anterior crossbite, removable appliances are inappropriate. In these circumstances, a fixed appliance with four brackets placed on the upper incisors and bands on the first molars (2 × 4 appliance) (Fig. 10.43) can be very effective. The bite can be opened with glass ionomer cement placed on the occlusal surface of the first molars. Simple fixed appliances offer a number of advantages over removable appliances:

- Bodily tooth movement;
- Less dependent on patient compliance;
- Rapid correction of an anterior crossbite;
- Multiple tooth movement;

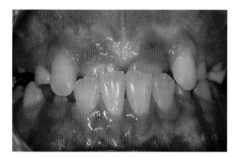

Figure 10.43 Correction of an anterior crossbite with a 2 × 4 fixed appliance.

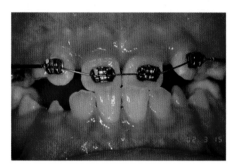
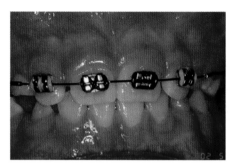

- Space possibly created for tooth movement if necessary; and
- Possible tooth extrusion for creating a positive overbite.

Skeletal problems in the mixed dentition

Skeletal discrepancies can also manifest during the mixed dentition and will often respond well to early intervention. However, the potential advantages associated with early correction need to be considered in relation to the disadvantages of long-term treatment, maintaining the stability of correction during subsequent facial growth and the fact that a shorter course of treatment in the late mixed or early permanent dentition will almost certainly achieve the same result.

Class II malocclusion

Class II malocclusions are amenable to early treatment using functional appliances; however, the timing of treatment should be carefully considered. Several large randomized controlled trials have shown little difference in outcome, in terms of both overall growth and the final occlusal result, between patients who underwent an early phase of treatment to reduce an overjet in the mixed dentition and those who received comprehensive treatment in the late mixed and early permanent dentition (see Chapter 8). Whilst overjet correction can be rapid in the mixed dentition, a significant problem is the length of time this correction must be retained whilst waiting for a patient to enter the permanent dentition, prior to a final stage of fixed appliance orthodontic treatment to detail the occlusion. The only significant difference would appear to be the overall treatment time; patients who undergo early correction ultimately spend longer in treatment. As a general rule, the most effective time for undertaking

> **Box 10.7 Indications for treatment of class II discrepancies in the mixed dentition**
>
> - Class II females with a significant skeletal discrepancy.
> - An increased overjet, which is a source of teasing and bullying.
> - An increased overjet, which is at risk of trauma (often associated with gross lip incompetence and marked maxillary protrusion).

correction of a class II malocclusion is during the adolescent growth spurt, as this will optimize mandibular growth whilst limiting the overall treatment time. However, several exceptions do exist (Box 10.7) and these relate primarily to reducing the risk of trauma and improving self-esteem.

Removable appliances
If the upper labial segment is proclined and spaced, a removable appliance with an active labial bow can be used to reduce an overjet (see Fig. 8.13). This should be worn full-time until the overjet is reduced and then as a retainer at night. In the presence of maxillary excess or a class II buccal segment relationship, headgear may also be needed in conjunction with the removable appliance.

Functional appliances
Functional appliances are very effective at overjet reduction. There can be problems associated with retention of tooth-borne appliances in the mixed dentition, as the first molars are often not fully erupted and can be difficult to crib effectively. The use of an activator-type appliance can help overcome this.

Class III malocclusions
A reduced or reverse overjet in the mixed dentition is usually a sign of an underlying class III skeletal relationship and this will tend to worsen with age. Treatment decisions are often delayed at this stage to monitor further growth and to better determine the extent of the skeletal problem; however, early treatment may be considered in patients with the following features:
- Skeletal class I, or only mildly class III;
- An average or reduced lower face height; and
- A large anterior displacement on closing.

A class III malocclusion on a skeletal I base with a significant forward mandibular displacement is sometimes referred to as a 'pseudo class III malocclusion', because the incisor relationship does not reflect the underlying skeletal relationship (see Fig. 6.17). This type of class III malocclusion is very amenable to early orthodontic treatment, but creating a positive overbite as well as overjet is crucial for stability following correction. When the overbite is reduced or there is an anterior openbite, it is more sensible to monitor growth into adolescence before final treatment decisions are made.

Functional appliances
Functional appliances are most commonly used to correct class II malocclusion; however, numerous appliances have also been described for the treatment of class III cases. These are only really able to treat the milder class III cases described above. This is largely because their effects are restricted to inducing the following tooth movements:

- Upper incisor proclination;
- Lower incisor retroclination; and
- Backward and downward rotation of the mandible.

A class III version of the Fränkel Functional Regulator (FR III) is most commonly used, but this appliance is bulky, prone to breakage and difficult to wear. More recently, a class III twin block, with the blocks reversed in comparison to the class II version, has been described (Fig. 10.44).

Fixed appliances

A 2 × 4 appliance can be used to correct a class III incisor relationship. If proclination of the upper labial segment is required, a compressed loop or pushcoil can be placed in the buccal segments.

Protraction headgear

Extraoral force can be utilized in an attempt to move the maxilla forwards in class III cases, applied by attaching heavy elastics from either a removable or fixed appliance to a facemask, which rests on the patient's forehead and chin for anchorage (Fig. 10.45). If worn for 12 to 14 hours each day, a significant anterior skeletal displacement of the maxilla is possible, making this approach the most appropriate for patients with maxillary hypoplasia (Fig. 10.46). This technique is theoretically more effective when combined with rapid maxillary expansion, because the expansion will disrupt the maxillary sutures and allows greater anterior displacement of the maxilla by the headgear. Greater skeletal change is seen in pre-adolescent patients, which essentially means those in the early mixed dentition. However, long-term results are dependent on further growth and patients with a vertical growth pattern or mandibular prognathism will often tend to outgrow any early positive effects of treatment. In addition, these appliances are some of the most demanding to wear in terms of patient compliance.

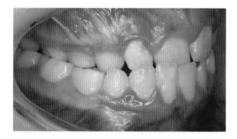

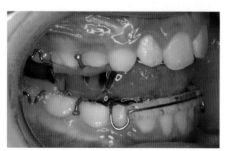

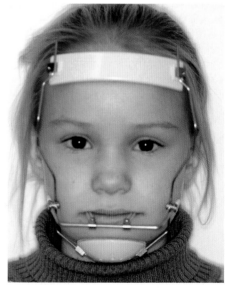

Figure 10.44 Reverse twin block for class III malocclusion.

Figure 10.45 Facemask therapy to induce protraction of the maxillary dentition.

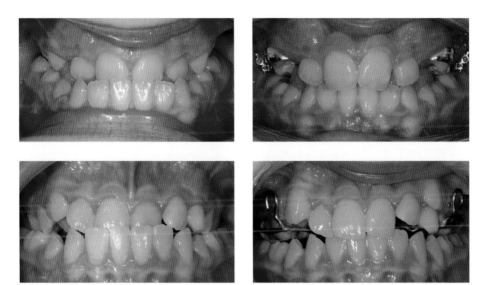

Figure 10.46 Considerable improvement can be achieved in a class III malocclusion treated with reverse headgear and palatal expansion. However, long-term stability is less predictable.

Abnormalities of tooth structure

Defects in the enamel or dentine of the tooth can give rise to varying degrees of discolouration and loss of structure. These anomalies can be caused by local and systemic environmental factors or genetic disease.

Enamel defects
The enamel of deciduous teeth begins to calcify at around 4 months in utero and is complete by the end of the first year of life. In the permanent dentition, this process occurs between 4 months and around 8 years of age (excluding third molars). A range of local and systemic factors can disturb enamel formation, which can lead to chronological hypoplasia and hypocalcification of the tooth crown (Table 10.7).

- Deciduous teeth are vulnerable to maternal and fetal conditions that can affect their development in utero:
  - A neonatal line is usually present in the enamel of deciduous teeth. This line is caused by an alteration in the order of enamel prisms and reflects metabolic changes that take place at birth. The neonatal line is rarely visible to the naked eye but can be more marked in children who are born prematurely, have a traumatic birth or suffer from illness during the early neonatal period.
  - Systemic upset during the first year of life can also affect the deciduous enamel.
- In the permanent dentition, localized trauma or infection associated with the deciduous teeth can often affect enamel formation, particularly in the incisor region.
- A number of systemic disorders during early childhood can also disturb enamel formation in the permanent dentition.

Table 10.7 Anomalies of enamel and dentine

Enamel defects

Localized factors

- Infection
- Trauma

Systemic factors

- Endocrine disorders
- Infections
- Drugs
- Nutritional deficiency
- Haematological disorders
- Neonatal illness
- Postnatal illness
- Fluoride ingestion

Dentine defects

Localized factors

- Infection
- Trauma

Systemic factors

- Rickets
- Ehlers-Danlos syndrome
- Hypophosphatasia
- Nutritional deficiency
- Drugs (Tetracycline)

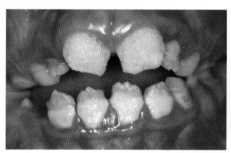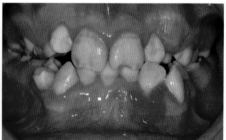

Figure 10.47 Amelogenesis imperfecta. Left panel courtesy of Joanna Johnson.

Amelogenesis imperfecta (OMIM 104510)

Amelogenesis imperfecta (AI) is a collective term for a group of inherited conditions characterized primarily by abnormal enamel formation in either dentition (Fig. 10.47). AI can be inherited as an autosomal dominant, autosomal recessive or sex-linked trait and has a prevalence that can range from 1 : 1,000 to 1 : 14,000, depending upon the population. The predominant enamel phenotype is either:

- Hypoplastic (normally mineralized but the matrix is deficient, resulting in thin enamel); or

Table 10.8   Classification of amelogenesis imperfecta[a]

Type I hypoplastic

- IA hypoplastic, pitted, autosomal dominant
- IB hypoplastic, local, autosomal dominant
- IC hypoplastic, local, autosomal recessive
- ID hypoplastic, smooth, autosomal dominant
- IE hypoplastic, smooth, X-linked dominant
- IF hypoplastic, rough, autosomal dominant
- IG enamel agenesis, autosomal recessive

Type II hypomaturation

- IIA hypomaturation, pigmented, autosomal recessive
- IIB hypomaturation
- IIC snow-capped teeth, X-linked
- IID autosomal dominant

Type III hypocalcified

- IIIA autosomal dominant
- IIIB autosomal recessive

Type IV hypomaturation–hypoplastic with taurodontism

- IVA hypomaturation–hypoplastic with taurodontism, autosomal dominant
- IVB hypoplastic–hypomaturation with taurodontism, autosomal dominant

[a]Witkop (1988).

- Hypomineralized (either hypomature or hypocalcified, or a combination of the two).

The classification of AI is complex, being based historically upon phenotype (Table 10.8). However, as knowledge of the genetic basis underlying this condition has improved, the classification has been adapted (Wright, 2006).

Dentine defects
In addition to systemic factors, localized environmental factors such as infection and trauma can interfere with dentinogenesis (Table 10.7).

Inherited conditions affecting dentine
A number of genetic conditions exist that can affect the dentine within teeth, either in isolation or in addition to other structures within the body (MacDougall et al, 2006) (Table 10.9). All of these conditions exhibit an autosomal dominant pattern of inheritance and can be classified as:

- Dentine dysplasia; or
- Dentinogenesis imperfecta.

Dentinogenesis imperfecta (DGI) represents the most common group of inherited dentine disorders (Fig. 10.48) and there are three essential subgroups, types I–III:

- Type I is associated with osteogenesis imperfecta or brittle bone disease and is caused by mutation in the *COLA1* or *COLA2* gene, both of which are essential for

Table 10.9 Genetic defects affecting dentine

- Dentine dysplasia type I (OMIM 125400) (rootless teeth)
- Dentine dysplasia type II (OMIM 125420)
- Dentinogenesis imperfecta
  - Type I (osteogenesis imperfecta)
  - Type II (OMIM 125490) (hereditary opalescent dentine)
  - Type III (OMIM 125500) (Brandywine staining)

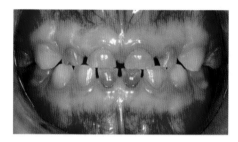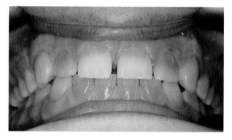

Figure 10.48 Dentinogenesis imperfecta in the deciduous and permanent dentitions. Courtesy of Evelyn Sheehy.

type I collagen formation in bones and dentine. The deciduous and permanent teeth are affected by discolouration, attrition and pulp canal obliteration.

- Type II (OMIM 125490) is seen in around 1 : 7,000 Caucasians and also affects teeth in both dentitions, causing translucent, amber and bluish grey discolouration, enamel chipping and marked attrition. The crowns are bulbous and the pulp canals also become obliterated.
- Type III (OMIM 125500) affects certain subpopulations of people, including Native American Indians and European Caucasians. Both dentitions can be affected by so-called 'shell teeth', which lose enamel and have poorly mineralized dentine, leading to multiple pulp exposures.

Orthodontic management of AI and DGI
Children affected by AI or DGI will require long-term multidisciplinary dental management. The appearance of affected teeth is often poor, with early loss of enamel leading to dentine exposure and subsequent sensitivity, which in turn can result in poor oral hygiene and a significant caries risk. All these factors make orthodontic treatment potentially difficult, this problem being compounded by a known association between AI and the presence of anterior open bite. When considering orthodontic treatment for the more severe cases:

- Removable appliances should be used where possible;
- Care needs to be taken if direct bonding is undertaken because bracket failure or removal can lead to enamel fracture;
- Orthodontic bands can be used where possible; and
- Oral hygiene and diet control must be carefully monitored during treatment.

Further reading

BECKER A (2007). *The Orthodontic Treatment of Impacted Teeth*, 2nd edn (London: Informa Healthcare).

BURDEN D, HARPER C, MITCHELL L, ET AL (1997). Management of unerupted maxillary incisors. Faculty of Dental Surgery of the Royal College of Surgeons of England. Available at URL:http://www.rcseng.ac.uk/fds/clinical_guidelines

HUSSAIN J, BURDEN D AND MCSHERRY P (2003). The management of the palatally ectopic maxillary canine. Faculty of Dental Surgery of the Royal College of Surgeons of England. Available at URL:http://www.rcseng.ac.uk/fds/clinical_guidelines

COBOURNE M, WILLIAMS A AND MCMULLEN R (2009). A guideline for the extraction of first permanent molars in children. Faculty of Dental Surgery of the Royal College of Surgeons of England (http://www.rcseng.ac.uk/fds/clinical_guidelines).

WINTER GB (2001). Anomalies of tooth formation and eruption. In: Welbury RR (ed) *Paediatric Dentistry* (Oxford: Oxford University Press).

References

BISHARA SE (1992). Impacted maxillary canines: a review. *Am J Orthod Dentofacial Orthop* 101:159–171.

BJERKLIN K AND BENNETT J (2000). The long-term survival of lower second primary molars in subjects with agenesis of the premolars. *Eur J Orthod* 22:245–255.

BRIN I, BECKER A AND SHALHAV M (1986). Position of the maxillary permanent canine in relation to anomalous or missing lateral incisors: a population study. *Eur J Orthod* 8:12–16.

BROOK AH (1984). A unifying aetiological explanation for anomalies of human tooth number and size. *Arch Oral Biol* 29:373–378.

COBOURNE MT (2007). Familial human hypodontia—is it all in the genes? *Br Dent J* 203:203–208.

ERICSON S AND KUROL J (1986). Radiographic assessment of maxillary canine eruption in children with clinical signs of eruption disturbance. *Eur J Orthod* 8:133–140.

ERICSON S AND KUROL J (1988). Early treatment of palatally erupting maxillary canines by extraction of the primary canines. *Eur J Orthod* 10:283–295.

FERGUSON JW (1990). Management of the unerupted maxillary canine. *Br Dent J* 169:11–17.

HARRISON JE AND ASHBY D (2001). Orthodontic treatment for posterior crossbites. *Cochrane Database Syst Rev*, CD000979.

JACOBS SG (1999). Localization of the unerupted maxillary canine: how to and when to. *Am J Orthod Dentofacial Orthop* 115:314–322.

JARVINEN S (1978). Incisal overjet and traumatic injuries to upper permanent incisors. A retrospective study. *Acta Odontol Scand* 36:359–362.

JUMLONGRAS D, BEI M, STIMSON JM, ET AL (2001). A nonsense mutation in MSX1 causes Witkop syndrome. *Am J Hum Genet* 69:67–74.

KJELLGREN B (1947). Serial extraction as a corrective procedure in dental orthopaedic therapy. *Trans Eur Orth Soc* 134–160.

KOCH G, HALLONSTEN AL, LUDVIGSSON N, ET AL (1987). Epidemiologic study of idiopathic enamel hypomineralization in permanent teeth of Swedish children. *Comm Dent Oral Epidemiol* 15:279–285.

KOKICH VG (2004). Surgical and orthodontic management of impacted maxillary canines. *Am J Orthod Dentofacial Orthop* 126:278–283.

KUROL J (1981). Infraocclusion of primary molars: an epidemiologic and familial study. *Community Dent Oral Epidemiol* 9:94–102.

KUROL J (2006). Impacted and ankylosed teeth: why, when, and how to intervene. *Am J Orthod Dentofacial Orthop* 129:S86–90.

KUROL J AND BJERKLIN K (1982). Ectopic eruption of maxillary first permanent molars: familial tendencies. *ASDC J Dent Child* 49:35–38.

LAMMI L, ARTE S, SOMER M, ET AL (2004). Mutations in AXIN2 cause familial tooth agenesis and predispose to colorectal cancer. *Am J Hum Genet* 74:1043–1050.

LEONARDI M, ARMI P, FRANCHI L ET AL (2004). Two interceptive approaches to palatally displaced canines: a prospective longitudinal study. *Angle Orthod* 74:581–586.

LUNDY HJ AND RICHARDSON ME (1995). Developmental changes in alignment of the lower labial segment. *Br J Orthod* 22:339–345.

MACDOUGALL M, DONG J AND ACEVEDO AC (2006). Molecular basis of human dentin diseases. *Am J Med Genet A* 140:2536–2546.

MOHLIN B AND THILANDER B (1984). The importance of the relationship between malocclusion and mandibular dysfunction and some clinical applications in adults. *Eur J Orthod* 6:192–204.

NEAL JJ AND BOWDEN DE (1988). The diagnostic value of panoramic radiographs in children aged nine to ten years. *Br J Orthod* 15:193–197.

NGAN DC, KHARBANDA OP AND DARENDELILER MA (2004). Considerations in the management of transposed teeth. *Aust Orthod J* 20:41–50.

NIEMINEN P, ARTE S, PIRINEN S, ET AL (1995). Gene defect in hypodontia: exclusion of MSX1 and MSX2 as candidate genes. *Hum Genet* 96:305–308.

PARKIN N, BENSON PE, SHAH A ET AL (2009). Extraction of primary (baby) teeth for unerupted palatally displaced permanent canine teeth in children. Cochrane Database Syst Rev 2: CD004621.

PARKIN N, BENSON PE, THIND B ET AL (2008). Open versus closed surgical exposure of canine teeth that are displaced in the roof of the mouth. Cochrane Database Syst Rev 4: CD006966.

PECK L, PECK S AND ATTIA Y (1993). Maxillary canine-first premolar transposition, associated dental anomalies and genetic basis. *Angle Orthod* 63:99–109; discussion 110.

PECK S (1998). On the phenomenon of intraosseous migration of nonerupting teeth. *Am J Orthod Dentofacial Orthop* 113:515–517.

PECK S, PECK L AND KATAJA M (1994). The palatally displaced canine as a dental anomaly of genetic origin. *Angle Orthod* 64:249–256.

PECK S, PECK L AND KATAJA M (1998). Mandibular lateral incisor-canine transposition, concomitant dental anomalies, and genetic control. *Angle Orthod* 68:455–466.

PITTS NB, CHESTNUTT IG, EVANS D, ET AL (2006). The dentinal caries experience of children in the United Kingdom, 2003. *Br Dent J* 200:313–320.

POWER SM AND SHORT MB (1993). An investigation into the response of palatally displaced canines to the removal of deciduous canines and an assessment of factors contributing to favourable eruption. *Br J Orthod* 20:215–223.

SANDLER PJ, ATKINSON R AND MURRAY AM (2000). For four sixes. *Am J Orthod Dentofacial Orthop* 117:418–434.

SARNAS KV AND RUNE B (1983). The facial profile in advanced hypodontia: a mixed longitudinal study of 141 children. *Eur J Orthod* 5:133–143.

SIMONS AL, STRITZEL F AND STAMATIOU J (1993). Anomalies associated with hypodontia of the permanant lateral incisors and second premolar. *J Clin Pediatr Dent* 17:109–111.

SLETTEN DW, SMITH BM, SOUTHARD KA, ET AL (2003). Retained deciduous mandibular molars in adults: a radiographic study of long-term changes. *Am J Orthod Dentofacial Orthop* 124:625–630.

STEWART DJ (1978). Dilacerated unerupted maxillary central incisors. *Br Dent J* 145:229–233.

TYROLOGOU S, KOCH G AND KUROL J (2005). Location, complications and treatment of mesiodentes—a retrospective study in children. *Swed Dent J* 29:1–9.

VAN DEN BOOGAARD MJ, DORLAND M, BEEMER FA AND VAN AMSTEL HK (2000). MSX1 mutation is associated with orofacial clefting and tooth agenesis in humans. *Nat Genet* 24:342–343.

VASTARDIS H, KARIMBUX N, GUTHUA SW, SEIDMAN JG ET AL (1996). A human MSX1 homeodomain missense mutation causes selective tooth agenesis. *Nat Genet* 13:417–421.

WALKER L, ENCISO R AND MAH J (2006). Three-dimensional localization of maxillary canines with cone-beam computed tomography. *Am J Orthod Dentofacial Orthop* 128:418–423.

WITKOP CJ JR (1988). Amelogenesis imperfecta, dentinogenesis imperfecta and dentin dysplasia revisited: problems in classification. *J Oral Pathol* 17:547–553.

WRIGHT JT (2006). The molecular etiologies and associated phenotypes of amelogenesis imperfecta. *Am J Med Genet A* 140:2547–2555.

The majority of orthodontic treatment is carried out in the late mixed or permanent dentition. This allows for comprehensive treatment within a finite and realistic time-frame, whilst optimizing adolescent growth and compliance. In this chapter the management of malocclusion in the permanent dentition will be discussed in terms of different occlusal traits. Although separated for clarity, an individual patient will often present with more than one of these. Therefore, treatment planning will routinely incorporate more than one aim. The final section in this chapter will look at the rationale and management of retention following active treatment.

Tooth–arch size problems

A discrepancy between the overall tooth size and arch dimension can lead to either dental arch crowding or spacing, depending upon whether there is too much or too little space for the teeth.

Crowding

Crowding and malalignment of the anterior teeth are some of the commonest problems encountered in the treatment of malocclusion, and patients are often very conscious of them. Crowding is usually recorded in millimetres and treatment will depend upon both the severity and position within the dental arch. In order to align crowded teeth space will need to be created. As a general rule, mild crowding requires up to 4-mm of space to relieve, moderate crowding between 5 and 8-mm and severe crowding 9-mm or more.

Mild crowding

If crowding is mild the removal of teeth can leave excessive space, which if closed with fixed appliances will often result in over-retraction of the labial segments. Therefore, unless this is an aim of treatment, mild crowding can usually be treated without extractions. A number of techniques that can provide space in the dental arches without the need for extraction exist.

Molar distalization

Moving the first permanent molars distally can create space. This is technically difficult in the mandibular arch and rarely attempted, but it is possible in the maxilla and appropriate for mild crowding, where the buccal segment relationship is up to half a unit class II. The most predictable technique, with the least associated anchorage loss, is extraoral traction mediated by the wearing of headgear (Fig. 11.1) (Sfondrini et al, 2002).

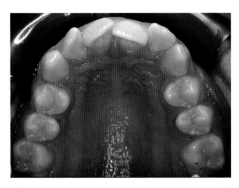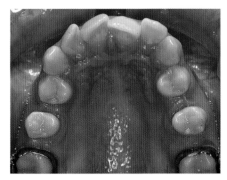

Figure 11.1 Molar distalization in the maxillary arch using headgear.

- Extraoral traction is effective in average or low angle cases, using cervical or straight-pull headgear. This will also aid in bite opening through some simultaneous extrusion of the maxillary molars.
- Care should be exercised in high angle cases because molar extrusion can result in further opening of the maxillary–mandibular planes angle. In such cases, high or occipital pull headgear should be used, although distalization is generally more difficult.
- Headgear will need to be worn for 12 to 14 hours per day with a bilateral force of at least 400 g to achieve molar distalization.
- Headgear can be run directly to the first molars via headgear tubes on molar bands. This can be supplemented with a removable appliance such as the *acrylic-cervical-occipital* (ACCO) (see Fig. 8.18), incorporating an anterior bite plane and palatal springs mesial to the first molars to provide 24-hour force.
- Headgear can alternatively be attached directly to a removable appliance with a midline expansion screw or coffin spring (see Fig. 8.17).
- As the molars move distally along the arch the transverse dimension increases. Therefore any distalization is usually accompanied by some expansion across the maxillary molars. This can be achieved by expanding the inner bow of the facebow when running directly to molar bands or by use of an expansion screw or spring incorporated in a removable appliance.
- Even with good compliance the average distal molar movement that can be achieved is about half a unit (Atherton et al, 2002).

The biggest problems with the use of headgear are the dependence upon good compliance and favourable growth for success. In an attempt to overcome problems associated with compliance, numerous appliances have been designed to distalize the maxillary buccal segments without the need for headgear and are accordingly described as 'non-compliance' appliances. Most use the palate for anchorage, with a distalizing force applied directly to the maxillary first molars via either palatal springs or compressed coils. Although effective, all will tip the molars to some extent and result in anchorage loss in the form of an increase in overjet. To avoid this, implants can be

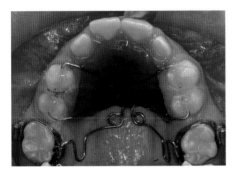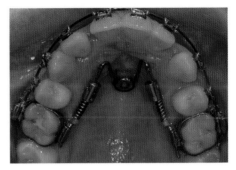

Figure 11.2 Distalization of the maxillary first molars using cantilever springs from an acrylic plate supported by the palate (a pendulum appliance) (left) or with compressed coil spring supported by a palatal implant (right). Right figure courtesy of David Tinsley.

used to support the anchorage further and these have been shown to be effective (Fig. 11.2) (Sandler et al, 2008).

Maintenance of the leeway space
The greater mesiodistal dimension of the second deciduous molars in comparison to the second premolar teeth can provide some additional space for the relief of crowding (Brennan & Gianelly, 2000). This can be done if the position of the first permanent molars is held just prior to exfoliation of the deciduous molars by fitting a lingual arch (see Figs 9.19 and 10.3). In the mandibular arch this provides approximately 2 to 2.5-mm of space per quadrant and in the maxilla around 1 to 1.5-mm.

Lip bumper
A lip bumper is a mandibular fixed appliance consisting of a 1.0-mm stainless steel wire attached to bands cemented to the first permanent molars. The wire passes along the buccal and labial sulci of the dentition, so that the labial portion sits in front of the lower incisors (Fig. 11.3). The wire can be encased in acrylic to increase its dimensions and is positioned so that the pressure normally applied to the mandibular dentition from the lower lip and cheeks is now applied to the appliance. This results in:
* Uprighting and distal movement of the lower molars;
* Forward movement of the lower incisors; and
* Some transverse arch expansion.

These appliances are most effective before the lower second permanent molars erupt or if they are extracted; however, as they act to allow passive expansion of the lower arch dentition, following removal relapse is common without permanent retention.

Interproximal enamel reduction
The removal of enamel from the interproximal regions can also be used to generate up to 1-mm of space per contact point in the buccal segments and 0.75-mm in the labial segments (Sheridan, 1985). This can be an effective way of gaining a precise

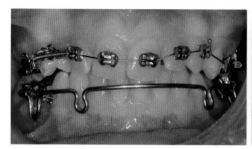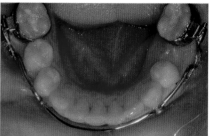

Figure 11.3 Lip bumper.

amount of space in mildly crowded cases with no apparent long-term damage to the teeth (see Fig. 7.19).

Active arch expansion

The active expansion of teeth is only recommended in the maxillary arch in the presence of a crossbite and in these cases a small amount of space can be generated for the relief of crowding. A variety of appliances for expanding the lower dentition to create space in the arch have been described. However, the instability of these procedures, particularly across the intercanine region, makes this practice unsatisfactory.

Moderate crowding

Unless the labial segments are to be proclined significantly, a moderate space requirement usually dictates the need for extractions. The extraction choice is dependent upon the position of the crowding and the anchorage requirements to achieve the treatment aims, particularly in relation to a need for incisor retraction. If there is an increased overjet to reduce as well as crowding, the space required necessitates the removal of teeth as far forward in the arch as possible, which normally means first premolars. If incisor retraction is undesirable, second premolars should be extracted.

By timing extractions appropriately, significant alignment can result without active orthodontic treatment, especially if first premolars are being extracted to relieve labial segment crowding only. In the maxillary arch the canines often erupt buccally; if first premolars are removed as the canines erupt, they will move distally and erupt into the line of the arch. In the mandibular arch, if the canines are mesially angulated, removal of first premolars will allow some uprighting of the canines into the extraction spaces. This will relieve crowding in the labial segments and allow spontaneous alignment of labiolingually displaced teeth (Stephens, 1989). Rotated teeth are less likely to align without active treatment. All spontaneous alignment will occur in the first six months following extraction and after this, fixed appliances are often required to fully align the teeth. However, well-timed extractions can result in a shorter overall treatment duration and occasionally negate the need for further treatment.

Severe crowding

If the crowding is severe, extraction is almost always necessary and often in combination with anchorage support. This is most important in the maxillary arch where there is a greater tendency for the buccal teeth to move mesially and hence space to be

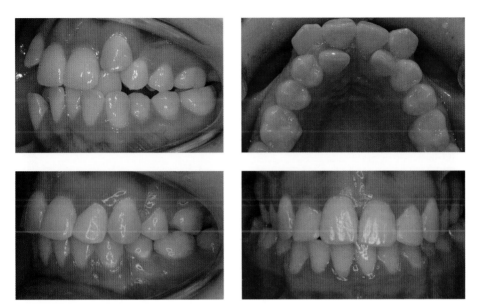

Figure 11.4 A severely crowded case treated by the loss of all first premolars and upper first permanent molars. Courtesy of Paul Scott.

lost. Various techniques for anchorage support are available and these are described in Chapter 5.

If more space is required than can be provided by the loss of premolars, not only does anchorage need to be supported but extra space will need to be created. This can be done by distalization of the buccal segments using extraoral traction or a temporary anchorage device (TAD), or occasionally by the extraction of more than one tooth per quadrant (Fig. 11.4).

Spacing

The main cause of spacing in the dental arches is a discrepancy of tooth size in relation to arch length. This can be the result of localized or generalized microdontia, hypodontia or an increased jaw dimension.

Tooth size–arch length discrepancy

One of the commonest manifestations of a tooth size–arch length discrepancy is a midline diastema in the maxilla, often associated with diminutive lateral incisors. A small midline diastema is often seen during normal dental development prior to eruption of the maxillary canines, but this will usually close on eruption of these teeth. However, a larger diastema can persist into the permanent dentition and can be a cause of concern to the patient. Fixed appliances are usually required to close the space, possibly with some buildup of the adjacent teeth if they are small.

The labial frenum has been considered to be a primary aetiological factor in the persistent midline diastema, due to the insertion of fibrous tissue into alveolar bone between the central incisors, and frenectomy suggested if the diastema is going to be closed (Edwards, 1977). However, this does not result in greater closure or a reduced potential for the diastema to reopen in the longer term following active treatment. Commonly, a frenum will remodel superiorly on closure of the space, and therefore if a frenectomy is performed, it can be carried out after the diastema is closed (Bergstrom et al, 1973; Shashua & Artun, 1999). For those cases where the frenum does not remodel and is unsightly or is causing problems, frenectomy is indicated. The closure of any diastema, irrespective of adjunctive surgical procedures, will be very prone to open up again after treatment and will require permanent retention.

Hypodontia
With the exception of third molars, hypodontia most commonly affects the maxillary lateral incisor and mandibular second premolar teeth in most populations. Localized hypodontia, when only one or two of these teeth are missing, is often encountered and commonly associated with spacing in the dental arches. Generally there are two treatment options:
- Space closure; and
- Space opening and maintenance for prosthetic replacement.

Maxillary lateral incisors
Whether the space is opened or closed for congenitally absent maxillary lateral incisors depends primarily upon the underlying malocclusion and whether space requirements in the lower arch justify the need for extraction. The size, shape and colour of the adjacent canine is also important, although this can be modified. General guidelines for management of congenitally absent maxillary incisors include:
- In class I cases if the lower arch is crowded consider extraction of premolars in the lower arch and space closure in the upper arch, substituting the upper lateral incisors with the permanent canines;
- In class II cases space from the missing teeth can be used to reduce the overjet and correct the incisor relationship; and
- In class III cases space closure will tend to retract the upper labial segment and worsen the incisor relationship. Therefore it is generally better to open space.

Space closure   When planning the substitution of a maxillary lateral incisor with a canine, this tooth may need to be adjusted to optimize the aesthetic result (Fig. 11.5) and there are several ways this can be achieved (Table 11.1). The first premolar distal to the canine should also be slightly rotated in a mesiopalatal direction to hide the palatal cusp and increase the amount of labial surface on show anteriorly to more accurately mimic a canine.

Space creation   Creating space for a missing maxillary lateral incisor will mean that the patient is reliant upon a prosthesis for the rest of their life and it is important that they understand the implications of this. Generally, the choice of prosthesis will be between an adhesive bridge or implant (Fig. 11.6). In the younger patient a simple denture or retainer incorporating the tooth can provide a useful temporary prosthesis. In patients where implant replacement is being considered, careful planning is required

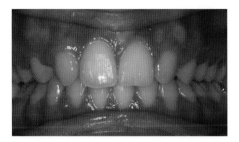 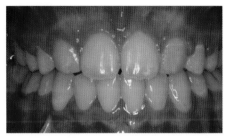

Figure 11.5 Maxillary canines substituting for the lateral incisors. On the left, there has been no modification of the canines. On the right, the crown tips have been built up with composite.

Table 11.1 Optimizing dental aesthetics when a maxillary canine is substituting for a lateral incisor

- Localized vital bleaching or veneering;
- Extrusion of tooth to lower the gingival margin;
- Reshaping the tip by grinding or composite buildup;
- Reducing the buccal and palatal bulge; and
- Reducing the width.

---

to ensure adequate bone and space are available (Table 11.2). Unless sufficient space already exists in the arch, space will actively need to be created. This usually involves fixed appliances and the use of compressed coil springs.

Mandibular second premolars

The aesthetic implications of congenitally absent mandibular second premolars are less important than those associated with the maxillary lateral incisor; however, they also require careful management.

- If space is required to relieve crowding in the lower arch, any retained second deciduous molars should be removed as part of the extraction profile and the space closed.

- In the absence of crowding in the lower arch, space closure may lead to over-retraction of the labial segments. If the long-term prognosis of the second deciduous molars is good, they can be retained. A small degree of infraocclusion can be managed by occlusal buildup with composite. The size discrepancy between a second deciduous molar and second premolar can create problems in achieving a good fit of the buccal occlusion. If the second deciduous molars are associated with a poor prognosis they will have to be removed and the space restored if closure is not practical. Problems for implant placement may arise due to a loss in alveolar width following extraction (Ostler & Kokich, 1994).

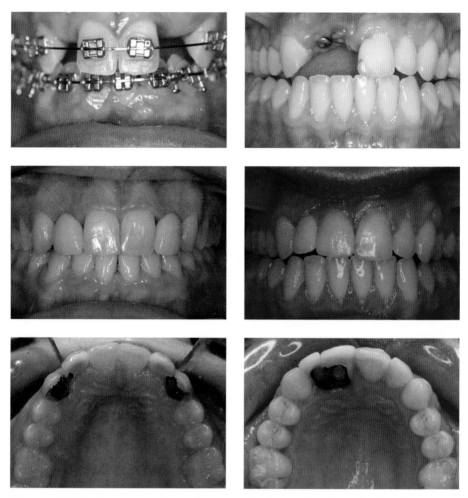

Figure 11.6 Replacement of the maxillary lateral incisors with adhesive bridges (left panels). Replacement of the UR1 and UR2 with implant restorations (right panels).

Table 11.2 Considerations when creating space for the implant replacement of missing teeth

Care must be taken that adequate space is created between the roots of adjacent teeth. This invariably requires bodily movement and fixed appliances. In addition, enough bone must be present buccolingually.
- Implants cannot be placed until around 18 years of age when vertical alveolar bone growth has ceased; otherwise, the implant and supragingival restoration will appear to submerge.
- If space for the prosthetic tooth is created too early and retained, there will be a reduction in width in the alveolus especially on the labial side, potentially compromising the position of the implant (Beyer et al, 2007).

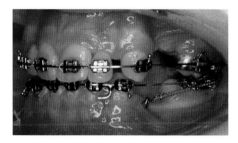

Figure 11.7 Temporary anchorage device to facilitate space closure in the lower arch. Courtesy of Paul Scott.

Generalized hypodontia

Where there is more than one missing tooth in each quadrant, treatment becomes more complex and will involve space redistribution with fixed appliances and prosthetic replacement of missing teeth. This treatment needs to be planned and executed within a multidisciplinary specialist team. Depending on how many teeth are missing and their position, anchorage management can be a problem, although recent advances in the use of temporary anchorage devices can help overcome this (Fig. 11.7). There is also an association between hypodontia and microdontia, meaning that existing teeth may require buildup to achieve the aesthetic and occlusal aims of treatment.

Anteroposterior problems

Anteroposterior problems usually manifest as an increased or reverse overjet, where there is a discrepancy between the dental arches. Protrusion of both upper and lower dentitions will result in bimaxillary protrusion or proclination. Conversely, retroclination of the dentition can result in bimaxillary retrusion, development of a class II division 2 incisor relationship and an increased overbite (discussed in vertical problems).

Increased overjet

An increased overjet is associated with a class II malocclusion and there are essentially two options for its reduction:
- Retraction of the upper labial segment; and
- Advancement of the lower labial segment.

Which option is chosen will depend on a number of factors, which relate primarily to the skeletal and soft tissue pattern, and patient age:
- Skeletal relationship—a class II malocclusion is usually associated with a class II dental base relationship and where this is the case, the majority of patients will have a degree of mandibular retrognathia (McNamara, 1981). The more severe the skeletal discrepancy, the more difficult it will be to reduce the overjet by orthodontic tooth movement alone and the greater potential compromise to the soft tissue profile. Treatment aimed at encouraging favourable growth should always be considered in a growing child with a skeletal discrepancy either using functional appliances or headgear.
- Soft tissue profile—the drape of the upper lip is in part determined by the position of the upper incisors. If these teeth are retracted the upper lip will follow, although it will not move as far as the teeth. If the upper incisors are proclined and the upper lip protrusive, as can occur when the lower lip rests behind the upper labial segment, retraction of the upper incisors will be beneficial particularly as the lower

lip will tend to uncurl and lengthen, adopting a more favourable position in front instead of behind the upper incisors. If the upper incisors are upright or retroclined, excessive retraction of the upper labial segment may result in flattening of the upper lip and excessive opening of the nasolabial angle, which can compromise the soft tissue profile.

- Age of the patient—in an adolescent patient mandibular growth can be utilized to reduce an increased overjet, especially during the pubertal growth spurt. Functional appliances can achieve this and are described in Chapter 8. In adult patients facial growth has essentially stopped and orthodontic correction of an increased overjet can only be achieved by tooth movement, either retraction of the upper labial segment or proclination of the lower. There is an anatomical limit to how far the upper labial segment can be retracted and proclination of the lower labial segment is prone to relapse. Therefore in certain cases, especially those with a severe underlying skeletal discrepancy, orthodontics combined with orthognathic surgery will be the treatment of choice.

Mechanotherapy for reducing an overjet

The options for reducing an increased overjet range from simple incisor tipping mediated by a removable appliance, functional appliances that attempt alteration of dental and skeletal relationships, fixed appliances to tip and move teeth bodily or orthognathic surgery to reposition the jaws.

- Removable appliances—if the upper labial segment is proclined and spaced, particularly when the lower lip rests behind it, an increased overjet can be reduced by simply tipping the upper incisors back. A removable appliance with an activated labial bow is an effective way of doing this (see Fig. 8.13).
- Functional appliances—in a growing patient, growth can be utilized to reduce an overjet and an effective way of doing this is the use of a functional appliance. Although there is little evidence that this will result in significantly increased mandibular growth beyond what might be expected naturally, this approach can utilize growth early on in treatment. These appliances are most effective during the pubertal growth spurt and, if successful, will result in effective overjet correction and reduced anchorage demand later on in treatment because there is no longer an overjet to reduce. However, this must be offset by the greater compliance required and the overall extension of treatment time (see Chapter 8).
- Fixed appliances—if bodily retraction of the upper labial segment is required, it necessitates the use of fixed appliances. Space will need to be created by either distal movement of the buccal segments or mid-arch extractions. Once space is available, the labial segment can be retracted to reduce the overjet. Treatment aims can be facilitated by the following:
  - If extractions are required in both arches to relieve crowding, extract further forward in the upper arch than the lower arch (Fig. 11.8).
  - If the lower arch is well aligned or treatment is planned without extraction, consider loss of upper premolars and treat to a class II molar relationship (Fig. 11.9).
  - Use class II intermaxillary elastics to support anchorage.

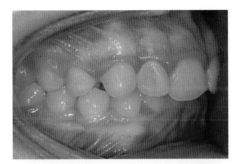

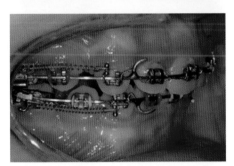

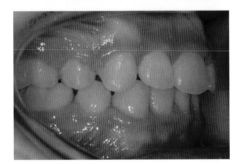

Figure 11.8 Class II division 1 malocclusion with an increased overjet treated by extraction of upper first premolars, lower second premolars and fixed appliances. Courtesy of Saba Quereshi.

When using an edgewise bracket system the incisors are moved backwards bodily on a heavy rectangular wire. This can be done using space closing loops, although when using a preadjusted system, sliding mechanics are generally used. A stretched elastomeric module or nickel titanium coil spring is connected between the terminal molar and hooks situated on the archwire in the labial segment (Fig. 11.10). This will result in the archwire shortening as it slides through the brackets in the buccal segment and is often facilitated by the use of class II elastics. If anchorage has been correctly planned, bodily retraction of the incisors and a reduction in the overjet will take place. When using the Begg or Tip-Edge appliance the overjet is reduced early in treatment by tipping the teeth with light class II elastics (Fig. 11.10). The teeth are later uprighted using auxiliary springs.

- Orthognathic surgery—once growth has ceased the only way to reduce an overjet is by orthodontic tooth movement. If there is a significant skeletal discrepancy

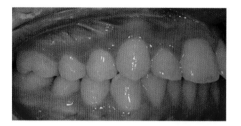

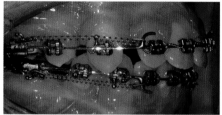

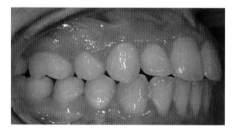

Figure 11.9 Class II division 1 malocclusion treated by extraction of upper first premolars only, treating to a class II buccal segment relationship.

Figure 11.10 Overjet reduction using a preadjusted edgewise appliance and intra-arch traction provided by nickel titanium coil springs (upper) or a Tip-Edge appliance and class II intermaxillary elastic traction (lower).

tooth movement alone may result in an unacceptable compromise to the patient's soft tissue profile. Therefore a combined orthodontic–orthognathic solution may have to be considered. Considering that mandibular retrognathia is a common aetiological factor in many significant class II malocclusions and that surgical setback of the maxilla to any great extent is difficult to achieve, this usually consists of mandibular advancement (see Chapter 12).

Reduced or reverse overjet

A reduced or reverse overjet is associated with a class III malocclusion and the options for correction include:

- Advancement of the upper labial segment; and
- Retraction of the lower labial segment.

Anatomical limitations mean that there is less scope for the retraction of lower incisors and advancement of the uppers using orthodontic mechanics. Therefore, the more severe class III cases are more reliant on surgical intervention. Whether a class III case can be treated by orthodontic tooth movement alone will depend significantly on the degree of existing incisor compensation for the skeletal pattern (Table 11.3). The upper incisors are often already proclined and the lowers retroclined and for orthodontic treatment to be successful it is important that this is minimal; otherwise, it limits the potential for further movement of these teeth aimed at correcting the class III incisor relationship.

Table 11.3 Features of a class III malocclusion that would indicate it is suitable for orthodontic camouflage treatment

- Skeletal class I or mild class III relationship;
- Minimal dentoalveolar compensation;
- Anterior displacement with patient able to achieve an edge-to-edge incisor relationship in retruded contact position (RCP);
- Average or increased overbite; and
- Patient past the adolescent growth spurt.

Table 11.4 Skeletal factors contributing to the development of a class III malocclusion[a]

- Short anterior cranial base;
- Long posterior cranial base;
- Acute cranial base angle;
- Shorter more retrusive maxilla; and
- Longer more prognathic mandible

[a] Guyer et al (1986).

The stability of incisor correction will depend in part on whether a positive overbite can be achieved at the end of treatment. Stability will also depend on future adolescent growth because any increase in mandibular prognathism will tend to worsen the class III incisor relationship. If there is any doubt, it is better to monitor growth in patients with a class III malocclusion before final treatment decisions are made, which can be done using serial cephalometric lateral skull radiographs taken a year apart (Table 11.4).

Mechanotherapy for correcting a class III incisor relationship
Correcting a reduced or reverse overjet with simple upper incisor tipping can be mediated by a removable appliance, whilst bodily tooth movement or lower incisor retraction will require fixed appliances. In more severe cases, orthognathic surgery to reposition the jaws will be required in combination with orthodontic treatment. The adverse nature of facial growth and difficulty in addressing the reduced maxillary or increased mandibular growth seen in many class III cases means the use of growth modification is more problematic in these patients. Functional appliances and protraction headgear, if used, are usually commenced in the mixed dentition. Options in the permanent dentition include:

- Removable appliances—a removable appliance can be used to push one or two maxillary incisors over the bite to correct an anterior crossbite if they are retroclined and a positive overbite can be achieved at the end of treatment to hold the corrected position (see Fig. 8.15).
- Fixed appliances—comprehensive treatment usually involves bodily movement of the incisors in both arches and therefore fixed appliances are more appropriate.

Figure 11.11 Class III malocclusion treated by extraction of lower first premolars, upper second premolars and fixed appliances.

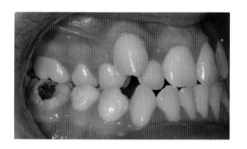

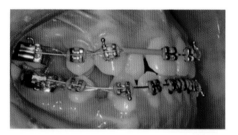

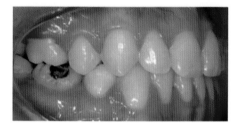

The aim is to create a positive overjet and overbite at the end of treatment and this can be facilitated by the following:

- If extractions are required in both arches to relieve crowding, extract further forward in the lower than in the upper arch (Fig. 11.11).
- If the upper arch is well-aligned but space is required to align and retrocline the lower incisors, extraction of a single lower incisor can be an option (see Fig. 7.12).
- Closing space on a round wire in the lower arch will facilitate retroclination of the lower incisors.
- Use of class III intermaxillary elastics will help procline the upper incisors and retrocline the lowers.

Orthognathic surgery and class III malocclusion

If there is a moderate or severe skeletal III skeletal base relationship, especially if the lower face height is increased and there is a reduced overbite, correction will almost certainly require a combination of orthodontics and surgery. A class III malocclusion is usually not due to a single factor, but a combination of morphological traits; therefore one surgical procedure does not fit all, and the surgical plan will need to be tailored to each individual case (see Table 11.4). There is also the tendency for a class III malocclusion to worsen with age, as mandibular growth persists. Surgery should be delayed until all adolescent growth has ceased, which will be the late teens. This does not mean that a crowded maxillary arch cannot be treated in the interim if this is a concern to the patient or teeth are ectopic (Fig. 11.12), even if it involves extractions. If the upper labial segment is left in the correct position in relation to the dental base it will not compromise any further surgical treatment although the patient will not have an ideal incisor relationship until definitive treatment is carried out. In the mandibular arch, extractions are best avoided in growing patients who look like they may need orthognathic surgery. Any retroclination of the lower labial segment will need to be undone as part of the presurgical orthodontic preparation and this is difficult following mid-arch extractions without reopening the extraction sites.

Bimaxillary proclination
Bimaxillary proclination or protrusion occurs when both the maxillary and mandibular incisor dentitions are perceived to be forwards in relation to their dental bases and the cranial base. It can occur in relation to an underlying skeletal discrepancy, with an associated increase or reduction in the overjet. If the skeletal base relationship is class I, the overjet is often within a normal range despite the labial segment proclination. As the incisors are proclined there will be a tendency to a reduced overbite and in extreme cases an anterior open bite.

Bimaxillary protrusion is a common finding in patients of African-Caribbean and Chinese descent and should therefore be considered part of the normal clinical spectrum of variation in these patients. However, in extreme cases it can cause unacceptable protrusion and incompetence of the lips, for which treatment is sought. This will usually involve retraction of the anterior teeth, necessitating mid-arch extractions and the use of fixed appliances. Using round wires and allowing the teeth to tip means that even very proclined teeth can be uprighted, which will improve lip competence and profile. However, as the teeth occupy a position of balance between the pressures from the tongue on one side and the lips and cheek on the other, any significant change in the position of the incisors will be unstable. Therefore permanent retention is usually required.

Vertical problems
Vertical problems usually manifest as either an increase or decrease in the incisor overbite. This can range from a small increase or decrease in either direction to an increased and complete overbite, or frank open bite.

Increased overbite
An increased overbite occurs when the incisors have erupted past each other and is often, although not always, associated with reduced vertical facial proportions. An increased overbite is a common feature of class II division 2 malocclusion and its reduction will be necessary to establish a class I incisor relationship.

It is much easier to correct an increased overbite in a growing patient because growth of the mandibular condyles can help compensate for any posterior dental extrusion that may be used to facilitate overbite reduction. In addition, correction of the inter-incisal angle is important for the stability of overbite reduction, as the establishment of an occlusal stop is essential to prevent the incisors from erupting past each other and the overbite increasing again following treatment. This is especially relevant for class II division 1 cases associated with proclined upper incisors because unless maxillary incisor inclination is corrected, an occlusal stop will not be established and the overbite will relapse (Houston, 1989) (Fig. 11.13). Management of deep overbite in cases with a low maxillary–mandibular planes angle is also made easier with a non-extraction approach. If teeth are extracted as space is closed towards the end of the treatment, overbite control becomes difficult as the incisors will tend to upright, which can lead to the overbite deepening again.

Mechanotherapy for correcting an increased overbite

There are essentially four ways to reduce a deep overbite associated with an increased curve of Spee in the lower arch using conventional orthodontic mechanics: buccal segment extrusion (relative incisor intrusion in a growing patient), incisor intrusion or incisor proclination (Fig. 11.14).

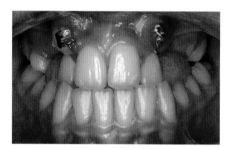
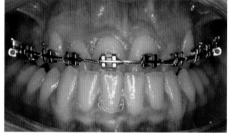

Figure 11.12   A 14 year-old class III case with impacted maxillary canines (left panel). The canines were aligned with a fixed appliance following the extraction of upper first premolars (right panel). No attempt was made to camouflage the underlying malocclusion and a reverse overjet was created. Once facial growth is complete, fixed appliances will be used to achieve full decompensation and orthognathic surgery carried out to definitively correct the malocclusion (Courtesy of Poh Then).

Figure 11.13 Creating the correct interincisal relationship to avoid relapse of overbite reduction following treatment. Simple tipping of the upper incisors to reduce an increased overjet in the presence of an increased overbite is not appropriate treatment because no occlusal stop is created. The upper incisors can retrocline and the lower incisors over-erupt, resulting in a worsening of the overbite (upper panel). The key to stable overbite reduction is moving the upper incisor root into the correct position behind the plane of the lower incisor edge (lower panel).

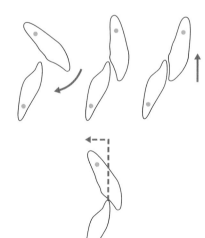

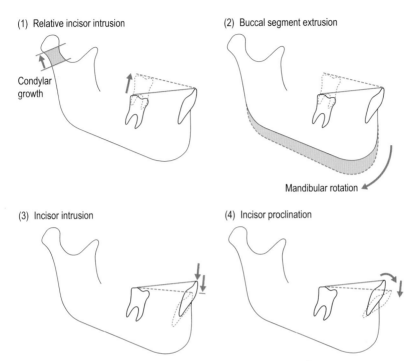

(1) Relative incisor intrusion

Condylar growth

(2) Buccal segment extrusion

Mandibular rotation

(3) Incisor intrusion

(4) Incisor proclination

Figure 11.14 Levelling the curve of Spee in the mandible. (1) Relative incisor intrusion. (2) Buccal segment extrusion. (3) Incisor intrusion. (4) Incisor proclination.

- Buccal segment extrusion—extrusion of the lower buccal segments whilst maintaining lower incisor eruptive position, is a very effective way of reducing an increased overbite. This is particularly true in a growing patient, where these tooth movements will produce relative incisor intrusion because vertical growth at the condyle helps compensate for any increase in the vertical dimension induced by the molar extrusion (Fig. 11.14 (1)). In an adult, there is little or no growth potential at the condyle and buccal segment extrusion will simply result in a downward and backward rotation of the mandible, steepening of the occlusal plane and an increase in the lower face height (Fig. 11.14 (2)). This will reduce the overbite but tends to worsen any underlying skeletal class II relationship and is prone to relapse following treatment. For these reasons, overbite reduction can be more difficult in adult patients.

  Buccal segment extrusion can be achieved using a removable appliance with a flat anterior bite plane. The appliance opens up the bite and allows eruption of the buccal segments, levelling the curve of Spee and reducing the overbite (Fig. 11.15). Many functional appliances have a similar bite-plane effect if the acrylic of the appliance is removed over the lower premolars and molars to allow eruption of these teeth.

  Using an edgewise-fixed appliance with a continuous archwire can also achieve buccal segment extrusion, although this will also be accompanied by some incisor

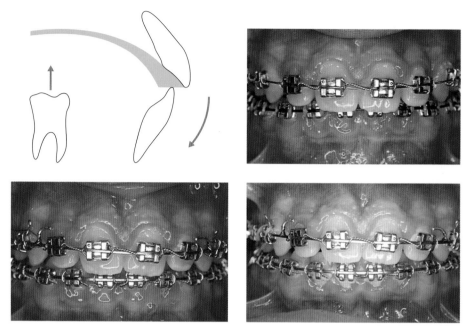

Figure 11.15 Overbite reduction can be achieved with a removable appliance by incorporating a flat anterior bite plane (upper left panel). Fixed appliances can reduce an increased overbite by placing a reverse curve of Spee in the lower archwire (upper right, lower left and lower right panels showing progressive overbite reduction; and see Fig. 9.30).

intrusion. These changes can be accentuated by using a rectangular stainless steel archwire with a reverse curve of Spee (Fig. 11.15). The lower second molars are generally included to increase vertical anchorage and aid these movements. Care must be taken, as there will also be a tendency for the lower incisors to procline, which will assist bite opening, but may not desirable or stable. Therefore it is often necessary to place lingual crown torque in the labial section of the archwire to counter this. The judicial use of class II inter-maxillary elastics will also assist in overbite reduction as the vertical component of force will tend to extrude the mandibular molars. Class II inter-maxillary elastics are integral in the Begg and Tip-Edge appliances which aim to reduce an increased overbite early on in treatment by the use of rigid round steel arches that bypass the premolar teeth to create a long range of action and light forces. An intrusive force is applied to the labial segments from the archwire by tip-back or anchor bends placed into the molar tubes and an extrusive force applied to the molars by the use of light class II elastics. Together this is very effective at reducing an increased overbite (see Fig. 9.29).

- True intrusion of the incisors—in cases with a high maxillary–mandibular planes angle and a class II malocclusion, molar extrusion can result in an undesirable downward and backward rotation of the mandible, especially in non-growing patients. A deep overbite in these cases, although not common, should be

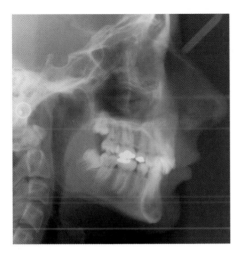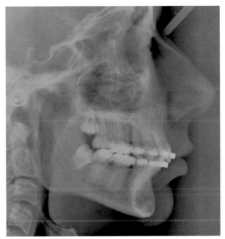

Figure 11.16 Proclination of the labial segments to reduce an increased overbite in a class II division 2 malocclusion.

reduced by intrusion of the incisor teeth (Fig. 11.13 (3)). Absolute intrusion of the incisors is mechanically difficult to achieve and requires fixed appliances. The general principle is to establish an anchorage unit in the buccal segments and intrude the incisors with a utility or bypass arch pitched against the buccal teeth (see Fig. 9.31). The utility archwire when passive will lie above the incisors in the gingival sulcus. By tying this archwire into or above the incisor brackets an intrusive force will be applied, which can achieve around 1 to 2-mm of incisor intrusion (Ng et al, 2005). Direct high-pull headgear applied to the upper incisors will also result in intrusion but unless the forces are kept light, this can increase the risk of root resorption. More recently, the use of micro-implants has been described to intrude anterior teeth, whilst intrusion can also be achieved using segmental surgery.

- Proclination of the incisors—a deep overbite can also be reduced by incisor proclination and an associated reduction in the inter-incisal angle (Fig. 11.13 (4)). As a general rule, lower incisor proclination is unstable and there will be a tendency for these teeth to return to their pre-treatment position, with a potential return of the increased overbite. However, where the lower labial segment is markedly retroclined, such as a class II division 2 malocclusion, some proclination of the lower incisors may be necessary to establish a class I incisor relationship with an acceptable inter-incisal angle (Fig. 11.16). This can effectively be achieved with fixed appliances, especially in the presence of crowding. By engaging the initial aligning archwire fully, the teeth will align by proclination and this can be supplemented further by placing a rectangular stainless steel wire in the lower arch once the teeth are aligned with a reverse curve of Spee. Any significant proclination will invariably require long-term or permanent retention following appliance removal to prevent relapse of the overbite.

Anterior open bite

An anterior open bite is associated with a lack of vertical incisor overlap. It may be localized, affecting only a few teeth; or it may be caused by a divergence of the skeletal planes. Treatment is often required because the patient has trouble incising food due to the lack of an anterior occlusion. Speech may also be a concern, as an anterior open bite can be associated with lisping. While treatment can improve both the occlusion and function, there is no guarantee that speech will improve as speech patterns are established early in life, long before establishment of the permanent dentition.

When planning treatment it is important to establish the aetiology (Table 11.5). In the presence of an anterior open bite, the tongue will come forwards between the incisors to fill the gap and create an anterior seal during swallowing. For many years it was thought that this tongue activity or 'tongue thrust' was the primary aetiological factor in the development of anterior open bite. It is now recognized that in the vast majority of cases this is an adaptive behaviour. If the main aetiological factor is a digit-sucking habit, as long as this ceases at an appropriate time, there can be complete and stable resolution of the anterior open bite. The main problems arise with anterior open bites that are skeletal in origin.

Mechanotherapy to correct an anterior open bite

There are essentially three ways that a skeletal open bite can be treated:

- Extrusion of the labial segments—an anterior open bite occurs when the labial dentition is at the limits of its eruptive potential. Therefore any further mechanical eruption or extrusion will be inherently unstable and is not advised unless it is related to a digit-sucking habit which has prevented eruption of the incisors. Occasionally, towards the end of fixed appliance therapy, a small anterior open bite can be resolved and occlusal settling achieved by the short-term use of anterior elastics (Fig. 11.17).

- Distal tipping of the molar dentition—it has been noted that the buccal dentition, especially the molars, is more upright or mesially angulated in the presence of an anterior open bite. A technique whereby the molars are tipped distally using multilooped wires with divergent curves of Spee built into them has been described (Kim, 1987). Heavy anterior elastics are used to stop the anterior open bite getting worse and bring the incisors together as the molars tip distally. This is further facilitated by removal of the terminal molars. As the mandible works on a hinge the removal of terminal molars, which are closer to the hinge access, should help close down an anterior open bite by removing the posterior occlusal contact.

Table 11.5 Aetiology of anterior open bite

- Transitional, as the permanent incisors are erupting;
- Secondary to a habit such as digit sucking;
- Secondary to local pathology such as a supernumerary tooth preventing eruption of the maxillary incisors;
- Secondary to generalized pathology such as poor soft tissue tone associated with muscular dystrophy or cerebral palsy; and
- Skeletal.

- Vertical control or intrusion of buccal segments—this is difficult to achieve with orthodontic tooth movement. The aim is to reduce posterior dental heights, which will result in a forward rotation of the mandible and closing down of the anterior open bite. Because the molars are closer to the condylar hinge, even a small amount of intrusion should result in a greater closure anteriorly. Numerous techniques that attempt to achieve this have been described (Table 11.6). Similarly, any extrusion of the molars will worsen the anterior open bite. It is important to avoid the use of class II and class III elastics in such cases. If intermaxillary traction is required, the elastics should be short and not run to the molars.

In a growing child, the use of high-pull headgear, especially when there is a skeletal class II base relationship, will control posterior vertical growth of the maxilla. This will theoretically redirect mandibular growth in a more anterior than vertical direction. The headgear can be run directly either to bands on the upper first molars or to a removable appliance with posterior capping (an intrusion splint) (Fig. 11.18). Headgear can also be used in combination with a functional appliance to try and correct an increased overjet when there is a reduced overbite and a vertical growth pattern. The main problem with this approach is that vertical growth continues throughout adolescence and therefore to be truly effective, headgear will have to be worn until adolescent growth has stopped.

In adults growth will have essentially ceased. Therefore, treatment of an anterior open bite will necessitate intrusion of the buccal segments. Although implants and microscrews potentially provide an exciting new way of achieving this, at present the most predictable and stable way of correcting an anterior open bite in an adult is by surgical impaction of the maxilla (see Fig. 12.27). This will reduce the posterior dental height, allowing the mandible to auto-rotate and close the anterior open bite.

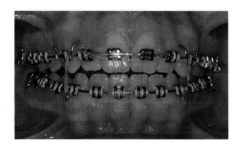 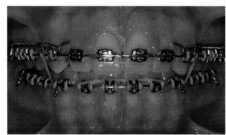

Figure 11.17 Anterior elastic to close an anterior open bite during the final stages of treatment with a fixed appliance.

Table 11.6   Treatment modalities to correct an anterior open bite

- High-pull headgear;
- Posterior bite blocks;
- Repelling magnets;
- Implants; and
- Surgical impaction of the maxilla.

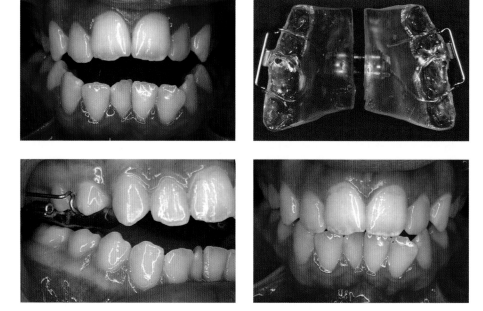

Figure 11.18 Anterior open bite treated with high-pull headgear attached to a buccal intrusion splint.

Transverse problems

The displacement of a tooth palatally in the maxilla or buccally in the mandible may result in a localized crossbite and is usually a reflection of crowding. Although a removable appliance with a palatal spring can be used to tip these teeth buccally, if space is created the tooth will usually need to be bodily moved, necessitating the use of fixed appliances. When there is a transverse discrepancy between the dental arches, a crossbite can affect all the teeth in the quadrant.

Buccal posterior crossbite

Posterior crossbite can be unilateral or bilateral, depending upon whether one or two sides of the dental arch are affected.

- Where the discrepancy is small and mostly dental in origin, a displacement affecting the mandibular dentition can often be elicited on closing from initial contact into the intercuspal position (ICP), resulting in a unilateral posterior crossbite and dental centreline discrepancy.
- A skeletal asymmetry can produce a unilateral crossbite without displacement; however, if the discrepancy is large a bilateral crossbite may occur. This is commonly found in severe class III malocclusion and is both a reflection of the transverse discrepancy and the relative anteroposterior positioning of the jaws.

The greater the skeletal contribution to a crossbite, the more difficult it is to correct. A skeletal crossbite with no associated displacement of the mandible on closing is often best accepted, especially if it is bilateral. Attempting orthodontic correction in these cases may result in the creation of a unilateral crossbite with a displacement,

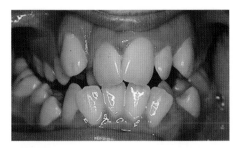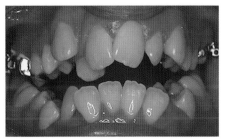

Figure 11.19 Increase in the vertical dimension and reduction in overbite following expansion of the maxillary dental arch.

which is occlusally less acceptable. As it is very difficult to constrict the mandibular arch, any treatment will usually involve expansion of the maxillary arch. Various techniques can be used to achieve this, but all will produce considerable tipping of the maxillary buccal teeth, with the exception of surgical expansion. On expansion, there will be a relative extrusion of these palatal cusps as the teeth are tipped. This can be a problem in patients with a reduced overbite, as this will worsen due to displacement of the mandible downwards and backwards (Fig. 11.19). Therefore caution should be exercised when expanding patients with an increased vertical pattern of growth and the use of techniques to control this, such as high-pull headgear in combination with expansion, should be considered.

Mechanotherapy to correct a posterior crossbite
The following techniques can be used to produce maxillary expansion:
- Removable appliances are effective for expansion particularly in the mixed dentition using a midline expansion screw which the patient activates.
- Fixed palatal expanders such as the quadhelix can be used for dental expansion; whilst rapid maxillary expansion (RME) can produce a significant component of skeletal expansion in growing patients.
  - The quadhelix appliance (see Fig. 9.20) is cemented to bands on the first molars and activated by expanding approximately a molar width. This will produce slow dental expansion, mostly by tipping the teeth buccally. It is therefore contraindicated when skeletal expansion is needed or when the maxillary molars are already tipped buccally. As active arch expansion has a high potential for relapse, the maxillary arch should be overexpanded so expansion is continued until the palatal cusps of the maxillary molars occlude on the lingual inclines of the buccal cusps of the mandibular molars. If no further treatment is planned, the quadhelix should be left in place for a further three months as a retainer.
  - RME is undertaken over a period of 2 to 4 weeks with the patient activating the appliance between one and four times a day, producing up to 1-mm of expansion a day (Fig. 11.20 and see Fig. 9.21). This generates large forces that in a child or adolescent will split the maxillary suture, resulting in initially mostly skeletal expansion. A transient midline diastema usually develops, but the maxillary arch should be overexpanded as relapse is inevitable. The appliance

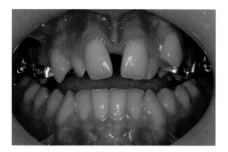

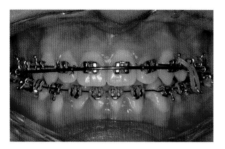

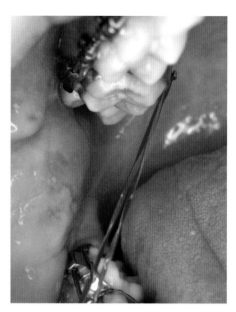

Figure 11.20 Maxillary expansion using RME (upper panel) and a buccal expansion arch (lower panel).

Figure 11.21 Cross elastics.

is then left in place following the active phase of treatment to maintain the expansion for at least three months. Despite this there is considerable relapse, with much of the skeletal expansion being lost. Even so, up to 10-mm of expansion is possible using this technique. In an adult the interdigitation of the maxillary suture makes it harder to achieve skeletal expansion without surgery.

- Fixed appliances incorporating expanded heavy stainless steel archwires will result in expansion of the dental arch. Rectangular wires should be used to prevent buccal tipping of the molars and maintain torque control in the buccal segments. Alternatively, an auxiliary buccal arch constructed from 0.9-mm steel can be placed in the molar headgear tubes and expanded (Fig. 11.20). Cross-elastics can also be run from the palatal aspect of the maxillary teeth and buccal aspect of mandibular teeth to correct crossbites (Fig. 11.21). As well as a transverse force component, these will also produce a vertical force and as such, is contraindicated in patients where extrusion of teeth in the buccal segments should be avoided. If an archwire with a larger arch form is chosen from the outset of treatment and twinned with a low friction bracket system, significant expansion and change in arch form is possible. However, there is no evidence that this is any more stable than any other method of expansion.

Irrespective of what type of expansion is undertaken, relapse potential is high. This can be reduced by establishing good intercuspation of the buccal dentition at the end of treatment, but a long period of retention will usually be required. Vacuum-formed retainers, if used, should be reinforced with a wire placed in the palate.

Lingual posterior crossbites

Localized lingual posterior crossbites can also occur, particularly when crowding causes a maxillary premolar to be displaced buccally. Complete lingual posterior crossbites are less common and usually associated with an underlying skeletal class II discrepancy. In a child, a functional appliance can be used to correct this relationship, and by doing so this may help correct the lingual crossbite. In an adult, fixed appliances can be used with cross-elastics and an expanded mandibular archwire. However, orthodontic expansion of the mandibular arch to any significant extent is problematic. If there is a skeletal class II base relationship, mandibular advancement surgery may help correct the lingual crossbite. Surgical techniques using distraction osteogenesis for widening the mandibular arch have also been described.

Relapse and retention

Following active orthodontic treatment the majority of patients will require a period of retention. This is a phase of treatment aimed at stabilization and maintenance of the achieved orthodontic correction, allowing settling of the occlusion and preventing or minimizing subsequent relapse.

Relapse

Relapse is a partial or full return of the pre-treatment features of a malocclusion following active treatment. Numerous longitudinal studies have shown the re-emergence of crowding, especially of the lower incisors following orthodontic treatment (Little et al, 1981, 1988). This is an almost universal finding that can occur many years following treatment, with a large degree of individual variation. It is impossible to gauge susceptibly in individual cases, although greater incisor irregularity may be expected following non-extraction expansion of the lower arch, rather than treatment involving premolar extraction (Little et al, 1990). Other occlusal features especially prone to relapse following treatment include rotations and spacing. Overall, a number of factors can potentially contribute to orthodontic relapse.

Periodontal and gingival tissues

Following orthodontic tooth movement, the tissues of the periodontal ligament and gingivae remodel to the new position of the tooth. Whilst collagen fibres in the periodontal ligament take between three to four months to remodel, those in the gingival tissues take slightly longer, at around six months. The slowest turnaround occurs in the elastic supracrestal fibres, which take up to one year. This has important implications for teeth that were rotated, as this slow remodelling is implicated in the very high relapse rate for rotational correction. The retention regime for these teeth can be supplemented by supracrestal fibrotomy (or pericision), a surgical procedure involving sectioning of the supracrestal fibres. This is carried out under local anaesthetic, once the rotation has been orthodontically corrected. A surgical blade is inserted into the gingival sulcus, severing the supracrestal and transeptal fibres. It has been shown to reduce rotational relapse in the maxillary incisor region with no loss of periodontal attachment (Edwards, 1988). However, this procedure should not be done on the mid-labial portion of any tooth with a narrow zone of attached gingivae or thin plate of alveolar bone, particularly the lower incisors. An alternative technique is simply to divide the interdental papilla. Overcorrection of rotated teeth early in treatment and maintaining them in their new position for a significant period before appliances are removed is also recommended which will allow for some relapse.

Soft tissues

To a large extent the soft tissues define the limitations of orthodontic tooth movement. Any change in the position of the teeth can move them out of the zone of soft tissue balance and increase the chance of relapse. For this reason the arch form, particularly of the lower arch, is not amenable to any significant change. If expanded during treatment, especially across the intercanine width, this will be very prone to relapse. Similarly, labiolingual movement of the lower incisors to any great degree is notoriously prone to relapse.

Vertically, the lower lip position is very important in the stability of overjet reduction. If the lips are competent following treatment and the lower lip rests labially to the upper incisors, there is greater stability. This is in part dependent on growth of the soft tissues, which grow vertically more than the underlying skeletal bases during the preadolescent period. This results in an increase in lip competence, especially in boys whose lips grow later and to a greater extent than girls (Nanda, 1990).

An endogenous tongue thrust is primarily neurological in origin, resulting in anterior position of the tongue and excessive force exerted on swallowing. Although this phenomenon is real, it is very rare and most abnormal tongue activity is adaptive. To create an anterior seal on swallowing with an anterior open bite, the tongue will invariably come forwards to fill the gap. If the anterior open bite is corrected, the tongue activity is normalized and the result will be stable. However, if a true tongue thrust is present, no amount of treatment will guarantee stability, as the primary aetiological factor will remain (Fig. 11.22).

Occlusion

Teeth retained by the occlusion are often stable. Correction of an anterior crossbite with a positive overbite following treatment requires no retention. It is also a widely held belief that a well-interdigitated class I occlusion aids stability at the end of treatment and there is some evidence for this (Kahl-Nieke et al, 1995). This is certainly true for overbite reduction and buccal segment correction but there is little evidence that it will prevent relapse or reappearance of incisor crowding. Occlusal forces themselves act in an anterior direction, and have been postulated to be causative in the develop-

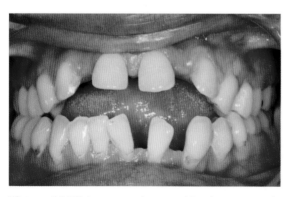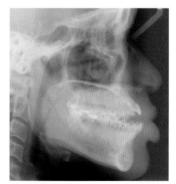

Figure 11.22 Large anterior open bite due to an endogenous tongue thrust.

ment of lower incisor crowding (Southard et al, 1990); however, the short duration of these forces makes this unlikely.

Growth

Facial growth continues throughout life, generally in the same direction as that occurring during adolescence, but to a much smaller degree (Behrents, 1985). Facial growth is not linear but rotational, especially mandibular growth. This can lead to forces being placed on the teeth from either soft tissues or the occlusion as the dentition compensates to maintain the occlusal position. This can manifest most notably as late lower incisor crowding, as the lower labial segment uprights to compensate for mandibular growth. This is thought to be a major factor in late lower incisor crowding seen in both orthodontically treated and untreated individuals.

In class III malocclusion, mandibular growth can result in the reappearance of a reverse overbite following early correction. This is one of the main reasons for monitoring growth in class III cases during adolescence before final treatment decisions are made.

Retention

Planning the retention phase of orthodontic treatment is part of the treatment planning process and allows the patient to make an informed decision about their treatment (Box 11.1). Retention should be discussed prior to the commencement of active treatment. The following factors need to be considered:

- Original malocclusion;
- Growth pattern;
- Type of retainer; and
- Duration of retention.

Original malocclusion

If the original malocclusion was severe, a small amount of relapse following treatment may be acceptable, as the overall aesthetic improvement will remain good. However, if the patient only presented with a mild malocclusion, any relapse may be unacceptable. This is especially true when mild labial segment crowding is treated. Numerous strategies for improving the stability of lower incisors following alignment have been devised. One of these is interproximal enamel reduction. Removing a small amount of enamel creates broader, flatter contact points between these teeth and theoretically reduces the chance of them slipping past each other and becoming crowded (Boese, 1980a, b). Despite these added precautions, all patients need to be made aware of the relapse potential prior to beginning treatment and the necessity for long-term or even permanent retention.

Growth pattern

Following treatment the original growth pattern will re-impose itself and continue to a greater or lesser degree throughout life. This is true for both sagittal and vertical growth. Thus, a corrected class III incisor relationship will relapse if there is unfavourable mandibular growth and an anterior open bite, which will reappear with continued vertical growth. Retention should therefore be involved in maintaining the skeletal correction. If a functional appliance or headgear was used to control growth during the active treatment phase it should ideally be continued during the retention phase, at least until adolescent growth is complete. This of course is very much compliance-based and provides a good argument against starting treatment too early where there is a skeletal discrepancy.

Type of retainers
Retainers are appliances designed to maintain the position of the teeth following orthodontic treatment. Retainers can be either removable or fixed.

Removable retainers
Removable retainers can be taken out of the mouth by the patient and therefore rely on good compliance. They are generally easy to maintain and do not compromise oral hygiene although like all removable appliances, they can affect speech. Although many different types of retainer have been described, the main types include the following:

- Hawley retainers are simple, robust and retentive; consisting of Adams cribs on the first molars and a labial bow around the incisors. The labial bow can be fitted (contoured around the incisors) or acrylated (with an acrylic facing) to improve retention and rotational control of the incisors (Fig. 11.23). Hawley retainers will allow some occlusal settling and in first premolar extraction cases, the labial bow

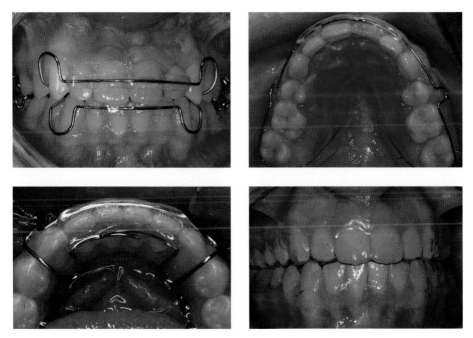

Figure 11.23 Hawley retainers with acrylated labial bows and a prosthetic tooth replacing the UL2 (upper-left); Begg retainer with acrylated labial bow (upper-right); Barrer spring-loaded retainer (lower-left); Essix-type vacuum-formed retainer (lower-right).

can be soldered directly to the first molar cribs, which avoids the wire crossing the extraction spaces and allowing them to reopen. A bite plane can also be incorporated to maintain overbite reduction.

- Begg retainers have the labial bow extending around the distal aspect of the terminal molar (Fig. 11.23). They allow occlusal settling, as no wire work crosses the occlusion. These retainers are less retentive than Hawley retainers and the labial bow is more prone to distortion.
- Spring or Barrer retainers carry acrylated bows both labially and lingually (Fig. 11.23). The original appliance extended only to the canines; however, due to the risk of swallowing or aspiration, a modification which includes cribs on the first molars has been described. These retainers can be used to realign minor lower incisor relapse if the teeth are realigned on the working model by the technician.
- Vacuum-formed retainers are clear thermoplastic retainers (Fig. 11.23). They are easy to construct by heating a sheet of clear plastic, which is then sucked down onto a dental cast by a vacuum. They provide good aesthetics and better control of incisor alignment than Hawley type retainers (Rowland et al, 2007), but they are not as robust. They can be extended just from canine to canine or back to the second molars, in which case they will not allow any occlusal settling after treatment. A palatal wire should be incorporated if used in cases where there has been significant maxillary expansion. Vacuum-form retainers can also be used for active

tooth movement. The teeth can be aligned on a working model from which the vacuum-formed retainer is constructed. Once fitted, if there is space for the teeth to move minor irregularities can be corrected with this type of appliance. Vacuum retainers should not be worn for eating or drinking, as they can act as a reservoir for fluids, increasing the risk of decalcification in the presence of a cariogenic diet.

Fixed retainers
Fixed retainers usually consist of a wire cemented or bonded to the teeth, which the patient cannot remove. These retainers are used when long-term or permanent retention is required, particularly for the lower incisors, and the wire usually extends from canine to canine. They can also be used for the upper incisors to prevent reopening of a midline diastema, but a higher failure rate can occur in this region, especially with an increased overbite. Early designs were made from plain wires with steel pads at each end bonded to the canines. This design was very good at maintaining the lower intercanine width but less effective at preventing rotational relapse of incisors not bonded to it. Later fixed retainers consisted of flexible multistrand stainless steel wires bonded to the lingual surfaces of the teeth with composite (Zachrisson, 1977) (Fig. 11.24). These are well tolerated, allow some physiological movement of the teeth, do not compromise on aesthetics and can provide excellent retention. They do not interfere with speech and are less reliant upon compliance than removable retainers. Fixed retainers do not seem to produce any long-term periodontal problems, although calculus can build up around them, particularly in the lower incisor region. Their placement is time-consuming and technique-sensitive and a back-up removable retainer should also be supplied to the patient to preserve tooth position if the fixed retainer fails.

Duration of retention
The duration of retention required following orthodontic treatment is variable. However, the only way to permanently guarantee stability of tooth position is to retain it indefinitely.

No retention
This is the exception rather than the rule, and is only applicable in cases where the occlusion will hold the correction or where no active treatment was undertaken:
● Anterior crossbite, with positive overbite and overjet following correction; and
● Spontaneous alignment following extractions and no active treatment.

Figure 11.24 Bonded upper retainer.

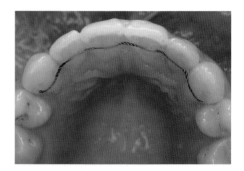

Medium-term retention

Medium-term retention usually means a period that allows reorganization of the soft tissues and periodontal ligament, and for adolescent growth and dental development to be completed, including eruption of the third molars. In reality this means retention into the late teenage years or early twenties and is usually indicated in most routine cases. Most retention regimes are fairly arbitrary and there is no evidence that there is any great difference in a period of full-time as opposed to part-time or nocturnal wear following removal of the active appliances. A period of full-time wear may result in less chance of the patient forgetting to wear the retainer, but when compliance is not a concern, removable retainers can be worn on a part-time basis from the end of active treatment.

Permanent retention

The only way to prevent any change in tooth alignment following active treatment is by long-term or even permanent retention. Certain occlusal traits are very prone to relapse following correction and these include:

- Severe rotations;
- Midline diastema and spacing; and
- Periodontally compromised teeth with bone loss.

In certain situations as part of the treatment plan, teeth may be purposely moved into areas where they will be prone to relapse:

- Proclination of the lower labial segment;
- Expansion of lower intercanine width;
- Alignment of palatally displaced maxillary lateral incisors in the absence of a positive overbite at the end of treatment;
- Correction of an anterior open bite by extrusion of incisors; and
- Correction of an overjet with lip incompetence at the end of treatment.

In such cases, permanent retention will be needed to maintain the position of the teeth usually in the form of a fixed retainer. It is important that this is discussed with the patient before they commence treatment and it should be part of the consent process.

Further reading

MCLAUGHLIN RP, BENNETT JC, TREVISI HJ (2001). *Systemised Orthodontic Treatment Mechanics* (St Louis: Mosby).

MELROSE C AND MILLETT DT (1998) Towards a perspective on orthodontic retention? *Am J Orthod Dentofacial Orthop* 113:507–514.

PROFFIT WR, FIELDS HW, SARVER DM (2007). *Comtemporary Orthodontics*, 4th edn (St Louis: Mosby-Elsevier).

References

ATACK N, HARRADINE N, SANDY JR, ET AL (2007). Which way forward? Fixed or removable lower retainers. *Angle Orthod* 77:954–959.

ATHERTON GJ, GLENNY AM AND O'BRIEN K (2002). Development and use of a taxonomy to carry out a systematic review of the literature on methods described to effect distal movement of maxillary molars. *J Orthod* 29:211–216; discussion 195–196.

BEHRENTS RG (1985). The biological basis for understanding craniofacial growth during adulthood. *Prog Clin Biol Res* 187:307–319.

BERGSTROM K, JENSEN R AND MARTENSSON B (1973). The effect of superior labial frenectomy in cases with midline diastema. *Am J Orthod* 63:633–638.

BEYER A, TAUSCHE E, BOENING K, ET AL (2007). Orthodontic space opening in patients with congenitally missing lateral incisors. *Angle Orthod* 77:404–409.

BOESE LR (1980a). Fiberotomy and reproximation without lower retention 9 years in retrospect: part II. *Angle Orthod* 50:169–178.

BOESE LR (1980b). Fiberotomy and reproximation without lower retention, nine years in retrospect: part I. *Angle Orthod* 50:88–97.

BRENNAN MM AND GIANELLY AA (2000). The use of the lingual arch in the mixed dentition to resolve incisor crowding. *Am J Orthod Dentofacial Orthop* 117:81–85.

EDWARDS JG (1977). A clinical study: the diastema, the frenum, the frenectomy. *Oral Health* 67:51–62.

EDWARDS JG (1988). A long-term prospective evaluation of the circumferential supracrestal fiberotomy in alleviating orthodontic relapse. *Am J Orthod Dentofacial Orthop* 93:380–387.

GUYER EC, ELLIS EE 3rd, MCNAMARA JA JR, ET AL (1986). Components of class III malocclusion in juveniles and adolescents. *Angle Orthod* 56:7–30.

HOUSTON WJ (1989). Incisor edge-centroid relationships and overbite depth. *Eur J Orthod* 11:139–143.

KAHL-NIEKE B, FISCHBACH H AND SCHWARZE CW (1995). Post-retention crowding and incisor irregularity: a long-term follow-up evaluation of stability and relapse. *Br J Orthod* 22:249–257.

KIM YH (1987). Anterior openbite and its treatment with multiloop edgewise archwire. *Angle Orthod* 57:290–321.

LITTLE RM, RIEDEL RA AND ARTUN J (1988). An evaluation of changes in mandibular anterior alignment from 10 to 20 years postretention. *Am J Orthod Dentofacial Orthop* 93:423–428.

LITTLE RM, RIEDEL RA AND STEIN A (1990). Mandibular arch length increase during the mixed dentition: postretention evaluation of stability and relapse. *Am J Orthod Dentofacial Orthop* 97:393–404.

LITTLE RM, WALLEN TR AND RIEDEL RA (1981). Stability and relapse of mandibular anterior alignment-first premolar extraction cases treated by traditional edgewise orthodontics. *Am J Orthod* 80:349–365.

MCNAMARA JA JR (1981). Components of class II malocclusion in children 8–10 years of age. *Angle Orthod* 51:177–202.

NANDA SK (1990). Growth patterns in subjects with long and short faces. *Am J Orthod Dentofacial Orthop* 98:247–258.

NG J, MAJOR PW, HEO G AND FLORES-MIR C (2005). True incisor intrusion attained during orthodontic treatment: a systematic review and meta-analysis. *Am J Orthod Dentofacial Orthop* 128:212–219.

OSTLER MS AND KOKICH VG (1994). Alveolar ridge changes in patients congenitally missing mandibular second premolars. *J Prosthet Dent* 71:144–149.

ROWLAND H, HICHENS L, WILLIAMS A, ET AL (2007). The effectiveness of Hawley and vacuum-formed retainers: a single-center randomized controlled trial. *Am J Orthod Dentofacial Orthop* 132:730–737.

SANDLER J, BENSON PE, DOYLE P, ET AL (2008). Palatal implants are a good alternative to headgear: a randomized trial. *Am J Orthod Dentofacial Orthop* 133:51–57.

SFONDRINI MF, CACCIAFESTA V AND SFONDRINI G (2002). Upper molar distalization: a critical analysis. *Orthod Craniofac Res* 5:114–126.

SHASHUA D AND ARTUN J (1999). Relapse after orthodontic correction of maxillary median diastema: a follow-up evaluation of consecutive cases. *Angle Orthod* 69:257–263.

SHERIDAN JJ (1985). Air-rotor stripping. *J Clin Orthod* 19:43–59.

SOUTHARD TE, BEHRENTS RG AND TOLLEY EA (1990). The anterior component of occlusal force. Part 2. Relationship with dental malalignment. *Am J Orthod Dentofacial Orthop* 97:41–44.

STEPHENS CD (1989). The use of natural spontaneous tooth movement in the treatment of malocclusion. *Dent Update* 16:337–338, 340–342.

ZACHRISSON BU (1977). Clinical experience with direct-bonded orthodontic retainers. *Am J Orthod* 71:440–448.

12 Adult orthodontics

An increasing number of adults are undergoing orthodontic treatment and this is a global trend. Adult dental health has improved significantly over the past few decades in the UK, with more teeth being retained for longer in this population. This has been accompanied by an increasing preoccupation with personal appearance and in particular, the importance of an attractive smile. As a result of the media and increasing use of the Internet, adults are more aware of the aesthetic improvements that can be achieved with orthodontic treatment and it has become more socially acceptable for them to wear fixed orthodontic appliances. Improvements in socioeconomic status and personal wealth have meant that the finances are increasingly available for them to seek out and embark on such treatment.

Why do adults undertake orthodontic treatment?

An adult may be motivated primarily by a desire to improve their dental appearance and may request orthodontic treatment. Amongst this group will be those who either refused or were not given the opportunity of treatment during their childhood, and those who may have received treatment but have been left dissatisfied with the result, often because of subsequent relapse or an inappropriate original treatment plan (Fig. 12.1). Routine orthodontics can be readily carried out in these patients, but the scope of increasingly complex treatment can be more limited in comparison to that which might be achieved in a growing child or adolescent. Moreover, adults can also present with other age-related problems that must be considered when providing orthodontic treatment (Box 12.1).

Alternatively, orthodontic treatment may not be sought directly by an adult, but prescribed as one component of a specific treatment plan:

- To facilitate restorative or periodontal treatment;
- For surgical correction of a jaw discrepancy to optimize the proposed surgical movements and ensure a stable and functional postsurgical occlusion;
- To use intraoral mandibular advancement appliances as part of a non-surgical treatment regime in the treatment of obstructive sleep apnoea.

Orthodontics as an adjunct to restorative treatment

Adults can often present with an incomplete dentition, permanent teeth having been lost prematurely as a result of caries, periodontal disease or trauma. This can lead to alterations in position of the remaining teeth due to drifting, tipping, rotation or

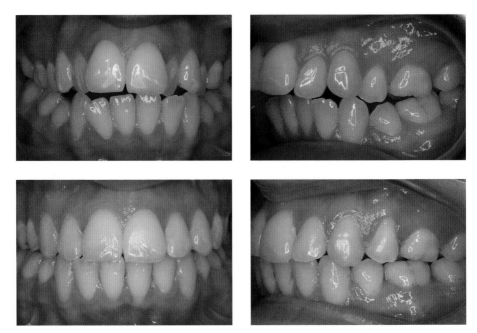

Figure 12.1 This adult patient was unhappy with the appearance of their teeth. Orthodontic treatment as a child had involved the loss of four premolars and fixed appliances to correct their class II division 1 malocclusion. Unfortunately, the incisor relationship was not fully corrected, which left a residual overjet that has almost certainly worsened. In addition, there has also been relapse in the incisor alignment within both dental arches (upper panels). Definitive treatment as an adult involved fixed appliances and bimaxillary surgery to correct the underlying skeletal discrepancy and produce a well-aligned class I occlusion (lower panels).

overeruption (Fig. 12.2). Whilst there are obvious negative aesthetic consequences associated with tooth loss and alterations in the position of adjacent teeth, occlusal instability and functional problems can also occur and contribute to:

- Excessive tooth wear;
- Pulpal involvement, loss of vitality and periodontal destruction associated with teeth in traumatic occlusion; and
- Temporomandibular dysfunction.

In the oral rehabilitation of adult patients affected by tooth loss, orthodontic treatment may be required as part of their multidisciplinary management in a variety of situations:

- Space closure to improve aesthetics and obviate the need for restorative treatment;
- Uprighting of abutment teeth to remove occlusal interferences or provide space for an adjacent restoration (Fig. 12.3);
- Intrusion of overerupted teeth to remove occlusal interferences or provide space in the opposing arch for the placement of a restoration;
- Extrusion of teeth to increase crown length and allow coronal restoration; and
- Simple alignment to remove occlusal interferences or permit coronal restoration.

A number of features associated with adult patients can make orthodontic treatment more challenging and these all need to be taken into consideration when planning and embarking upon treatment (Nattrass & Sandy, 1995).

Growth
Adults are non-growing individuals which will reduce the scope of treatment available in comparison to that for a child or adolescent.
- Growth modification is not possible: a skeletal discrepancy will have to be either accepted or corrected with surgery.
- A lack of vertical condylar growth makes overbite correction more challenging. To avoid an increase in the vertical dimension, tooth intrusion is required and this is difficult (see Fig. 11.13).
- The midpalatal suture is essentially closed, which precludes any skeletal expansion of the maxillary arch without surgery.

Periodontal Tissues
The prevalence of periodontal disease and loss of attachment increases with age, becoming more common in adults. An adult patient should undergo a complete clinical and radiographic assessment of their periodontal status before embarking on orthodontic treatment (Johal & Ide, 1999). Previous attachment loss does not preclude orthodontics, but active periodontal disease will require treatment and evidence of stabilization before any appliances are placed (Table 12.1). An excellent standard of plaque control should be attained and then maintained throughout treatment, if necessary with professional supra- and subgingival scaling. Teeth with previous attachment loss and reduced bony support will also respond differently to orthodontic force:
- The centre of resistance moves apically (see Fig. 5.4) and tipping occurs more readily than bodily movement; and
- The relative anchorage value will reduce.
   Increasing age is associated with a reduction in vascularization and collagen turnover within the periodontium, with an overall reduction in bone volume. Initial tooth movement can be slower in adults and light forces should be used to avoid the risk of root resorption.

Restorations
Adult patients often have a heavily restored dentition, which can complicate the choice of orthodontic extractions and necessitate the bonding of appliances to ceramics or alloys. Root canal-treated teeth are amenable to orthodontic tooth movement as long as they are symptomless and correctly obturated (Drysdale et al, 1996).

Aesthetics
Whilst adult patients will accept fixed orthodontic appliances, they often request aesthetic tooth-coloured brackets, which can produce wear of opposing teeth, enamel fractures on debonding and increased friction. Lingual fixed appliances or transparent removable appliances can also be used, but these can represent a compromise in terms of efficient tooth movement.

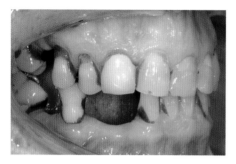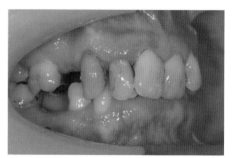

Figure 12.2 Tooth migration and tipping in adult dentitions compromised by tooth extraction.

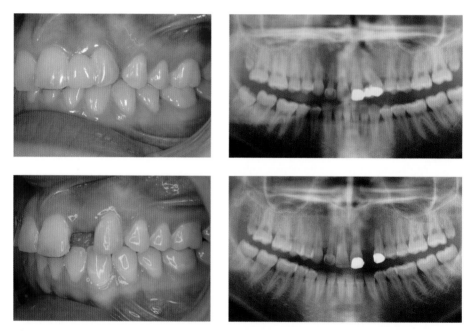

Figure 12.3 An adult patient with a congenitally absent UL2 was unhappy with the aesthetics of a resin-retained bridge bonded to the UL1 and UL3. The UL3 was markedly distally angulated, which precluded the placement of an implant restoration for the UL2. Following removal of the bridge pontic, orthodontic treatment was carried out to upright the UL3 and create space for an implant.

In many cases, adjunctive orthodontic treatment of this kind will not attempt definitive correction of a malocclusion; rather it will be restricted to moving only those teeth required for the specific treatment plan.

Orthodontics as an adjunct to periodontal treatment

Tooth migration can also occur as a consequence of attachment loss secondary to periodontal disease. In particular, the labial segments can procline significantly, resulting in an increased overjet, generalized spacing and extrusion with lengthening of the clinical crowns (Fig. 12.4). Orthodontic treatment can be carried out to retract or intrude these teeth and close spaces, but permanent retention is usually required to maintain the new position. Orthodontic intrusion can also reduce the clinical crown height and improve attachment levels if light forces are employed and associated with minimal tipping (Melsen, 2001). A prerequisite before embarking upon any orthodontic treatment in the periodontally compromised patient is stabilization of the disease process itself (Table 12.1).

Orthodontics and orthognathic surgery

A malocclusion associated with any significant discrepancy in the dentofacial skeleton of an adult requires a combination of orthodontics and surgical repositioning of the jaws for definitive correction (Fig. 12.5). These skeletal problems can include:

- Anteroposterior disproportion associated with the size or position of the maxilla and mandible in class II and class III cases;
- Vertical disproportion, associated with excessive or reduced maxillary incisor tooth show, increased overbite or open bite;
- Transverse anomalies; and
- Asymmetries of the face and jaws.

Orthodontic camouflage may be possible in some cases, but this approach can be a compromise and limited by the extent of the skeletal discrepancy. Growth modification is not possible in an adult, but many of these malocclusions would be amenable to attempts at treatment with a functional appliance if diagnosed in a growing child

---

Table 12.1 Treatment targets in patients with active periodontal disease prior to embarking on orthodontic treatment[a]

- Smokers should stop the habit;
- Pocket reduction of 1 mm for those of depth 4–6 mm;
- Pocket reduction of 2 mm or more for those of depth > 6 mm;
- Bleeding and plaque scores less than 15%;
- Cleanable teeth and prostheses; and
- No root caries.

[a] Johal & Ide (1999).

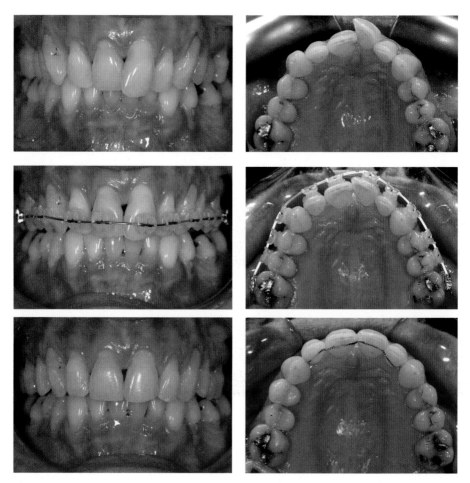

Figure 12.4 Rotation and extrusion of the UL1 as a result of periodontal disease. The position of the UL1 was corrected with fixed appliances and permanent retention.

or adolescent. However, it should be remembered that these more severe forms of skeletal discrepancy are the ones least likely to respond to attempts at growth modification and often end up requiring a surgical approach.

Orthognathic surgery can involve a range of surgical movements, which achieve repositioning of the maxilla or mandible within the facial skeleton (Fig. 12.6). Surgery of this kind does not affect any inherent growth capacity that may reside in the jaws and for this reason it is only carried out once skeletal growth has ceased, in the adult. This is particularly important for class III cases with mandibular excess, where continued forward growth of the mandible after backward surgical repositioning can lead to the reappearance of a reverse overjet if the surgery is carried out before growth has ceased.

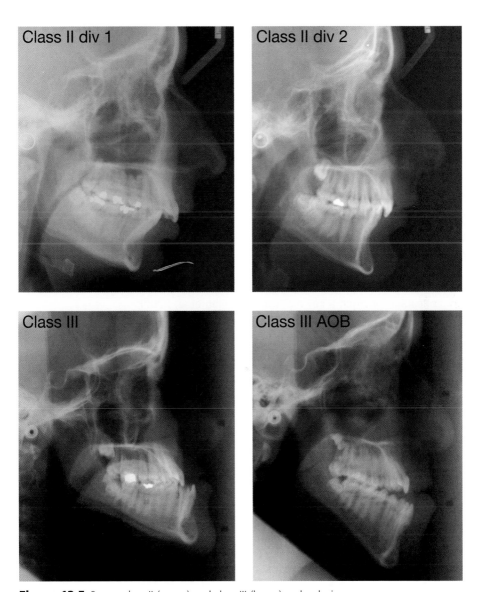

Figure 12.5 Severe class II (upper) and class III (lower) malocclusion.

Why do adults present for orthognathic surgery?

An adult patient will ultimately be advised that they require orthodontics and orthognathic surgery if the discrepancy in their skeletal base relationship is so severe that orthodontic camouflage either is not possible or would significantly compromise facial aesthetics.

Figure 12.6 Range of surgical movements. (1) The maxilla can be moved forwards, upwards and downwards. (2) The mandible can be moved forwards or backwards. (3) The chin can be moved forwards, backwards, upwards and downwards.

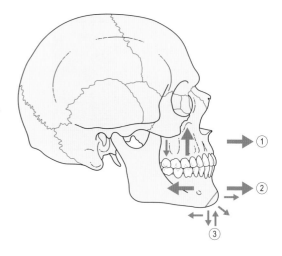

- Many are unhappy with the way they look and achieving a normal facial appearance is often a key motivation (Stirling et al, 2007);
- Some are more concerned with functional difficulties associated with their malocclusion, such as eating or, more rarely, speaking; and
- Others are simply unhappy with the appearance of their teeth.

It can often come as something of a shock to a patient who is primarily concerned with the appearance of their teeth to be told that not only do they need orthodontic treatment to correct their position, but facial surgery as well. In these instances surgical intervention may be declined and orthodontic treatment limited to tooth alignment alone, with the patient and orthodontist accepting the underlying skeletal discrepancy.

A minority of patients may exhibit a significant preoccupation with an imagined, relatively minor or non-existent defect in their facial appearance: a condition known as body dysmorphic disorder (Cunningham & Feinmann, 1998). Any suspicion of this should elicit referral for a more formal psychiatric assessment prior to embarking on any combined treatment.

Assessment of patients for combined treatment

The acquisition of records and principles of treatment planning for adults with marked skeletal discrepancies follows the same essential sequence as for any other patient. The primary objective is to position a well-aligned class I occlusion within a balanced and proportional facial skeleton. A fundamental difference between planning for surgical correction of a skeletal discrepancy and conventional orthodontic growth modification or camouflage is the extent of predictable change that can be brought about. Jaw movements of up to 1 cm can be achieved by the surgeon, which in combination with fixed appliance systems that allow precise tooth positioning, means that significant malocclusions can be corrected with great accuracy.

Patients should be assessed within the environment of a joint clinic that involves both surgeon and orthodontist. This allows a preliminary plan to be presented and explained to the patient, affords them the opportunity to ask any questions and come to an informed decision with regard to undertaking such treatment.

The orthodontist plays a predominant role in preparing a patient for orthognathic surgery. Once it is felt that the teeth are in a position to allow the required surgical movements to take place, the patient returns to the joint clinic and the surgery is definitively planned by orthodontist and surgeon.

Presurgical orthodontic treatment

There are two principle aims of presurgical orthodontic treatment:

- Eliminate any natural dentoalveolar compensation that might exist for a skeletal discrepancy and therefore allow complete surgical correction; and
- Coordinate the dental arches to produce a well-interdigitated, functional and stable occlusion in the final postsurgical position.

These aims are achieved within a number of overlapping phases, primarily during presurgical treatment through orthodontic tooth movement, although occasionally some surgical intervention may also be required, particularly for expansion (Box 12.2) or levelling of the maxillary arch. Surgically-assisted expansion is carried out before the definitive osteotomy, whilst surgically-assisted levelling usually takes place with it (Table 12.2). Some controversy exists regarding the amount of orthodontic treatment

---

Box 12.2   Surgically-assisted rapid maxillary expansion

In cases associated with severe maxillary hypoplasia, considerable expansion is often required in the maxillary arch and in adults this may not be attainable with traditional methods of orthodontic expansion alone. Surgically-assisted rapid maxillary expansion (SARME) is a form of distraction osteogenesis, which utilizes orthopaedic expansion of the maxilla in combination with partial osteotomy or corticotomy to facilitate expansion, followed by bony infill. The corticotomy can involve separation through the zygomatic buttress, midpalatal suture or pterygoid plates; whilst the orthopaedic force is applied through a tooth or bone-born expansion appliance. The advantages of this technique are that it affords considerable expansion of the maxilla (see Figure below) and reduces the likelihood of relapse; although compelling evidence regarding long-term stability is currently lacking. The main disadvantage is the requirement for surgical intervention, which in patients requiring a definitive osteotomy will mean two separate surgical procedures.

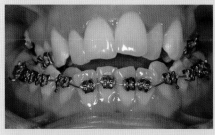 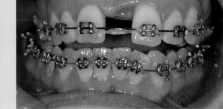

Surgically-assisted rapid maxillary expansion.

Table 12.2 Phases of orthodontic treatment for orthognathic patients

- Alignment;
- Levelling:
  - With orthodontic mechanics prior to surgery;
  - With segmental surgery; or
  - With orthodontic mechanics following surgery;
- Arch coordination.
  - With orthodontic expansion of the maxilla;
  - With surgically-assisted expansion of the maxilla;
- Finishing.

Box 12.3 How much orthodontic treatment is required prior to surgery?

There are different schools of thought regarding the amount of orthodontic treatment that should be carried out prior to surgical jaw correction. Conventionally, most tooth movement is achieved before surgery:

- Allowing accurate and maximal correction of the skeletal problem; and
- Requiring only a short period of postsurgical orthodontic treatment to detail the occlusion.

An alternative philosophy advocates completing only minimal tooth movement before carrying out the surgery as early as possible. The advantages of this approach include the following:

- Improved facial aesthetics are achieved earlier in treatment;
- Subsequent tooth movement is more predictable and achievable within a class I skeletal environment;
- Local metabolic changes associated with postsurgical healing facilitate more effective tooth movement; and
- Surgical repositioning is rarely completely accurate and therefore the sooner postsurgical orthodontic treatment can be instigated, the better.

Whilst these arguments and proposed advantages have some validity they are marginal and conventional wisdom would suggest achieving maximal occlusal decompensation prior to surgery.

that should be completed prior to surgery (Box. 12.3), but conventional planning requires full decompensation.

Alignment of the dental arches

Orthodontic alignment of the dental arches will be necessary. Space requirements will need to be assessed and if these are high, tooth extraction may be needed (Box 12.4). However, in surgical cases the planned anteroposterior and vertical position of the upper and lower incisors can significantly influence these requirements.

Box 12.4   Extractions and orthognathic surgery

Extractions may be required to provide space for tooth alignment and levelling, incisor decompensation or access for segmental osteotomy cuts. However, it is important to note that tooth movements required for orthodontic camouflage are often directly opposite to those necessary for decompensation prior to surgery, and extraction-based camouflage treatment should be approached with some caution in individuals with significant skeletal discrepancy. A good illustration is extraction of premolars in the mandibular arch of a class III case. These will often be required to provide space for retroclination of the lower incisors if orthodontic camouflage is planned; however, if this treatment proves to be unsuccessful and surgical decompensation is subsequently required, the lower incisors will need to be proclined. If premolars have previously been extracted, this will lead to considerable space opening up in the buccal segments. For this reason, particularly in class III cases, if there is any suspicion that orthognathic surgery may be required, mandibular premolar extractions should be avoided and any treatment decisions delayed until facial growth has ceased.

- Class II cases may require extraction in the mandibular arch if there is any degree of crowding, particularly if this is combined with a requirement to upright or intrude the incisors. Proclination of the mandibular incisors is usually undesirable because it will reduce the amount of potential forward surgical movement of the mandible. In the maxillary arch of class II cases, crowding is generally less common, incisor movement rarely requires significant space (quite the contrary in a class II division 2 malocclusion) and some arch expansion is often desirable; therefore extractions are rarer. If the incisors are retroclined, space will be generated as they are moved forwards to create an overjet necessary to facilitate mandibular advancement.
- Class III cases do not usually require extractions in the mandibular arch, crowding is generally rare because of the increased arch length associated with an enlarged mandible and space is often generated as a result of the incisor proclination required for decompensation. In contrast, space is often at a premium in the maxilla, arch length can be reduced because of a small and narrow upper jaw and there is commonly crowding. To make matters worse, the incisors often require some retroclination, which requires space, and therefore premolar extractions are often needed.

Altering the labiolingual position of the incisors

The final labiolingual position of the incisor teeth is important because it will dictate the amount of surgical movement that can take place in the anteroposterior dimension. Any existing dentoalveolar compensation that would restrict this movement needs to be corrected prior to surgery. Inevitably, these incisor movements can lead to considerable worsening of the malocclusion during this period and the patient should be made aware of this before treatment begins (Fig. 12.7).

- Class II cases often require maximal forward movement of the mandible and this is achieved by ensuring an overjet is present. Retroclination of lower and occasion-

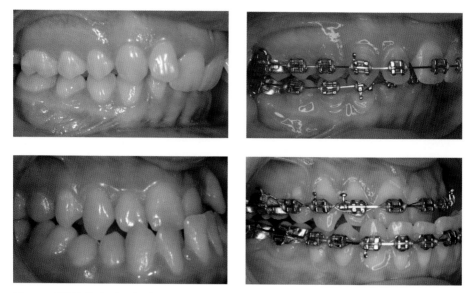

Figure 12.7 Orthodontic decompensation will create an overjet in a class II division 2 malocclusion (upper) and increase a reverse overjet in a class III malocclusion (lower).

ally some proclination of the upper incisors can be required in class II division 1 cases, whilst in class II division 2 cases a significant amount of upper incisor proclination is usually needed.

- Class III cases are often associated with the opposite situation. The upper incisors are proclined, whilst the lowers are retroclined and presurgical orthodontic treatment mechanics are required to reverse these positions and produce a reverse overjet.

Arch levelling

An excessive or reduced curve of Spee in either the maxillary or mandibular arch will require levelling if good interdigitation of the teeth is to be achieved in the final occlusion. This can take place at one of three time points during treatment and the choice of mechanics will be dictated by the method of levelling employed.

Arch levelling prior to surgery

A decision to level the arches using orthodontic treatment mechanics prior to surgical treatment usually take place in the absence of severe discrepancies in either of the occlusal planes. Levelling can be achieved with incisor intrusion, molar extrusion, a combination of these two movements, or more rarely, incisor proclination.

- With mandibular surgery alone, levelling a curve of Spee with incisor intrusion will result in the lower face height being maintained following surgery and is usually planned for patients with acceptable vertical proportions.
- In the patient requiring posterior impaction of the maxilla to correct an open bite, care should be taken if orthodontic levelling of a reduced curve of Spee in the maxillary arch will involve excessive extrusion of the incisors. Following surgery,

any vertical relapse of these teeth will result in a tendency towards reopening of the open bite.

Arch levelling during segmental surgery
Occasionally, the vertical discrepancy is so severe that segmental jaw surgery is indicated to achieve arch levelling. This is more common in the maxilla in association with a markedly reduced curve of Spee and anterior open bite. If a decision is made to correct this with segmental surgery, the orthodontist will use segmented archwires to level the teeth within segments and ensure that the vertical discrepancy is maintained prior to surgery. Space will be required between teeth adjacent to the planned segments to allow for vertical osteotomy cuts and premolar extractions are often required to create this (Fig. 12.8).

Arch levelling following surgery
Class II cases with a reduced lower anterior face height are often associated with an increased curve of Spee in the mandibular arch. It is desirable to increase the lower face height in these cases as the mandible is advanced and this is achieved by maintaining the curve of Spee prior to surgical movement. The lower incisor position ensures an increase in face height as the mandible is advanced and the arch is subsequently levelled by extrusion of posterior teeth during the postsurgical period. This technique is known as a 'three-point landing' because in the initial postsurgical position there is only tooth contact between the incisors and posterior molars (Fig. 12.9). Clearly, in these cases it is important that the orthodontist maintains the curve of Spee in the mandible prior to surgical repositioning.

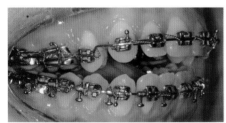 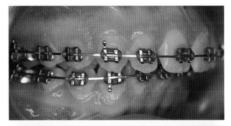

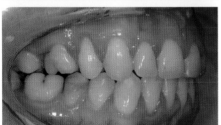 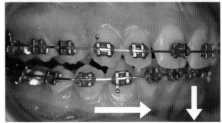

Figure 12.8 Segmental arch mechanics prior to maxillary segmental surgery to correct an anterior open bite (upper panel pre-surgery and lower panel following surgery and appliance removal).

Figure 12.9 A three-point landing maintains a curve of Spee in the mandibular arch and allows an increase in face height as the mandible is advanced. The posterior open bites are closed down after surgery.

Transverse arch coordination

The final stage of orthodontic preparation ensures that the dental arches are coordinated in the transverse plane following surgical movement. In the proposed surgical position, there should be an absence of crossbites and good interdigitation of the buccal segments from the canine teeth back. Transverse coordination is almost always achieved prior to surgical movement.

- Class II cases requiring mandibular advancement often need some expansion of the maxillary arch to compensate for the relative increase in the transverse dimension of the mandibular buccal segments as they move forwards. This is usually achieved by dental expansion with orthodontic archwires or in more severe cases, expansion with a quad helix or rapid maxillary expansion appliance.
- Class III cases are often characterized by a narrow maxilla, which will require expansion even though the relative anteroposterior surgical movements between maxilla and mandible may favour transverse coordination. Depending upon the degree of maxillary constriction, this can be achieved with orthodontic or occasionally, surgically-assisted expansion (see Box 12.2).

Final surgical planning

The presurgical orthodontic phase of treatment is usually regarded as being complete when the orthodontist has achieved the following goals:

- Alignment of all the teeth, with rigid rectangular stainless steel archwires present in both dental arches;
- Correct incisor position in the anteroposterior and vertical dimensions; and
- Demonstration by 'snap' dental casts of arch coordination in a class I occlusal relationship.

This is confirmed following examination of the patient on a joint clinic with a new set of comprehensive records: in particular, a cephalometric lateral skull radiograph and profile photograph. Together with the patient, these records are used to plan in detail the surgical movements required to correct the malocclusion (Box 12.5) and simulate their effect on the soft tissue facial profile. These predictions can be carried out manually by hand (Fig. 12.10) or with the aid of computer software (Fig. 12.11). In the case of manual prediction, the orthodontist carries out the proposed jaw movements on a cephalometric radiograph and reproduces the soft tissue changes using profile outlines, templates or superimposed photographs (Hunt and Rudge, 1984). Computer prediction programmes allow this process to be carried out electronically, which theoretically should produce more accurate profile prediction, although this is not necessarily the case (Eckhardt and Cunningham, 2004). However, a problem with all these methods is that the soft tissues do not respond to the surgical movements in a simple ratio and changes can vary in different regions of the face and between individuals. More recently, three-dimensional surgical planning has been advocated, but whether this is any more accurate than planning based on the profile, remains to be seen (Hajeer et al, 2004).

Model surgery

Once the surgical movements have been planned, articulated study casts are required to allow the dental technician to simulate them in the laboratory (Fig. 12.12).

Box 12.5 Planning orthognathic treatment

Conventional orthognathic surgery can significantly alter the jaw relationship and appearance of the middle and lower face. More severe discrepancies involving the upper face are usually associated with craniofacial syndromes and may require osteotomies at the Le Fort II and III level. Specialist supra-regional units usually carry out combined treatment of this nature.

Clinical and cephalometric examination will highlight the primary source of any jaw discrepancy and allow a decision to be made regarding the essential jaw movements required. The precise directions and distances in millimetres are normally calculated following orthodontic decompensation when the patient is judged to be ready for surgery. Correct positioning of the maxillary dentition is a key factor. Any significant changes planned for the position of the upper incisor or molar dentition will require a maxillary osteotomy, either to move these teeth upwards, forwards, backwards or unilaterally to correct a centreline.

- Numerous cephalometric measurements have been advocated to describe the correct antero-posterior maxillary incisor position (see Chapter 6).
- Class III cases with maxillary retrusion will often require maxillary advancement.
- Vertically, around 3 to 4-mm of incisor crown should be visible below the upper lip at rest, increasing to show 75–100% on smiling (see Box 6.2). This relationship is influenced by upper lip length (which should be around 20-mm), and vertical development of the maxilla. In the presence of vertical maxillary excess, maxillary impaction will be required.
- The upper dental midline should be coincident with the facial midline.
- The maxillary dentition should be level in the transverse plane.

Once the maxillary incisor position has been decided, it will be necessary to place the mandibular incisors into a class I relationship, with coincident centrelines and a harmonious profile.

- Class II cases with mandibular deficiency will require advancement of the mandible.
- Class III cases with mandibular excess will require set-back of the mandible.
- If there is an anterior open bite or increased LAFH, a posterior impaction of the maxilla may be needed to reduce the vertical dimension. This will be associated with some mandibular autorotation, which may be sufficient to reduce the overjet in less severe class II cases—if it does not, then mandibular advancement will also be required. In class III cases, autorotation will worsen the incisor relationship and influence the required jaw movements.

Chin position is also important and may require either reduction or enhancement with a genioplasty.

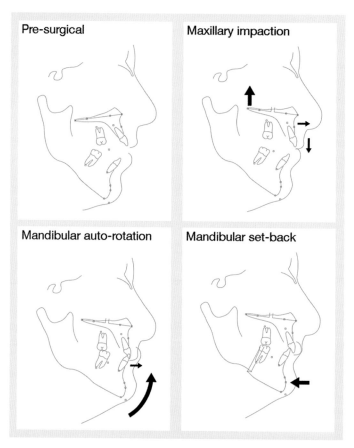

Figure 12.10 Hand tracing for cephalometric surgical prediction. Differential impaction of the maxilla to correct an anterior open bite. The maxillary molar dentition is moved upwards and the incisors downwards and forwards. Autorotation of the mandible following posterior maxillary impaction successfully closes down the open bite, but produces a class III incisor relationship. The mandible is therefore moved backwards with a sagittal split osteotomy to obtain a class I incisor occlusion (see the case treated in Fig. 12.28).

- For single jaw mandibular surgery, an acrylic wafer is constructed on models articulated in the planned final occlusal position. This provides a positional guide for the surgeon at operation.
- Surgery involving either the maxilla in isolation or the maxilla and mandible requires a facebow recording, which allows the technician to mount the maxillary dental cast on a semi-adjustable articulator. The mandibular dental cast is then articulated in the retruded contact position (RCP) and the mandibular hinge axis is reproduced. The technician simulates the planned maxillary osteotomy and constructs an

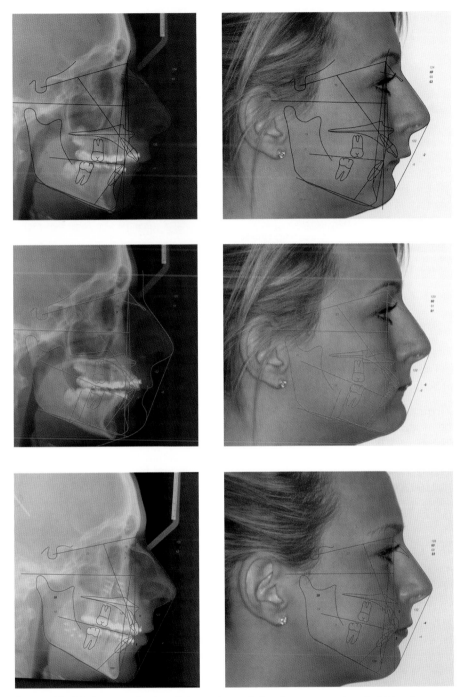

Figure 12.11 Computerized cephalometric prediction for a severe class II division 1 case. The pre-surgical cephalometric radiograph is digitized (upper left) and superimposed on the pre-surgical profile picture (upper right). The surgical movements are carried out using the cephalometric analysis – in this case, a differential maxillary impaction and sagittal split forward mandibular osteotomy (middle left) and the soft tissue prediction is produced by photomorphing (middle right). The actual post-surgical lateral skull radiograph and profile picture are shown in the lower panels. It should be remembered that these methods of prediction offer a guide and are not absolute.

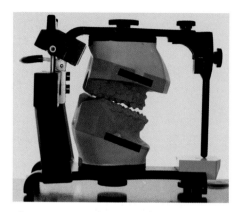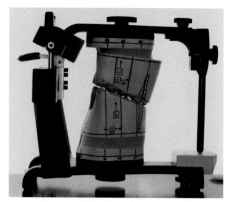

Figure 12.12 Model surgery.

intermediate wafer, which uses the original mandibular position. The surgeon uses this wafer as an aid to positioning the maxilla during surgery, which is why an accurate reproduction of the condylar axis is required.

- For bimaxillary surgery, the technician will also construct a final wafer for the surgeon, which reproduces the planned final occlusal position of the mandible.

Surgical movements

The maxillofacial surgeon is responsible for repositioning the jaws in accordance with the surgical plan. Advances in anaesthetic and surgical techniques mean that there is now increased scope to position the jaws optimally within their soft tissue envelope (see Fig. 7.3). The use of bimaxillary surgery to reposition both the maxilla and mandible has made surgical compromise less common and increased the range of malocclusions that can be corrected. Rigid internal fixation, mediated by small bone plates and screws (Fig. 12.13), has reduced postoperative discomfort, improved safety for the patient by avoiding the need for postoperative maxillomandibular fixation and improved long-term stability of the final result (Box 12.6).

Maxillary procedures

A number of surgical procedures are commonly carried out to alter the position, width and occlusal plane of the maxilla.

Le Fort I osteotomy

The entire maxilla can be moved in anteroposterior, vertical or transverse directions as a single unit with a Le Fort I osteotomy. These movements can be carried out using a single vector, or with a combination to produce differential changes in position.

Le Fort I involves disarticulating the maxilla from the skull by cutting along the lateral outer wall through the base of the zygomatic buttress, extending anteriorly to the piriform fossa and posteriorly to the pterygoid plates (Fig. 12.14). Internally, the nasal septum and lateral wall of the nasal cavity are freed, with the maxilla being finally mobilized by separating it from its attachment at the pterygoid plates. The surgeon achieves superior vertical repositioning by removing bone in the region of these cuts, whilst inferior movements require grafting into the intervening space.

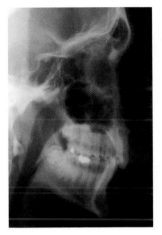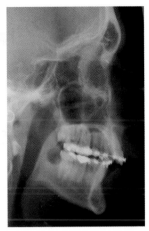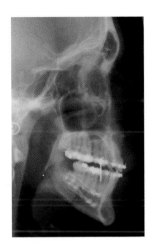

Figure 12.13 Rigid internal fixation following bilateral sagittal split osteotomy.

The maxilla can be moved forwards or upwards by anything up to 10-mm and these movements are generally stable; backward repositioning is also possible, but the changes that can be achieved are less, at around 5-mm. Inferior repositioning of the maxilla is notoriously unstable and generally avoided.

Segmental maxillary surgery

Segments of the maxilla can also be moved by the surgeon, either as an isolated procedure or, more commonly, in combination with Le Fort I osteotomy:

- Anterior subapical osteotomy (Wunderer, Cupar or Wassmund) (Fig. 12.15) achieves isolated movement of the canine and incisor teeth, for either reduction of an overjet or correction of a vertical discrepancy, usually anterior open bite;
- Posterior subapical osteotomy (Schuchardt) (Fig. 12.16) is occasionally used for isolated correction of a unilateral posterior crossbite; and
- Following Le Fort I osteotomy, the maxilla can also be divided bilaterally to facilitate correction of a transverse discrepancy, usually expansion for a bilateral posterior crossbite; or segmented into three pieces for levelling an occlusal plane during the correction of a vertical discrepancy (Fig. 12.17).

These segmental procedures often require some room between relevant teeth, which provide surgical access for the necessary cuts within the alveolus. This is usually achieved by premolar extraction or less commonly, by increases in arch length and root paralleling mediated by the orthodontist (see Fig. 12.8).

Mandibular procedures

The body of the mandible can be advanced or moved backwards in relation to the ramus or this movement can incorporate the ramus. In addition, chin prominence can be adjusted with localized osteotomy along the inferior border.

Box 12.6 How stable is surgical correction of jaw position?

The University of North Carolina has followed up almost 1500 patients who have received surgical repositioning of the jaws for a minimum of one year postsurgery, with over 500 of these being reviewed for at least five years. This research programme has identified a hierarchy of stability in the immediate twelve-month postsurgical period, which is influenced primarily by the amount and direction of jaw movement (Proffit et al, 1996, 2007).

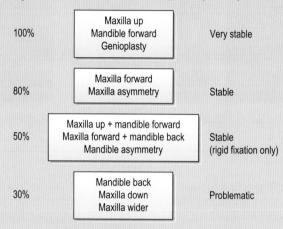

100%	Maxilla up / Mandible forward / Genioplasty	Very stable
80%	Maxilla forward / Maxilla asymmetry	Stable
50%	Maxilla up + mandible forward / Maxilla forward + mandible back / Mandible asymmetry	Stable (rigid fixation only)
30%	Mandible back / Maxilla down / Maxilla wider	Problematic

Stability of orthognathic surgical procedures in the first postsurgical year. Procedures are grouped as very stable (90% of patients judged to have an excellent result); stable (little or no change in around 80% of patients); stable with rigid fixation only (an excellent result in 90% of cases with rigid fixation and 60% of those without it); problematic (up to 50% pf patients have >2-mm change and 20% have >4-mm). Adapted from Proffit et al (2007).

- Highly stable procedures include superior repositioning of the maxilla, advancement of the mandible and genioplasty;
- Stable procedures include maxillary advancement and two-jaw surgery for the correction of class II (maxilla up, mandible forward), class III (maxilla forward, mandible back) and asymmetries; and
- Problematic procedures include isolated mandibular setback, inferior movement of the mandible and widening of the maxilla.

A different pattern of stability is evident after twelve months once surgical healing is complete.

- Mandibular advancement is associated with some decrease in length, although dentoalveolar adaptation prevents an increase in overjet in more than half these patients;
- Maxillary superior positioning will relapse by > 2-mm in a third of patients;
- Significant changes occur in jaw positions after bimaxillary surgery, but these are not necessarily reflected in changes of overjet or overbite; and
- Class III patients are more stable in the long-term than class II.

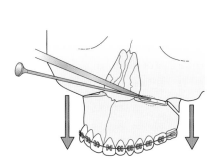

Figure 12.14 Le Fort 1 osteotomy.

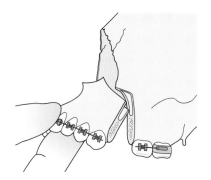

Figure 12.15 Anterior subapical osteotomy.

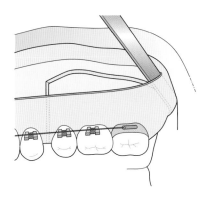

Figure 12.16 Posterior subapical osteotomy.

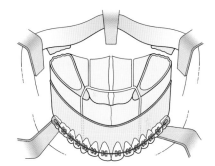

Figure 12.17 Segmented maxillary osteotomy.

Sagittal-split osteotomy

The bilateral sagittal-split osteotomy (BSSO) is used to move the mandible forwards or backwards in the treatment of retrognathia, prognathia or asymmetry (Fig. 12.18). A medially positioned cut is placed into cortical bone of the ramus just above the lingula; whilst a laterally placed cut is fashioned through cortical bone of the body in the region of the molar dentition. These cuts are then joined by splitting the mandible along a line extending through the cortex, which allows forward or backward movement of the body in relation to the ramus, but maintains patency of the neurovascular bundle.

The mandible can be moved in either a forward or backward direction using a BSSO. Both these movements demonstrate good stability, particularly mandibular advancement, although the upper limit is around 10-mm.

Vertical subsigmoid osteotomy

The vertical subsigmoid osteotomy is used primarily to move the mandible backwards for the correction of mandibular prognathism or asymmetry and involves a cut from

Figure 12.18 Sagittal-split osteotomy.

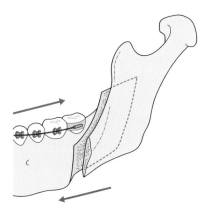

Figure 12.19 Vertical subsigmoid osteotomy.

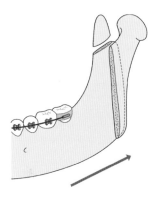

the sigmoid notch in front of the condyle, extending vertically down behind the neurovascular bundle, to the angle of the mandible (Fig. 12.19).

Genioplasty

The genioplasty is an osteotomy involving the inferior border of the chin and is achieved with a horizontal cut across this region (Fig. 12.20). The bony segment can be moved in an anterior or posterior direction to augment or reduce chin prominence, whilst vertical reduction can be used to diminish the height of the anterior mandible. Genioplasty can be used in isolation to correct mild problems of chin aesthetics, particularly assymetries; however, it is most commonly used as an adjunct to BSSO, either to reduce chin prominence or to increase it.

Anterior subapical osteotomy

The anterior subapical osteotomy is occasionally used to alter the position of the lower labial segment in the mandible and requires vertical cuts through the alveolus behind the canine teeth, which are joined by a horizontal cut underneath the root apices to free the anterior segment. The subapical osteotomy can be utilized in the correction

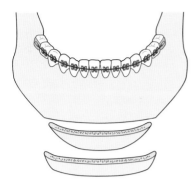

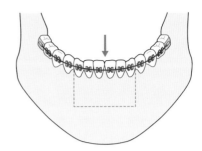

Figure 12.20 Genioplasty.

Figure 12.21 Anterior subapical osteotomy.

of anterior open bite and bimaxillary proclination or for levelling an excessive curve of Spee if this cannot be achieved orthodontically and the anterior face height needs to be maintained (Fig. 12.21).

Postsurgical orthodontic treatment

Postsurgical orthodontic treatment is usually initiated within two weeks of surgery if rigid fixation has been employed and often begins with removal of the final surgical wafer. Up to this point the final wafer in combination with intraoral elastics placed in theatre has maintained the occlusal position whilst normal function is re-established. This final period of orthodontic treatment is concerned with establishing ideal occlusal relationships and maximum interdigitation of the teeth. During this period, flexible archwires are placed by the orthodontist and elastic wear is prescribed according to the final adjustments required (Fig. 12.22). The duration of this treatment will depend upon the amount of tooth movement still required. In cases where arch levelling has been achieved either prior to or with surgery, the postsurgical phase is usually only concerned with final occlusal detailing. In contrast, postsurgical levelling can take a little longer, but in most cases a period of no more than six months of postsurgical orthodontic treatment will be required.

Distraction osteogenesis

Distraction osteogenesis (DO) in the craniofacial region is a technique that involves osteotomy of either the maxilla or mandible, followed by progressive mechanical separation of the bone fragments using a fixed expandable device (Box 12.7). An advantage of this technique is that it allows jaw movement in considerable excess to that which is achievable using conventional orthognathic surgery. For the treatment of patients with severe jaw deficiency, particularly those with a syndromic craniofacial disorder, DO can afford great potential for more stable correction of the skeletal discrepancy.

The success of DO when applied to the membrane-derived bones of the facial complex relies upon the applied tension across the initially soft callus of the fracture site resulting in the creation of new bone. An important principle is to allow a latent period of four to five days following the osteotomy, before any tension is applied. This

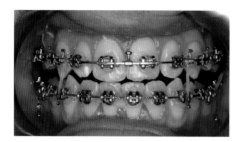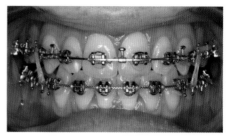

Figure 12.22 Postsurgical orthodontic elastics to close a bite down and achieve maximum intercuspation.

results in the production of a soft callus and optimal bone formation during distraction. Once the desired movement has been achieved, a period of consolidation is then required to allow maturation of the newly formed bone and stabilization of the new jaw position (Fig. 12.23). It is clearly important during DO to carefully control the vector of surgical movement.

Common malocclusions and their surgical treatment

Isolated mandibular deficiency often manifests as a class II division 1 malocclusion in the presence of a normal or increased lower face height and a class II division 2 incisor relationship with a reduced lower face height. The approach to surgical correction of these problems will involve forward movement of the mandible, usually achieved with a BSSO. However, the vertical relationship will also influence the treatment plan and if a significant increase in the lower face height exists, some posterior impaction of the maxilla may also be required to allow mandibular autorotation and a reduction in this dimension. If the face height is normal, the mandible will be brought forward with a level occlusal plane and maintenance of the existing vertical dimension (Fig. 12.24). If the face height is reduced, the curve of Spee is generally maintained in the mandible and the postsurgical face height increased with the osteotomy (Fig. 12.25). When moving the mandible forwards the chin position should also be considered; some reduction may be required if the chin point is prominent in the correct surgical position, or augmentation with marked micrognathia.

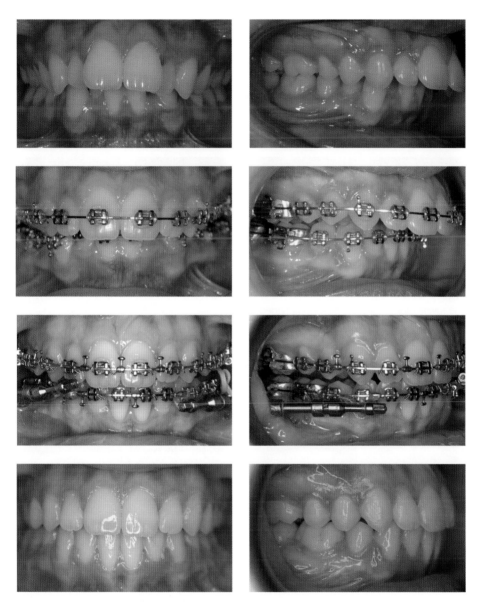

Figure 12.23 Distraction osteogenesis to correct a severe class II division 1 malocclusion. An overjet of 15-mm was reduced with forward distraction of the mandible.

Class III cases can be associated with varying amounts of maxillary retrusion and mandibular prognathism, either alone or in combination and will require corresponding anteroposterior movement of these jaws, often via Le Fort I and BSSO (Fig. 12.26). Significant variation in the lower face height can also be seen in combination with a class III malocclusion (see Fig. 12.5) and if excessive, may require maxillary impaction

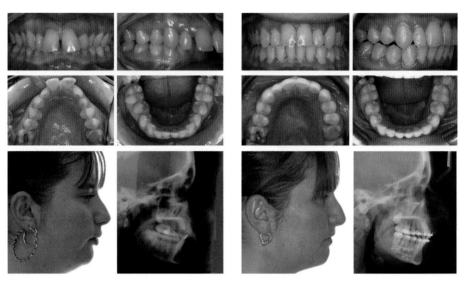

Figure 12.24 Correction of a class II division 1 malocclusion with a forward-sliding BSSO. The lower face height has been maintained.

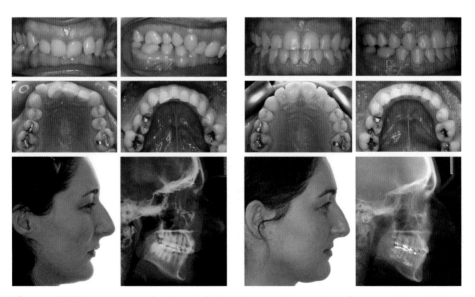

Figure 12.25 Correction of a class II division 2 malocclusion with a forward-sliding BSSO and three-point landing to increase the lower anterior face height.

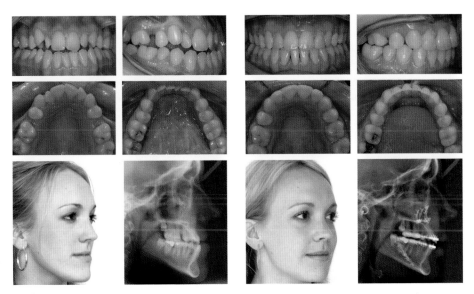

Figure 12.26 Correction of a class III malocclusion with a bimaxillary osteotomy. The maxilla was moved forwards and the mandible back. Presurgical orthodontics done by Saba Quereshi.

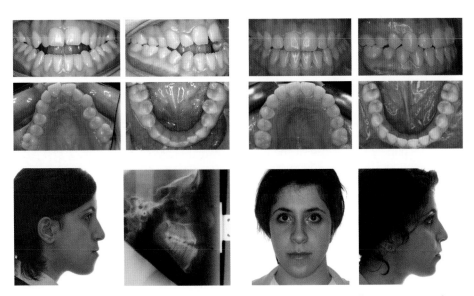

Figure 12.27 Correction of a class III AOB malocclusion with a bimaxillary osteotomy. The posterior maxilla was impacted and the mandible autorotated and moved back. Presurgical orthodontics carried out by Alastair Smith.

Figure 12.28 Differential impaction of the maxilla and sagittal split osteotomy of the mandible to correct a significant anterior open bite (for the surgical plan, see Fig. 12.10).

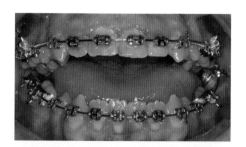

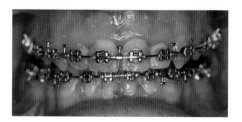

in combination with anteroposterior change. It should be remembered that maxillary impaction is also associated with mandibular autorotation, which can be beneficial in the correction of class II discrepancies but will tend to worsen a class III relationship.

Additional vertical problems, either in isolation or combined with an anteroposterior discrepancy, often require maxillary impaction. These can include problems of vertical maxillary excess and a 'gummy smile' or anterior open bite and may require either one-piece or segmental maxillary surgery to correct the vertical incisor position (see Figs 12.8 and 12.28).

Obstructive sleep apnoea

Obstructive sleep apnoea (OSA) is a complex disorder characterized by periodic cessations (apnoea) or interruptions (hypopnoea) in normal breathing during sleep and occurs secondary to collapse of the upper airway (Magliocca & Helman, 2005). OSA affects around 2% of the adult population and is distinct from simple snoring; being associated with clinical features that can manifest both nocturnally and during the day (Table 12.3). Importantly, untreated OSA can have implications for general health; a variety of long-term complications have been identified, including hypertension, cardiac arrhythmias, stroke, angina and depression. Definitive diagnosis involves an overnight sleep study or polysomnography in a dedicated hospital sleep unit.

The medical management of mild to moderate OSA involves a hierarchy of intervention aimed at improving the airway:

- Eliminating factors known to aggravate OSA (encouraging sleep in a lateral rather than supine position, abstinence from alcohol and weight loss);
- Continuous positive airway pressure (CPAP) maintains upper airway patency by applying pressured air via a nasal or oral mask worn nocturnally (Fig. 12.29); and
- Mandibular advancement splints can be worn nocturnally to increase the size of the pharyngeal airway.

Table 12.3 Signs and symptoms associated with OSA[a]

Nocturnal
- Drooling
- Xerostomia
- Restless sleep
- Apnoeas
- Choking or gasping

Daytime
- Excessive sleepiness
- Morning headaches
- Impaired concentration
- Depression
- Decreased libido
- Irritability

[a] Magliocca & Helman (2005).

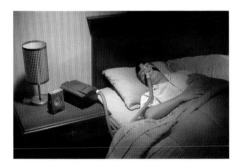

Figure 12.29 Continuous positive airway pressure in the treatment of sleep apnoea. Courtesy of Dr Ama Johal.

In more severe cases of OSA, surgical intervention may be required to enlarge the posterior pharyngeal space and provide long-term stabilization of the airway.

Mandibular advancement splints

CPAP has proved to be an effective treatment for OSA, but it can be associated with poor compliance because of the necessity to wear a bulky external appliance over the face at night. Mandibular advancement splints offer a viable alternative: worn nocturnally and increasing the pharyngeal airway by displacing the position of the mandible and tongue forwards (Johal & Battagel, 2001). These appliances can reduce snoring and improve the symptoms of OSA although some side effects, including excessive salivation or xerostomia, discomfort in the orofacial musculature and TMJ, occlusal alterations and occasionally even worsening symptoms associated with OSA, have been reported (Hoekema et al, 2004).

A variety of individual appliance designs are available (Fig. 12.30), but they can be broadly categorized as:

- Monobloc appliances, which consist of one piece and rigidly fix the mandible into an anterior position; and
- Bibloc appliances, composed of two interconnected pieces, which allow adjustable advancement of the mandible.

Figure 12.30 Monobloc appliance for treatment of sleep apnoea. Courtesy of Dr Ama Johal.

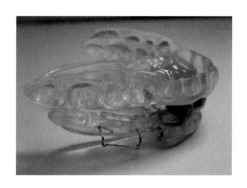

Further reading

ARNETT GW AND MCLAUGHLIN RP (2004). *Facial and Dental Planning for Orthodontists and Oral Surgeons* (Edinburgh: Mosby).
PROFFIT WR, WHITE RP JR AND SARVER DM (2003). *Contemporary Treatment of Facial Deformity* (Edinburgh: Mosby).
HARRIS M AND REYNOLDS IR (1991). *Fundamentals of Orthognathic Surgery* (London: Saunders).

References

CUNNINGHAM SJ AND FEINMANN C (1998). Psychological assessment of patients requesting orthognathic surgery and the relevance of body dysmorphic disorder. *Br J Orthod* 25:293–298.
DRYSDALE C, GIBBS SL AND FORD TR (1996). Orthodontic management of root-filled teeth. *Br J Orthod* 23:255–260.
ECKHARDT CE AND CUNNINGHAM SJ (2004). How predictable is orthognathic surgery? *Eur J Orthod* 26:303–309.
HAJEER MY, MILLETT DT, AYOUB AF, ET AL (2004). Applications of 3D imaging in orthodontics: part I. *J Orthod* 31:62–70.
HOEKEMA A, STEGENGA B AND DE BONT LG (2004). Efficacy and co-morbidity of oral appliances in the treatment of obstructive sleep apnea-hypopnea: a systematic review. *Crit Rev Oral Biol Med* 15:137–155.
HUNT NP AND RUDGE SJ (1984). Facial profile and orthognathic surgery. *Br J Orthod* 11:126–136.
JOHAL A AND BATTAGEL JM (2001). Current principles in the management of obstructive sleep apnoea with mandibular advancement appliances. *Br Dent J* 190:532–536.
JOHAL A AND IDE M (1999). Orthodontics in the adult patient, with special reference to the periodontally compromised patient. *Dent Update* 26:101–104, 106–108.
MAGLIOCCA KR AND HELMAN JI (2005). Obstructive sleep apnea: diagnosis, medical management and dental implications. *J Am Dent Assoc* 136:1121–1129; quiz 1166–1167.
MELSEN B (2001). Tissue reaction to orthodontic tooth movement—a new paradigm. *Eur J Orthod* 23:671–681.
NATTRASS C AND SANDY JR (1995). Adult orthodontics—a review. *Br J Orthod* 22:331–337.
PROFFIT WR, TURVEY TA AND PHILLIPS C (1996). Orthognathic surgery: a hierarchy of stability. *Int J Adult Orthodon Orthognath Surg* 11:191–204.
PROFFIT WR, TURVEY TA AND PHILLIPS C (2007). The hierarchy of stability and predictability in orthognathic surgery with rigid fixation: an update and extension. *Head Face Med* 3:21.
STIRLING J, LATCHFORD G, MORRIS DO, ET AL (2007). Elective orthognathic treatment decision making: a survey of patient reasons and experiences. *J Orthod* 34:113–127; discussion 111.

13 Cleft lip and palate, and syndromes affecting the craniofacial region

A syndrome is the association of several clinically recognizable signs and symptoms, which can occur together in an affected individual. A large number of syndromic conditions involve the craniofacial region (Gorlin et al, 2001) and these can be broadly subdivided into:

- Those that occur as part of a characterized Mendelian disorder, resulting from a single gene defect;
- Those arising from structural abnormalities of the chromosomes;
- Those associated with known teratogens; and
- Those whose causation remains obscure and are therefore currently uncharacterized.

Single gene disorders are the result of specific gene mutations and are inherited according to Mendelian rules, with varying levels of penetrance and expressivity within pedigrees:

- Autosomal dominant;
- Autosomal recessive;
- X-linked dominant; and
- X-linked recessive.

Cytogenetics, or the study of chromosomal abnormalities, has also revealed a wide range of physical chromosomal alterations, including variations in both number and structure, which can cause perturbations of gene function and congenital malformations.

Teratogenic agents come in many forms and can include:

- Drugs (alcohol, phenytoin, thalidomide);
- Infections (cytomegalovirus, rubella, syphilis); and
- Physical agents (radiation, intrauterine mechanical restraint).

Identifying candidate genes for genetic conditions

Elucidating the genetic basis of an inherited condition is not a straightforward task. The human genome contains over 3 billion base pairs within the entire DNA sequence and some genetic disorders can arise from a change in only a single one of these. One of the main obstacles is the location and identification of the causative gene, a process that has become easier with advances in molecular biology and bio-informatics (Box 13.1).

For single-gene disorders, positional cloning aims to identify, or at least localize, the chromosomal region where a candidate disease gene may reside. Geneticists use markers within the genome that can be tracked through members of an affected pedigree and provide linkage to the candidate region for a particular condition:

> ### Box 13.1   The human genome project
>
> Publication of the draft human genome sequence (Lander et al, 2001; Venter et al, 2001) has provided an important global resource that will have an effect upon all our lives. Within the human genome there are approximately 30,000 genes distributed across the 23 chromosomes and access to this sequence information has important implications for molecular medicine. In particular, geneticists are now able to identify disease genes and position them within the genome much more easily. A candidate sequence can be entered into sophisticated online browsers and the whole human DNA sequence searched in a matter of minutes. This knowledge is also allowing the development of more rapid and specific tests for the presence of, or susceptibility to certain genetic diseases; which will lead to earlier diagnosis and hopefully treatment of these conditions. In addition, knowledge gained from the human genome will allow progress to be made in therapeutics, with the design of drugs that function at the molecular level and target the specific causes of the disease rather than simply controlling the effects. Finally, the sequence is also an invaluable resource for biologists, providing valuable insight into human evolution and diversity.

- The closer a marker is to a disease gene, the less often it will be separated during meiotic recombination, and therefore, the marker and the disease gene will tend to be inherited together through generations.

Modern geneticists use DNA polymorphisms as markers. These are identifiable sequence variations situated at specific positions within the genome. By identifying those most closely associated with a disease locus, a region of DNA at a specific point within the genome that might harbor the candidate gene for a particular disease is identified. Once the region has been narrowed down in this way, specific genes within the locus can be investigated.

Unfortunately, many disorders are multifactorial and do not behave in a simple Mendelian manner. These conditions have a more complex aetiological basis, being the combined product of:

- Numerous susceptibility genes that each makes a minor contribution to the condition; and
- Environmental influences.

A good example of a multifactorial condition that can affect the craniofacial region is nonsyndromic cleft lip and palate. For these conditions, populations rather than family pedigrees usually must be investigated, and more complex methods of genetic mapping are required. For this reason, there has been less success in elucidating the basis of multifactorial conditions than that of single-gene disorders.

Cleft lip and palate

Clefts involving the lip and/or palate (CLP) or isolated clefts of the palate (CP) are the commonest congenital anomaly to affect the craniofacial region in man (Fraser, 1970).

They represent a complex phenotype and reflect a failure of the normal mechanisms involved during early embryological development of the face. In human populations CLP and CP can be broadly subdivided into:

- Nonsyndromic, which occur in isolation; and
- Syndromic, which occur in combination with other physical and developmental anomalies.

Classification

A number of formal classifications have been described for CLP and CP; however, the clinical presentation of these conditions is so variable that a specific description of each individual case is more useful (Fig. 13.1).

- CLP can range from simple notching or isolated clefting of the upper lip with or without involvement of the alveolus, to complete unilateral or bilateral clefts of the lip, alveolus and hard/soft palate; and
- CP can range from a simple submucous cleft (a lack of continuity of the muscles across the palate) or bifid uvula to a complete cleft involving the primary and secondary palate.

Epidemiology

- In Caucasian populations, CLP is seen in approximately 1:1,000 live births, but racial differences occur, Asian races being affected most commonly (1:500) and African races least (1:2,500).
- Males are more commonly affected than females (approximately 2:1).
- Unilateral CLP represents around 80% of all facial clefts, with the left side being most commonly affected.
- In 70% of cases CLP is nonsyndromic, whilst the remaining 30% are syndromic.
- In Caucasian populations, CP is seen in around 1:2,000 live births (around half that of CLP), with no significant racial differences.
- Females are more commonly affected than males (approximately 4:1).
- In 50% of cases CP is nonsyndromic.

Aetiology

Whilst a number of causative genes have been identified for different types of syndromic CLP and CP (Table 13.1), the aetiology and pathogenesis of nonsyndromic forms are poorly understood. This is a reflection of the multifactorial nature of these conditions, being the result of genetic and environmental interactions affecting development of the face at specific time points during embryogenesis. It has been suggested that up to fourteen different genetic loci may be involved in nonsyndromic CLP, which means that very large and genetically pure sample sizes are required to identify specific causative genes (Lidral & Murray, 2004).

At the embryological level, perturbations in a variety of mechanisms during facial development are known to cause clefting (Fig. 13.2). A growing number of mutant mouse strains that exhibit CP (and to a lesser extent, CLP) have now been generated and these continue to provide a host of candidate genes for the human condition (Gritli-Linde, 2007; Jiang et al, 2006).

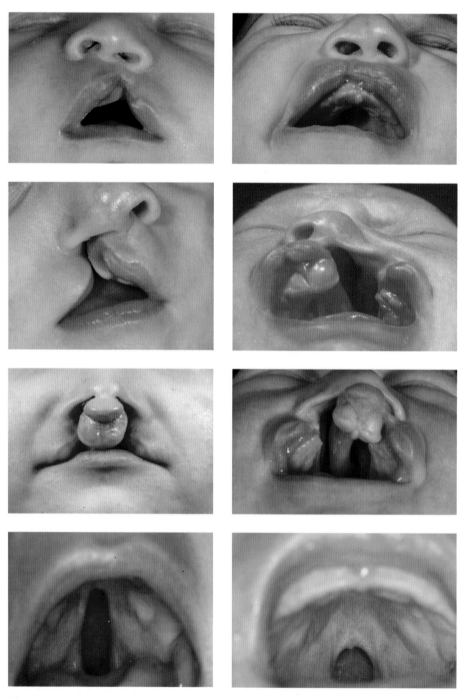

Figure 13.1 Orofacial clefting. Unilateral cleft lip (top row), unilateral cleft lip and palate (second row), bilateral cleft lip and palate (third row), isolated cleft palate (bottom row).

Table 13.1 Causative genes in syndromic CLP and CP

Syndrome	Gene	Protein product	Cleft phenotype
van der Woude	IRF6	Transcription factor	CLP
CLP–ectodermal dysplasia	PVRL1	Cell adhesion molecule	CLP
Clefting–hypodontia	MSX1	Transcription factor	CLP, CP
Opitz	MID1	Microtubular protein	CLP
Treacher Collins	TREACLE	Nucleolar phosphoprotein	CP
Stickler	COL2AI	Collagen	CP

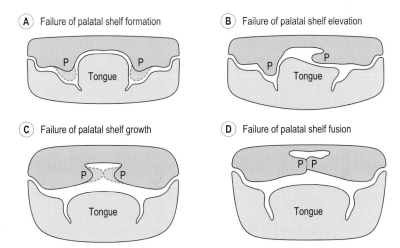

Figure 13.2 Embryonic causes of cleft palate. Redrawn from Chai Y and Maxon RE Jr. (2006) Recent advances in craniofacial morphogenesis. *Dev Dyn*, 235:2353–75.

Treatment

A child born with orofacial clefting will require complex long-term treatment, depending upon the severity of the cleft, and there may be lifelong implications for those individuals unfortunate enough to be affected. The principle objectives of treatment are to establish:

- Good facial appearance;
- Good orofacial function during speech, eating and swallowing;
- An aesthetic, functional and stable occlusion; and
- Good hearing.

If these objectives are achieved, they maximize the chances of an affected child growing up and developing normally within their social environment.

The clinical management of children born with clefting is most effective when carried out by a fully integrated team, in a centralized unit that treats a high number of patients (Box 13.2). The modern cleft team therefore includes a number of key

> ### Box 13.2 Providing care for patients with orofacial clefting in the United Kingdom
>
> In the late 1980s, some concern was raised amongst healthcare professionals regarding the quality of care being provided for children born with CLP or CP in the UK. This was based principally upon the outcome of two studies:
>
> - The GOSLON (Great Ormond Street, London and Oslo) Yardstick was developed as a clinical tool that categorized dental arch relationships into five discrete categories. Using this yardstick, comparison between UK and Norwegian cleft centres demonstrated significant shortcomings in outcome associated with the UK centre (Mars et al, 1987).
> - A European, multicentre clinical audit of treatment outcome for complete unilateral CLP (Eurocleft) found the two UK centres that participated to be weakest on almost every aspect of care (Shaw et al, 1992).
>
> This concern led to the establishment of a Clinical Standards Advisory Group (CSAG) national investigation into cleft care in the UK. This study reported upon clinical outcome in a total of 457 5- and 12-year-old children affected by nonsyndromic unilateral CLP (Sandy et al, 1998). On the basis of this investigation, the CSAG Cleft Lip and Palate Committee made a number of recommendations regarding the future provision of cleft care in the UK:
>
> - Cleft care should be centralized, with expertise and resources concentrated in 8 to 15 national centres (instead of the 57 identified in the study).
> - A common nationwide database should be established for all cleft patients.
> - Training for specialist cleft clinicians should only be provided in cleft centres where high-volume and high-quality clinical experience was available.
>
> These recommendations reflected the findings that high-quality clinical outcome in cleft care was primarily associated with centralization of services; providing clinical operators that treated large numbers of patients the correct environment for high-quality training and the infrastructure to establish effective clinical audit and intercentre comparison. Inevitably, implementation of these recommendations has required a considerable reduction in the number of centres and personnel providing cleft care in the UK, a feat that has not been achieved without some opposition.

members, in addition to other specialists who may be involved with long-term care (Table 13.2).

Birth

Giving birth to a child affected by a cleft can be a distressing experience for the parents, particularly if this condition has not been diagnosed in utero (Fig. 13.3). A multitude of emotions can occur, including shock, anger, guilt, grief and even rejection. It is important that adequate support is given to the parents and that a bond is quickly established between the parents and child.

- The clinical nurse specialist from the regional cleft team provides initial support, help and advice as soon as possible after diagnosis.

Table 13.2 Members of the modern cleft team
• Cleft surgeon • Orthodontist • Speech therapist • Cleft nurse • ENT surgeon • Paediatrician • Paediatric dentist • Restorative dentist • Psychologist • Paedodontist • Audiologist • Geneticist • General dental practitioner • Nutritionist.

• Patient support groups such as the Cleft Lip and Palate Association (CLAPA) also play an important role in providing continued help and advice.

A baby born with CLP may experience difficulty in feeding at birth. CP produces an open communication between the oral and nasal cavities. Suckling can be slow because the baby will have difficulty generating adequate intraoral pressure and milk can be lost through the nose before it is swallowed. It is important to establish an effective feeding regime as soon as possible:

• Feeding is generally successful using an assisted feeding bottle with a standard orthodontic teat, which can be squeezed to generate the necessary pressure; and
• Breastfeeding is occasionally possible, but may need supplementary feeding from a bottle.

Presurgical orthopedics

A period of active presurgical orthopedic alignment of the cleft alveolar segments is occasionally carried out in the neonate to reduce the size of the cleft defect and facilitate surgical repair. Specialized facial strapping or orthodontic plates (Fig. 13.4) are used, which can be passive or active and help mould or reposition the divided facial and maxillary segments. In particular, these plates have been used for:

• Reducing protrusion of the premaxillary segment in bilateral CLP cases;
• Reducing the size of an alveolar cleft and approximating the lip margins in unilateral CLP; and
• Reducing the width of an isolated palatal cleft.

Presurgical orthopedic treatment is usually carried out at the discretion of the operating surgeon. There is currently little substantive evidence to suggest that any of these techniques provide long-term benefit for the dental arch relationship or facial appearance and their use remains controversial.

Surgical repair of cleft lip and palate

A number of individual surgical techniques for repairing the embryonic deficits associated with both the lip and palate have been described. However, evaluating which technique, sequence or timing will provide optimum results is difficult and currently no true consensus for any of these criteria exists (Roberts-Harry & Sandy, 1992; Sandy & Roberts-Harry, 1993).

Figure 13.3 Lip development can be monitored using ultrasound scanning. The external nares of the nose (outlined arrow) and both lips (white arrows) can be seen on this 16 week scan. The baby is on its side and development of these structures is normal.

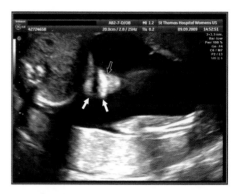

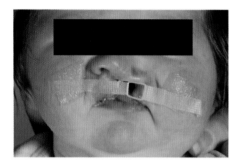 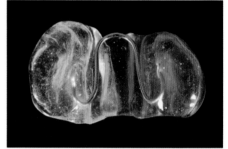

Figure 13.4 Orthopedic cleft appliance to approximate the lip segments prior to repair (left panel) and intraoral orthopedic appliance to approximate the palatal shelves. Courtesy of Christoph Huppa.

Early surgery does allow the child to establish good orofacial function as soon as possible and this is particularly important for the development of normal speech. However, surgical repair can be associated with scarring in the maxillary region, which can produce growth deficiencies in all three planes of space:

- Midline scar tissue can prevent transverse growth and produce crossbites; and
- Scar tissue within the tuberosity region can tether the maxilla to the sphenoid bone, preventing downward and forward growth and producing a class III skeletal pattern (Fig. 13.5).

It is clear from comparative studies that facial growth is compromised in operated cleft subjects when compared with those from unoperated samples, particularly those that have undergone palatal repair (Mars & Houston, 1990). The goal of surgical correction is to minimize any potential growth discrepancy, whilst maximizing the aesthetic and functional outcome.

Lip repair

Surgical repair of cleft lip is usually carried out between 3 and 6 months of age as a single procedure (Fig. 13.6), the exact age being dictated by surgeon preference. Classically, the rule of 'tens' has been used, with surgery only taking place once the child is at least 10 weeks old, 10 pounds in weight, and having a haemoglobin level of

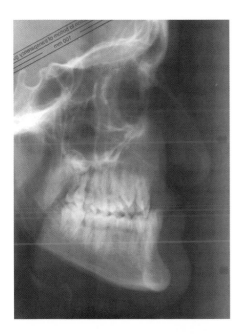

Figure 13.5 Maxillary hypoplasia in a patient with repaired cleft palate.

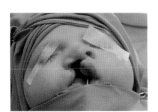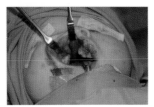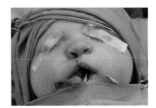

Figure 13.6 Primary surgery for unilateral cleft lip. Courtesy of Christoph Huppa.

10%. However, waiting until these criteria are achieved can delay surgery and it has been argued that this can cause problems with both parent–infant bonding and early growth and development. Indeed, advances in neonatal care and paediatric anaesthesia have made it possible to perform cleft surgery during the neonatal period, although there is currently no clear evidence to suggest that this is particularly advantageous (Schendel, 2000).

- The Millard rotation advancement repair is one of the commonest methods for the repair of cleft lip. This method effectively hides the horizontal scar in the base of the nostril, but is technically difficult to perform and often does not produce adequate lip length.
- The triangular flap of Tennison is easier to carry out and is more effective at lengthening the upper lip and preserving Cupid's bow, but this technique does place a horizontal scar within the lip, which can be unsightly.
- Current surgical practice advocates primary repair of cleft lip in conjunction with reconstructing the displaced underlying musculature, rather than simply rearrang-

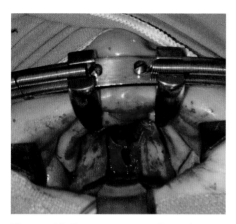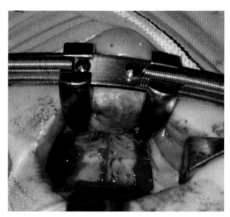

Figure 13.7 Primary surgery for cleft palate. Courtesy of Christoph Huppa.

ing skin flaps. This technique aims to reproduce normal anatomy within this region, leading to better appearance, function and enhanced growth of the underlying bony structures (Delaire, 1978).

Bilateral cleft lip is also repaired with a single procedure, involving simultaneous correction of the lip, nose and alveolus (Mulliken, 2000). The upper lip orbicularis oris muscle must be freed from each lateral cleft element and repaired in the midline anterior to the premaxilla.

Palate repair (palatoplasty)
The timing of palate repair represents a balance between maximizing the positive effects of early palate closure on feeding and speech development, whilst minimizing the potentially negative effects of inhibited maxillary growth and development as a result of surgical scarring.

Currently, repair of CP is normally undertaken between 9 and 12 months of age and usually involves a palatoplasty to move tissue towards the midline, with or without some lengthening of the palate to improve the posterior soft palate seal (Fig. 13.7).

Speech and language
Following repair of the palate, a speech and language therapist monitors speech development closely. Velopharyngeal insufficiency (VPI) is the result of an inadequately functioning soft palate, which may be unable to lift and produce a good seal with the posterior pharyngeal wall. VPI can produce:
- Nasal escape on pressure consonants (i.e. k, p, t); and
- Hypernasality.

The main problem is a lack of mobility in the soft palate, secondary to scarring from the palate repair. In combination with the dental abnormalities, malocclusion and hearing difficulties, which are all often seen in cleft children, VPI can also produce poor articulation, which results in significant difficulties with speech.

VPI is diagnosed by speech assessment and confirmed with videofluoroscopy or nasoendoscopy. Treatment involves surgery combined with speech and language therapy. Surgery is usually carried out as soon as VPI is diagnosed, around the age of

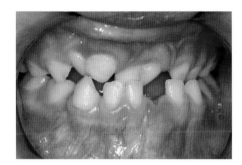

Figure 13.8 Incisor and buccal crossbite associated with unilateral CLP.

4 before the child begins school, and generally involves either a re-repair of the soft palate or pharyngoplasty. Pharyngoplasty aims to reduce hypernasality by narrowing the velopharyngeal space.

Middle ear disease
Otitis media is also a common finding in children with CP, disruption to the muscles of the soft palate affecting function of the eustachian tube. This can reduce the acuity of their hearing, causing further potential adverse effects on the development of speech and language. It is important that an audiologist monitors these children and if necessary, tympanostomy tubes (or grommets) are placed by an ear–nose–throat (ENT) surgeon.

Dental care during the deciduous dentition
It is important that a program of preventative dentistry is established during early dental development, particularly as many children affected by clefting are vulnerable to caries. Dietary advice should be provided, good oral hygiene established and fluoride supplementation instituted, if necessary.

There is occasionally delay in the eruption of deciduous teeth adjacent to the cleft and the deciduous lateral incisor can be absent, hypoplastic or even duplicated. Crossbites can occur in the buccal segments; however, orthodontic treatment is rarely indicated in the deciduous dentition.

Dental care during the mixed dentition
As the permanent teeth begin to erupt, crossbites affecting both the incisor and molar dentitions can occur and their severity often reflects the degree of disruption that has occurred to maxillary growth and development as a result of previous surgery. The maxillary incisors can also be crowded, rotated and tilted, particularly those adjacent to the cleft (Fig. 13.8).

Dental preventative measures should continue during the mixed dentition; in particular, the first molars should be fissure sealed and monitored to ensure these teeth do not become carious. It is particularly important in cleft cases to avoid the potential occlusal complications associated with early loss of deciduous teeth or first molars.

Alveolar bone grafting
The presence of a residual bony defect in the maxillary alveolus of children affected by complete clefts is a deformity associated with a number of functional and aesthetic problems, which can affect both the occlusion and local orofacial region:

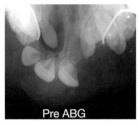
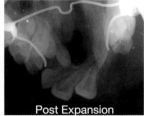
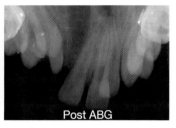

Pre ABG   Post Expansion   Post ABG

Figure 13.9 Upper anterior occlusal radiographs of a right-sided unilateral CLP prior to alveolar bone grafting (ABG), following orthodontic expansion and post ABG. Note that the UR2 and UR3 are beginning to erupt following the graft. Courtesy of Shivani Patel.

- Adjacent teeth are often displaced, rotated or tipped;
- Teeth in the region of the defect are unable to erupt (particularly the maxillary canine and if present, the lateral incisor);
- The bony defect can lead to collapse of the maxillary dental arch with a loss of alveolar contour;
- Bony support around the base of the nose can also be compromised, with flattening on the cleft side;
- In bilateral cases, there can be instability and mobility of the premaxillary segment; and
- Larger defects can be associated with oronasal fistulae (communications between the oral and nasal cavities in the anterior palate).

Alveolar or secondary bone grafting involves placing cancellous bone, usually harvested from the iliac crest, directly into the maxillary alveolar defect. This procedure is normally carried out at around 8–10 years of age, prior to eruption of the permanent canine, when root formation of this tooth is around two-thirds complete. A period of orthodontic treatment is usually required prior to graft placement to expand the collapsed maxillary arch and create surgical access, maximizing the amount of bone that can be placed (Fig. 13.9). This expansion is often achieved with a tri- or quadhelix appliance, followed by a period of retention with a palatal arch. During this phase of orthodontic treatment, some alignment of the maxillary incisors can be achieved by either extending the arms of the helix or using a simple fixed appliance, but care needs to be taken not to move any teeth into the cleft site where there is no bone, and if this is a concern, these teeth should be aligned after the bone graft.

Alveolar bone grafting has made a significant contribution to the oral rehabilitation of children with cleft palate (Table 13.3) (Bergland et al, 1986). Traditionally, orthodontic treatment was aimed at tooth alignment followed by expansion of the maxillary arch to create space in the region of the cleft for the placement of a denture or bridge. This approach was associated with a number of significant disadvantages:

- Aligning teeth in regions devoid of bone;
- Relying upon long-term tooth replacement with a dental prosthesis; and
- Considerable instability of the unsupported alveolar segments in the maxillary arch.

Grafting cancellous bone into the cleft allows teeth to erupt into this region and facilitates tooth movement, which means that orthodontic tooth alignment and space closure can be achieved (Fig. 13.10). Moreover, the timing of alveolar bone grafting means that it does not interfere with growth in the width and length of the anterior

Table 13.3 Advantages of alveolar bone grafting

- Allows the eruption of the canine tooth.
- Allows alignment and orthodontic space closure in the maxillary arch (particularly if there is absence of the lateral incisor tooth).
- Produces a stable, well-aligned and intact maxillary arch.
- Helps to stabilize the premaxillary segment, particularly in bilateral cases.
- Establishes good alveolar contour.
- Preserves vulnerable teeth adjacent to the cleft alveolus.
- Increases upper facial height.
- Closes fistulae in the anterior palate.
- Enhances support for the affected alar base.

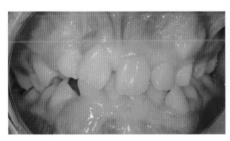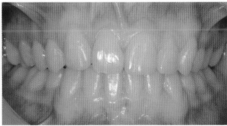

Figure 13.10 Definitive orthodontic treatment in a unilateral CLP patient following alveolar bone grafting. The UR2 is absent and the UR3 has been modified to resemble the UR2.

maxilla, because this is essentially complete by 8 years of age; whilst vertical development of the maxilla would appear to continue normally after the insertion of a bone graft.

Dental care during the permanent dentition
Once the permanent dentition is established a decision is made regarding the need for orthodontic treatment alone to correct any malocclusion, or a combination of orthodontics and orthognathic surgery. A key factor is the degree of maxillary and midfacial retrusion, but it should be remembered that these patients also exhibit a full range of mandibular growth patterns and mandibular prognathia can also be seen. A period of time monitoring further facial growth may be required before a final decision is made, but if surgery is indicated, presurgical orthodontic treatment will usually begin once facial growth is complete. Occasionally, in cases with severe maxillary retrusion, osteogenic distraction is employed to move the maxilla forwards in a younger, growing patient. This will provide some early improvement in the profile and reduce the size of the jaw movements that will be required for definitive orthognathic surgery in the late teenage years, once facial growth is complete.

In those cases that can be treated with orthodontics alone, there are often a number of specific problems that exist:
- Crowding associated with a narrow and retrusive maxillary arch (Fig. 13.11);
- Crossbites affecting teeth in the anterior and posterior maxilla; and
- Congenital absence or anomalies associated with teeth in the cleft region.

Orthodontic treatment with fixed appliances is usually indicated in these cases, often in conjunction with some maxillary expansion; but following the same general

Figure 13.11 Severe crowding secondary to maxillary hypoplasia in a patient with a repaired unilateral CLP.

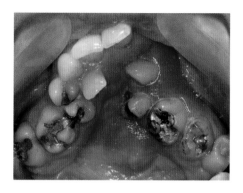

principles of treatment planning for any malocclusion. Correction of the severely rotated teeth and posterior crossbites often seen in these cases usually requires long-term retention.

Surgical revision

In young adults affected by complete clefts the nasal aesthetics can be poor; in particular, the nose can be asymmetric at the tip and alar base and may require some surgical revision. In addition, revision of any surgical scarring associated with the lip repair may also be required. These procedures are usually carried out following the completion of definitive orthodontic or combined treatment in the late teenage years.

Cleidocranial dysplasia

Cleidocranial dysplasia (CCD; OMIM 119600) is an autosomal dominant skeletal dysplasia characterized by defective ossification of both intramembranous and endochondral bones, in combination with severe dental anomalies. Mutations in the *RUNX2* (formerly *CBFA1*) gene situated on chromosome 6p12-21 have been identified as the cause of CCD (Lee et al, 1997; Mundlos et al, 1997). *RUNX2* encodes a transcription factor essential for the terminal differentiation of bone-forming osteoblasts. Mice generated with targeted disruption in *Runx2* have a complete absence of bone and they die at birth (Komori et al, 1997; Otto et al, 1997).

In humans, the bones most severely affected are those that develop in membrane:
- An absence, or hypoplasia of the clavicles, is common, allowing affected subjects to adopt the classic pose of approximated shoulders (Fig. 13.12);
- The skull exhibits features of delayed ossification, including the presence of wide-open sutures, persistence of the fontanelles and the development of multiple wormian bones, particularly within the lambdoid suture of older subjects;
- The presence of frontal bossing and midface hypoplasia, which leads to relative mandibular prognathism and produces a characteristic facial appearance; and
- Endochondral bones can also be affected, with shortening of the long bones of the axial skeleton and digits (brachydactyly). Together with the craniofacial features, this can give an overall clinical impression of mild achondroplasia (dwarfism).

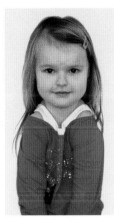
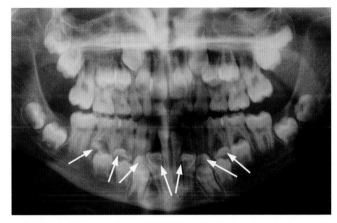

Figure 13.12 Clavicular hypoplasia allowing shoulder approximation (left) and multiple supernumerary teeth (right, arrowed), both features of cleidocranial dysplasia.

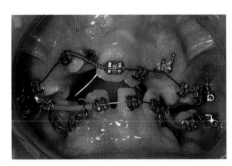
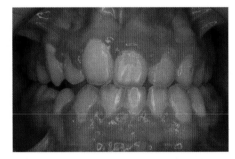

Figure 13.13 Multiple supernumerary teeth and delayed exfoliation of the deciduous dentition in a child with cleidocranial dysplasia. Treatment involved multiple exposures and mechanical traction of teeth.

The dental features of CCD include a triad of:
- Retained deciduous teeth;
- Multiple supernumerary teeth; and
- Failure of eruption affecting the permanent dentition.

The dental phenotype is highly penetrant and can produce considerable problems, usually manifesting as retention and progressive deterioration of the deciduous dentition with only variable degrees of permanent tooth eruption (Fig. 13.12) . Historically, the dental management of CCD has involved either prosthetic replacement of the permanent teeth, with or without judicious tooth extraction, or surgical repositioning and transplantation of affected teeth. A more coordinated approach combines deciduous and supernumerary tooth extraction with surgical exposure and bonding in an attempt to achieve as normal an occlusion as possible (Becker et al, 1997a, b). However, the impacted permanent teeth of individuals affected by CCD can be extremely resistant to orthodontic traction (Fig. 13.13).

Figure 13.14 Ectodermal Dysplasia.

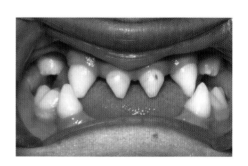

Ectodermal dysplasia

The ectodermal dysplasias (ED) represent a heterogeneous group of conditions characterized primarily by defective:

- Teeth;
- Hair;
- Nails; and
- Sweat glands.

The hypohidrotic or anhidrotic forms of ED are the most common and amongst these, X-linked recessive hypohidrotic ectodermal dysplasia (XLHED; OMIM 305100) is seen most frequently. Affected males have the following clinical features:

- Severe hypodontia, affecting both the deciduous and permanent dentitions, with those teeth that do form often being microdont and abnormally shaped (Fig. 13.14);
- Sparse and lightly pigmented scalp hair, which is usually lost prematurely to produce juvenile alopecia;
- Hypoplastic or aplastic sweat glands, which results in an inability to sweat (hypohidrosis) and impaired temperature regulation; and
- Split, dystrophic or abnormally keratinized nails.

Female carriers in the heterozygous state can also be affected by XLHED, but the clinical features are generally less severe.

An autosomal recessive form of hypohidrotic ectodermal dysplasia (ARHED; OMIM 224900), which is clinically indistinguishable from XLHED, also exists; however, in ARHED affected males and females can exhibit the full clinical spectrum of anomalies.

Autosomal dominant hypohidrotic ectodermal dysplasia (ADHED; OMIM 129490) has also been documented, but this is rare, only being described in a few family pedigrees.

These hypohidrotic forms of ED are caused by disruption to the ectodysplasin (EDA) signalling pathway. This pathway is active in organs that develop via reciprocal signalling between epithelium and mesenchyme and is essential for their normal development (Box 13.3). The EDA signal is initiated by binding of ligand to the EDA type 1 receptor (EDAR). This binding event results in recruitment of an EDAR-associated death-domain protein (EDARRAD). EDARRAD acts as an adapter within the cell cytoplasm, interacting with a number of molecules, which ultimately mediate activation of a signalling pathway called NFkB. XLHED is caused by mutation in the gene encoding the EDA ligand (*EDA1*) (Xq12-13.1) (Kere et al, 1996), whilst mutation in *EDAR* can cause both ADHED and ARHED (Monreal et al, 1999).

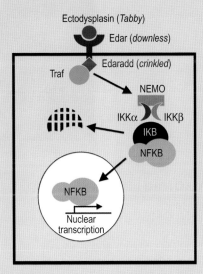

Ectodysplasin signalling pathway.

A number of naturally occurring, spontaneous mouse mutants mimic very accurately the features of human hypohidrotic ED. *Tabby*, *downless* and *crinkled* mutant mice have indistinguishable phenotypes from each other. These mouse mutants have absent or abnormally shaped teeth, a lack of sweat glands, regional alopecia and anomalies in the texture of coat hair; all features of hypohidrotic ED. The genes responsible for each of these mutants have been cloned; *Tabby* also resides on the X chromosome and is equivalent to human *EDA1*, *downless* to *EDAR* and *crinkled* to *EDARRADD*. Indeed, it was only after the positional cloning of *crinkled* in the mouse that the equivalent gene was identified in humans. Therefore, disruption within the same signalling pathway produces an almost identical phenotype in mouse and human.

Although teeth, hair and sweat glands would at first glance appear to be a very diverse group of structures, their embryonic origins are surprisingly similar. All these appendages develop from interactions between epithelial and mesenchymal tissues and the EDA signalling pathway plays a key role in this process. In the developing tooth *Tabby*, *downless* and *crinkled* have distinct expression domains in different regions of the epithelium. Whilst a lack of EDA signalling results in the hypodontia or anomalies of tooth shape seen in ED, the mouse has also been used to demonstrate that too much EDA signalling can produce the opposite phenotype: supernumerary teeth.

Figure 13.15 CT scan of a 10-year-old child with hemifacial microsomia.

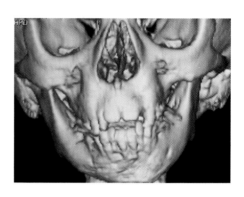

Hemifacial microsomia

Hemifacial microsomia (HFM; OMIM 164210) is a relatively common condition associated primarily with unilateral developmental defects in the orofacial region (Fig. 13.15). HFM occurs in around 1:5,600 children and is usually sporadic, although autosomal dominant familial cases have been reported.

A wide spectrum of clinical features are seen in association with HFM, but a common presentation is:

- Skeletal asymmetry of the facial region, associated with unilateral aplasia or hypoplasia of the mandibular ramus and condyle;
- A marked retrognathia, associated with mandibular asymmetry and canting of the occlusal plane; and
- A reduction in size or flattening of the facial bones.

These skeletal defects characteristically become more pronounced as facial growth progresses.

The soft tissues are also affected in cases of HFM:

- The pinna of the ear is often severely malformed or absent (microtia);
- Preauricular skin tags are common;
- The orbital palpebral fissures (the separation between the upper and lower eyelids) can be narrowed; and
- Epibulbar dermoids (benign tumours on the eyeballs) are often present unilaterally.

Less commonly, CLP, palatal and tongue muscle hypoplasia and velopharyngeal insufficiency are also present. A related condition is Goldenhar syndrome, which incorporates vertebral anomalies and epibulbar dermoids in combination with the features described above.

The aetiology of HFM is not fully understood, but a disruption during early development of the pharyngeal arches is consistent with the phenotype. Haemorrhage of the stapedial artery has been described as one possible mechanism (Poswillo, 1973) and a transgenic mouse line harbouring an insertional mutation within chromosome 10 has been shown to phenocopy the syndrome; this mouse demonstrates microtia, an asymmetric bite and anomalies of the external auditory canal, middle ear and maxilla (Cousley et al, 2002; Naora et al, 1994).

Linkage analysis in human populations has suggested the *GOOSECOID* (*GSC*) gene as a potential candidate gene for HFM (Kelberman et al, 2001). *GSC* encodes a transcription factor strongly expressed in the pharyngeal arches and mice lacking *Gsc* function have a number of craniofacial defects, including hypoplasia and a lack of coronoid and angular processes in the mandible, and defects in the maxillary, palatine and pterygoid bones (Rivera-Perez et al, 1995; Yamada et al, 1995).

Treacher Collins syndrome

Treacher Collins syndrome or mandibulofacial dysostosis (TCS; OMIM 154500) is a rare autosomal dominant disorder of facial development that occurs in around 1:50,000 live births (Fig. 13.16). The regions of the face affected are those derived from pharyngeal arches 1 and 2, but there can be considerable variation in the severity of clinical presentation, even amongst individuals within the same pedigree.

A characteristic facial appearance is common:
- Down-slanting palpebral fissures;
- Zygomatic, supraorbital and mandibular hypoplasia;
- Colobomas (areas of tissue deficiency) of the lower eyelids;
- Severe malformation of the ears, including the external ear, middle ear ossicles and atresia of the external auditory canal, which together often result in conductive hearing loss;
- Isolated cleft palate, present in around one-third of cases; and
- Usually a severely class II skeletal pattern with increased vertical proportions, due to mandibular deficiency and posterior mandibular growth rotation.

Individuals with TCS usually undergo extensive hard and soft tissue reconstruction during the first two decades of life. This treatment is aimed primarily at improving respiratory function and reconstructing the affected soft and hard tissues. The management of such cases requires a dedicated and multidisciplinary team approach (Kobus & Wojcicki, 2006).

A large-scale and collaborative effort identified *TCOF1* as the gene mutated in TCS (Dixon et al, 1996). *TCOF1* encodes the Treacle nucleolar phosphoprotein thought to have a key role in ribosomal biogenesis, which is essential for normal cell growth and differentiation. Unfortunately, efforts to study TCS using mouse models have been hampered because mice lacking the function of only one *Tcof1* allele have a TCS phenotype even more severe than that found in the human, depending upon their genetic background (Dixon & Dixon, 2004). These mice have a compromised production of mature ribosomes in cranial neuroepithelial and neural crest cells, which leads to diminished proliferation and a massive increase in programmed cell death associated with the early neural tube, and a reduction in neural crest cell migration into the early craniofacial region. Therefore, a primary defect in TCS is the production of neural crest cells that populate the first and second pharyngeal arches early in development; cells ultimately responsible for producing much of the facial skeleton (Box 13.4).

Pierre Robin syndrome

Pierre Robin syndrome or Robin sequence (PRS; OMIM 261800) (Fig. 13.17) occurs in around 1:10,000–20,000 and is characterized by a triad of:

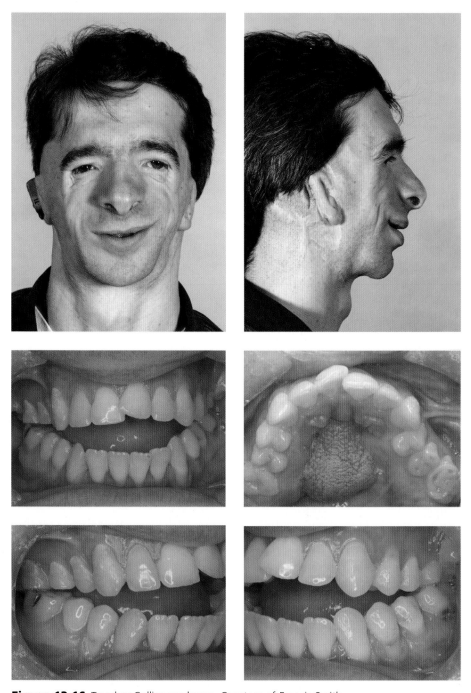

Figure 13.16 Treacher Collins syndrome. Courtesy of Francis Smith.

Box 13.4   Rescuing a mouse model of Treacher Collins syndrome

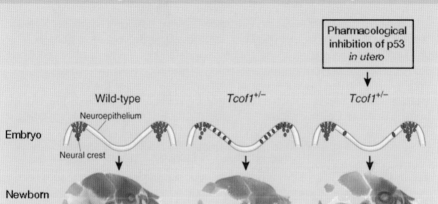

Rescue of cell death in the Treacher Collins mouse model by inhibition of p53. Normal neural crest cell proliferation, migration and craniofacial development in the wild type mouse (left). In the *Tcof1* mutant, premature death of neural crest cells results in hypoplasia of facial bones and the Treacher Collins phenotype (middle). Inhibition of p53 in the mutant prevents much of the premature death associated with neural crest cells and allows normal facial development to take place. Reprinted by permission from Macmillan Publishers Ltd: *Nature Medicine* (McKeown SJ and Bronner-Fraser M (2008). Saving face: rescuing a craniofacial birth defect. *Nat Med* 14:115–116).

A landmark collaborative study between groups led by Mike Dixon in the UK and Paul Trainor in the USA has recently demonstrated a rescue of the craniofacial defects associated with a mouse model of Treacher Collins syndrome (Jones et al, 2008). This investigation has raised the possibility of future therapeutic prevention of a serious inherited craniofacial birth defect.

The *Tcof1* heterozygous mouse models human Treacher Collins syndrome; reduced levels of a functional Treacle protein results in abnormal ribosome biogenesis, a lack of proliferation and premature death of precursor neural crest cells. The mechanism underlying this effect appears to be increased abundance of a protein called p53 (an important molecule for cell cycle regulation) secondary to its stabilization and prevention from degradation. If this stabilization of p53 ultimately causes the death of neural crest cells in the

Tcof1 embryo—what happens if p53 activity is inhibited? Importantly, could this rescue the phenotype if done at the correct stage of development?

Significantly, by injecting pregnant mice carrying the *Tcof1* mutation with a pharmacological inhibitor of p53 function these investigators were able to produce a marked rescue of the craniofacial defects in the newborn mice. This study demonstrates that an understanding of the molecular mechanisms underlying inherited disorders can provide opportunities for therapeutic intervention. However, some caution must be applied in the case of preventing human Treacher Collins syndrome as serious logistical problems still remain. This approach could only be used in families with identified mutations, not those cases arising spontaneously; any treatment would need to begin very early in the pregnancy—in the third week of gestation during neural crest migration; and finally, p53 is a potent tumour suppressor in many tissues and its inhibition can lead to spontaneous tumour development (McKeown & Bronner-Fraser, 2008).

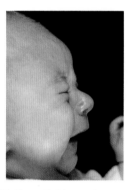
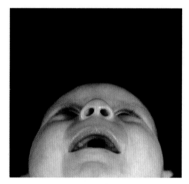

Figure 13.17 Pierre Robin syndrome.

- Mandibular micrognathia;
- Glossoptosis (posterior positioning of the tongue); and
- Isolated cleft palate.

Micrognathia is the primary aetiological factor, an excessively small mandible resulting in the tongue falling downwards and backwards into the pharynx, being compressed between the palatal shelves and preventing their closure. In addition to a large and U-shaped cleft palate, the tongue position can also cause life-threatening respiratory difficulty at birth, obstructing the epiglottis and preventing adequate inhalation of the lungs.

Several theories have attempted to explain why growth and development of the mandible is so restricted in PRS:

- Oligohydramnios or a reduced amniotic fluid pressure compressing the chin against the sternum and therefore restricting mandibular development (Poswillo, 1968);

- A lack of mandibular movement during embryogenesis (secondary to muscle weakness or hypotonia); and
- Generalized growth deficiency during embryogenesis.

It is likely that PRS may also contain a genetic component, as Robin sequence is seen in association with other syndromes: in particular, Stickler syndrome (OMIM 108300), the 22q11 deletion syndromes (see Box 2.1) and some extremely rare conditions featuring this sequence in combination with cardiac, neurological and axial skeletal defects.

In many cases of PRS, the upper airway obstruction presents as a medical emergency at birth, requiring neonatal nasopharyngeal intubation or tracheostomy. However, once the airway is stabilized and a feeding regime put in place, these infants usually thrive; with surgical repair of the cleft palate taking place during the first year of life. It has been suggested that compensatory growth of the mandible may occur during the first 5 years in cases of PRS, but this is controversial. Whilst mandibular skeletal growth certainly does occur in these subjects, there is evidence to suggest that these children are more likely to maintain a class II skeletal relationship (Daskalogiannakis et al, 2001).

Craniosynostosis

The craniosynostoses are a heterogenous group of disorders characterized by premature fusion of the cranial sutures (Fig. 13.18). This can occur in isolation or in association with other anomalies, in a number of well-characterized syndromes (Wilkie, 1997; Wilkie & Morriss-Kay, 2001).

Isolated craniosynostosis
Around 1:2,000 children are born with premature fusion of a cranial suture, most commonly the sagittal; but the coronal, metopic and lambdoid sutures can also be affected. These cases usually occur sporadically but can also be familial. The craniofacial features are dependent upon which suture is affected but usually involve distortion of the skull due to excessive compensatory growth in unaffected regions.

Apert syndrome
Apert syndrome (OMIM 101200) is characterized by craniosynostosis, midfacial malformations, symmetrical syndactyly of the hands and feet and mental retardation. This condition can occur sporadically or be inherited in an autosomal dominant manner, but is rare, occurring in around 1:65,000. Apert syndrome is characterized by a wide midline calvarial defect, which rapidly closes with bone and a coronal suture that fuses early in infancy. The principle craniofacial features include:
- Steep forehead;
- Hypertelorism;
- Ocular proptosis (forward displacement and entrapment of the eye from behind the eyelids) and downslanting palpebral fissures;
- Low-set ears;
- Maxillary hypoplasia, with an associated Byzantine-shaped maxillary arch and severe dental crowding;

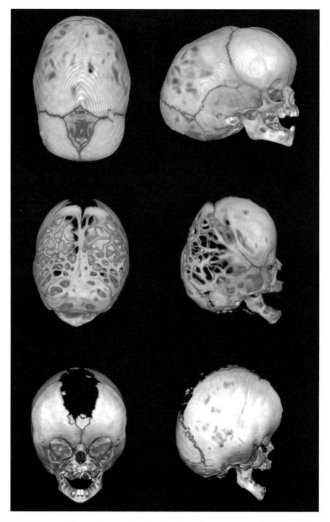

Figure 13.18 CT scans of craniosynostosis. The top images are of isolated sagittal suture synostosis with calvarial bone growth restricted in a transverse direction. Compensatory growth at the coronal and lambdoidal sutures has resulted in an elongated calvarium. The middle images are of Crouzon syndrome. There is synostosis of the sagittal and coronal sutures and maxillary hypoplasia. The lower images are of Apert syndrome. There is bilateral synostosis of the coronal suture, a wide midline defect in the calvarium and maxillary hypoplasia. Courtesy of Professor David Rice and Jyri Hukki.

- Lateral palatal swellings, which can give a pseudo-cleft appearance; and
- Cleft palate.

Crouzon syndrome

Crouzon syndrome (OMIM 123500) involves craniosynostosis, ocular proptosis and midfacial malformation, but the limbs are unaffected. It occurs with a similar prevalence to that of Apert syndrome and is also either sporadic or inherited in an autosomal dominant manner. Crouzon syndrome is characterized by the premature fusion of multiple sutures from an early age and is dominated by the following features:

- Brachycephaly (a wide head);
- Marked ocular proptosis;
- Maxillary hypoplasia and dental crowding; and
- Conductive hearing loss.

A number of other craniosynostosis syndromes, including Pfeiffer (OMIM 101600) and Saethre-Chotzen (OMIM 101400), exist. The majority of these conditions are associated with mutations in genes encoding receptors for the fibroblast growth factor family of signalling molecules (FGFRs), particularly *FGFR2*; and increased paternal age is a significant risk factor. These are often gain-of-function mutations, which lead to constitutive activity of the signalling pathway. FGF signalling is important during many stages of embryonic development, but the mutations associated with craniosynostosis clearly have a significant effect during the closely coordinated interactions that take place during formation of membrane bones within the skull.

Oral-Facial-Digital syndromes

The oral-facial-digital syndromes (OFD) represent a heterogeneous group of developmental disorders, which combine both oral and craniofacial abnormalities with anomalies affecting the digits. The best characterized is OFD-1 (OMIM 311200), which is inherited as an autosomal dominant X-linked condition and occurs in around 1:50,000 live births; only females are affected because it is lethal in the male heterozygous state.

OFD-1 is also characterized by a distinctive facies; there is:

- Frontal bossing;
- Midfacial hypoplasia;
- Broad nasal root;
- Wide-open eyes;
- Short upper lip; and
- Sparse and brittle scalp hair.

Within the oral cavity, an unusual and marked hyperplasia of the frenula occur, which results in a characteristic pattern of orofacial clefting (Fig. 13.19):

- A small midline cleft of the upper lip extending through the vermillion border is often present in combination with more severe clefting of the palate;
- A deep transverse cleft usually separates the primary and secondary palates, whilst a full-length cleft of the secondary palate, extending through the soft palate, is also present; and
- Frenula hyperplasia is also present in the mandibular region, resulting in clefting of the tongue in around half of cases.

The digits also present with a range of anomalies (Fig. 13.20), including:

- Curvatures (clinodactyly);
- Fusions (syndactyly); and
- Shortness (brachydactyly).

The *OFD1* gene has been identified and encodes a protein involved in the organization and assembly of primary cilia (Ferrante et al, 2001; Romio et al, 2004), small

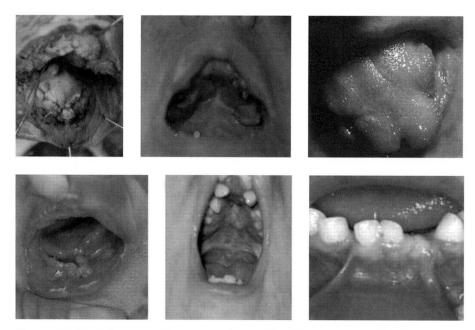

Figure 13.19 Oral abnormalities associated with OFD-1.These include multiple buccal frenulae, lingual hamartoma; cleft and lobulated tongue, tooth defects and cleft palate (repaired in both middle panels). Reproduced from Thauvin-Robinet C, Cossée M, Cormier-Daire V, et al (2006). Clinical, molecular, and genotype–phenotype correlation studies from 25 cases of oral–facial–digital syndrome type 1: a French and Belgian collaborative study. *J Med Genet* 43:54–61. With permission from BMJ Publishing Group Ltd.

contractile extensions found on the surface of many cell populations. It is becoming increasingly clear that cilia are important mediators of cell signalling during development and a recently generated mouse model of human OFD-1 suggests that normal cilia formation is defective under this condition (Ferrante et al, 2006).

Holoprosencephaly

Holoprosencephaly (HPE; OMIM 236100) is a clinically heterogeneous and complex developmental defect of the forebrain, in which the cerebral hemispheres fail to split into distinct halves (Muenke and Beachy, 2000). The underlying brain malformation can have a profound affect upon midline development of the face (Fig. 13.21). In the most severe form, the forebrain fails to divide and the face is characterized by cyclopia, with a single eye situated below a rudimentary proboscis and midline clefting of the lip and palate. HPE is one of the commonest causes of embryonic lethality, responsible for up to 1:250 miscarriages and seen in around 1:15,000 live births.

In some cases of HPE, the molecular defects have been identified; HPE-Type 3 (OMIM 142945) is caused by mutation in the sonic hedgehog (*SHH*) gene. *SHH*

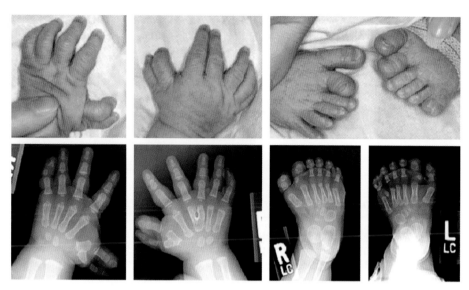

Figure 13.20 Limb abnormalities associated with oral-facial-digital syndrome include anomalies of the hands and feet, including polydactyly, with varying degrees of brachydactyly, syndactyly, and clinodactyly. Reproduced from Hayes LL, Simoneaux SF, Palasis S, et al (2008). Laryngeal and tracheal anomalies in an infant with oral-facial-digital-syndrome type VI (Váradi-Papp): report of a transitional type. *Ped Radiol* 38:994–998. With kind permission from Springer Science and Business Media.

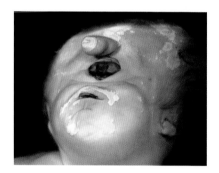

Figure 13.21 Severe alobar holoprosencephaly. Courtesy of the Gordon Museum, King's College London.

encodes an important signalling molecule, which is expressed in many regions of the embryo, including the prechordal plate (see Fig. 2.5). A lack of signalling in this region leads to a failure of forebrain subdivision and HPE. Mutations in the human *SHH* gene can also lead to a milder defect in midline facial development, the formation of only a solitary median maxillary central incisor (SMMCI) in the primary or secondary dentition (Fig. 13.22). This can occur as an isolated syndrome (OMIM 147250) or as a manifestation of HPE. Individuals with SMMCI have had offspring with HPE and therefore, SMMCI is a recognized risk factor and can be one of the mildest manifestations in autosomal dominant HPE (Nanni et al, 2001).

Figure 13.22 Single midline maxillary central incisor (SMMCI).

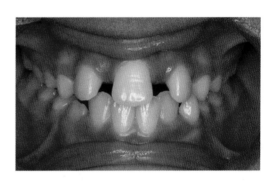

Fetal alcohol syndrome

The anomalies associated with the fetal alcohol syndrome (FAS) arise as a direct result of alcohol consumption during pregnancy (Jones et al, 1973). It is estimated that worldwide, FAS affects approximately 1 in 100 newborn children to varying degrees, making it the commonest cause of learning difficulty (O'Leary, 2004). The principle features of FAS include:

- Retarded somatic growth;
- A characteristic facies, including short flat nose, midfacial hypoplasia, thin vermilion border of the upper lip and an indistinct philtrum;
- Cleft palate (in more severe cases); and
- Dysfunction of the central nervous system (CNS).

The severity of this condition is in proportion to the quantity and timing of alcohol ingestion during gestation. In the most extreme cases, FAS represents a form of HPE. Moreover, whilst the exact mechanisms underlying alcohol teratogenicity are not fully understood, exposure of developing chick embryos to ethanol causes the death of neural crest cell populations in the craniofacial region.

Further reading

ONLINE MENDELIAN INHERITANCE IN MAN (OMIM). Available at URL:http://www.nslijgenetics.org/search_omim.html

EPSTEIN CJ, ERICKSON RP AND WYNSHAW-BORIS A (2004). *Inborn Errors of Development* (Oxford: Oxford University Press).

References

BECKER A, LUSTMANN J AND SHTEYER A (1997a). Cleidocranial dysplasia: Part 1—General principles of the orthodontic and surgical treatment modality. *Am J Orthod Dentofacial Orthop* 111:28–33.

BECKER A, SHTEYER A, BIMSTEIN E ET AL (1997b). Cleidocranial dysplasia: Part 2—Treatment protocol for the orthodontic and surgical modality. *Am J Orthod Dentofacial Orthop* 111:173–183.

BERGLAND O, SEMB G AND ABYHOLM FE (1986). Elimination of the residual alveolar cleft by secondary bone grafting and subsequent orthodontic treatment. *Cleft Palate J* 23:175–205.

COUSLEY R, NAORA H, YOKOYAMA M, ET AL (2002). Validity of the Hfm transgenic mouse as a model for hemifacial microsomia. *Cleft Palate Craniofac J* 39:81–92.

DASKALOGIANNAKIS J, ROSS RB AND TOMPSON BD (2001). The mandibular catch-up growth controversy in Pierre Robin sequence. *Am J Orthod Dentofacial Orthop* 120:280–285.

DELAIRE J (1978). Theoretical principles and technique of functional closure of the lip and nasal aperture. *J Maxillofac Surg* 6:109–116.

DIXON MJ (1996). Positional cloning of a gene involved in the pathogenesis of Treacher Collins syndrome. *Nat Genet* 12:130–136.

DIXON J AND DIXON MJ (2004). Genetic background has a major effect on the penetrance and severity of craniofacial defects in mice heterozygous for the gene encoding the nucleolar protein Treacle. *Dev Dyn* 229:907–914.

FERRANTE MI, GIORGIO G, FEATHER SA, ET AL (2001). Identification of the gene for oral-facial-digital type I syndrome. *Am J Hum Genet* 68:569–576.

FERRANTE MI, ZULLO A, BARRA A, ET AL (2006). Oral-facial-digital type I protein is required for primary cilia formation and left-right axis specification. *Nat Genet* 38:112–117.

FRASER FC (1970). The genetics of cleft lip and cleft palate. *Am J Hum Genet* 22:336–352.

GORLIN RJ, COHEN MMC Jr AND HENNEKAM RCM (2001). *Syndromes of the Head and Neck* (New York: Oxford University Press).

GRITLI-LINDE A (2007). Molecular control of secondary palate development. *Dev Biol* 301:309–326.

JIANG R, BUSH JO AND LIDRAL AC (2006). Development of the upper lip: Morphogenetic and molecular mechanisms. *Dev Dyn* 235:1152–1166.

JONES KL, SMITH DW, ULLELAND CN ET AL (1973). Pattern of malformation in offspring of chronic alcoholic mothers. *Lancet* 1:1267–1271.

JONES N, LYNN ML, GAUDENZ K ET AL (2008). Prevention of the neurocristopathy Treacher Collins syndrome through inhibition of p53 function. *Nat Med* 14:125–133.

KELBERMAN D, TYSON J, CHANDLER DC, ET AL (2001). Hemifacial microsomia: progress in understanding the genetic basis of a complex malformation syndrome. *Hum Genet* 109:638–645.

KERE J, SRIVASTAVA AK, MONTONEN O, ET AL (1996). X-linked anhidrotic (hypohidrotic) ectodermal dysplasia is caused by mutation in a novel transmembrane protein. *Nat Genet* 13:409–416.

KOBUS K AND WOJCICKI P (2006). Surgical treatment of Treacher Collins syndrome. *Ann Plast Surg* 56:549–554.

KOMORI T, YAGI H, NOMURA S, ET AL (1997). Targeted disruption of Cbfa1 results in a complete lack of bone formation owing to maturational arrest of osteoblasts. *Cell* 89:755–764.

LANDER ES, LINTON LM, BIRREN B, ET AL (2001). Initial sequencing and analysis of the human genome. *Nature* 409:860–921.

LEE B, THIRUNAVUKKARASU K, ZHOU L, ET AL (1997). Missense mutations abolishing DNA binding of the osteoblast-specific transcription factor OSF2/CBFA1 in cleidocranial dysplasia. *Nat Genet* 16: 307–310.

LIDRAL AC AND MURRAY JC (2004). Genetic approaches to identify disease genes for birth defects with cleft lip/palate as a model. *Birth Defects Res A Clin Mol Teratol* 70:893–901.

MCKEOWN SJ AND BRONNER-FRASER M (2008). Saving face: rescuing a craniofacial birth defect. *Nat Med* 14:115–116.

MARS M AND HOUSTON WJ (1990). A preliminary study of facial growth and morphology in unoperated male unilateral cleft lip and palate subjects over 13 years of age. *Cleft Palate J* 27:7–10.

MARS M, PLINT DA, HOUSTON WJ, ET AL (1987). The Goslon Yardstick: a new system of assessing dental arch relationships in children with unilateral clefts of the lip and palate. *Cleft Palate J* 24:314–322.

MONREAL AW, FERGUSON BM, HEADON DJ, ET AL (1999). Mutations in the human homologue of mouse dl cause autosomal recessive and dominant hypohidrotic ectodermal dysplasia. *Nat Genet* 22:366–369.

MUENKE M AND BEACHY PA (2000). Genetics of ventral forebrain development and holoprosencephaly. *Curr Opin Genet Dev* 10:262–269.

MULLIKEN JB (2000). Repair of bilateral complete cleft lip and nasal deformity—state of the art. *Cleft Palate Craniofac J* 37:342–347.

MUNDLOS S, OTTO F, MUNDLOS C, ET AL (1997). Mutations involving the transcription factor CBFA1 cause cleidocranial dysplasia. *Cell* 89:773–779.

NANNI L, MING JE, DU Y, ET AL (2001). SHH mutation is associated with solitary median maxillary central incisor: a study of 13 patients and review of the literature. *Am J Med Genet* 102:1–10.

NAORA H, KIMURA M, OTANI H, ET AL (1994). Transgenic mouse model of hemifacial microsomia: cloning and characterization of insertional mutation region on chromosome 10. *Genomics* 23:515–519.

O'LEARY CM (2004). Fetal alcohol syndrome: diagnosis, epidemiology, and developmental outcomes. *J Paediatr Child Health* 40:2–7.

OTTO F, THORNELL AP, CROMPTON T, ET AL (1997). Cbfa1, a candidate gene for cleidocranial dysplasia syndrome, is essential for osteoblast differentiation and bone development. *Cell* 89:765–771.

POSWILLO D (1968). The aetiology and surgery of cleft palate with micrognathia. *Ann R Coll Surg Engl* 43:61–88.

POSWILLO D (1973). The pathogenesis of the first and second branchial arch syndrome. *Oral Surg Oral Med Oral Pathol* 35:302–328.

RIVERA-PEREZ JA, MALLO M, GENDRON-MAGUIRE M, ET AL (1995). Goosecoid is not an essential component of the mouse gastrula organizer but is required for craniofacial and rib development. *Development* 121:3005–3012.

ROBERTS-HARRY D AND SANDY JR (1992). Repair of cleft lip and palate: 1. Surgical techniques. *Dent Update* 19:418–423.

ROMIO L, FRY AM, WINYARD PJ, ET AL (2004). OFD1 is a centrosomal/basal body protein expressed during mesenchymal-epithelial transition in human nephrogenesis. *J Am Soc Nephrol* 15:2556–2568.

SANDY J, WILLIAMS A, MILDINHALL S, ET AL (1998). The Clinical Standards Advisory Group (CSAG) Cleft Lip and Palate Study. *Br J Orthod* 25:21–30.

SANDY JR AND ROBERTS-HARRY D (1993). Repair of cleft lip and palate: 2. Evaluation of surgical techniques. *Dent Update* 20:35–37.

SCHENDEL SA (2000). Unilateral cleft lip repair—state of the art. *Cleft Palate Craniofac J* 37:335–341.

SHAW WC, DAHL E, ASHER-MCDADE C, ET AL (1992). A six-center international study of treatment outcome in patients with clefts of the lip and palate: Part 5. General discussion and conclusions. *Cleft Palate Craniofac J* 29:413–418.

VENTER JC, ADAMS MD, MYERS EW, ET AL (2001). The sequence of the human genome. *Science* 291:1304–1351.

WILKIE AO (1997). Craniosynostosis: genes and mechanisms. *Hum Mol Genet* 6:1647–1656.

WILKIE AO AND MORRISS-KAY GM (2001). Genetics of craniofacial development and malformation. *Nat Rev Genet* 2:458–468.

YAMADA G, MANSOURI A, TORRES M, ET AL (1995). Targeted mutation of the murine goosecoid gene results in craniofacial defects and neonatal death. *Development* 121:2917–2922.

Index

G